Forensic Mental Health Care

For Churchill Livingstone

Senior Commissioning Editor: Jacqueline Curthoys
Project Development Manager: Mairi McCubbin
Project Manager: Jane Shanks
Design Direction: George Ajayi

Forensic Mental Health Care

A Case Study Approach

Edited by

Dave Mercer BA(Hons) MA RMN PGCE
Lecturer, Department of Nursing, University of Liverpool, Liverpool, UK

Tom Mason BSc(Hons) PhD RGN RMN RNMH
Senior Lecturer, Department of Nursing, University of Liverpool, Liverpool, UK

Mick McKeown BA(Hons) RGN RMN DPSN(Thorn)
Lecturer, Department of Nursing, University of Liverpool; Practitioner,
North Mersey Community NHS Trust, Liverpool, UK

Ged McCann BPhil MPH RMN DPSN(Thorn)
County Development Officer for Mentally Disordered Offenders,
North Yorkshire Health Authority; Lecturer, University of York, York, UK

Foreword by

Ron Blackburn MA MSc PhD CPsychol FBPsS FIOP
Professor of Clinical and Forensic Psychological Studies,
Department of Clinical Psychology, Liverpool University, Liverpool, UK

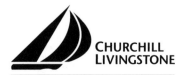

CHURCHILL
LIVINGSTONE

EDINBURGH LONDON NEW YORK PHILADELPHIA ST LOUIS SYDNEY TORONTO 2000

CHURCHILL LIVINGSTONE
An imprint of Harcourt Publishers Limited

© Harcourt Brace and Company Limited 2000

◢ is a registered trademark of Harcourt Publishers
Limited

First published 2000

ISBN 0 443 06140 8

British Library Cataloguing in Publication Data
A catalogue record for this book is available from the British
Library

Library of Congress Cataloging in Publication Data
A catalog record for this book is available from the Library
of Congress

Note
Medical knowledge is constantly changing. As new
information becomes available, changes in treatment,
procedures, equipment and the use of drugs become
necessary. The editors, the contributors and the publishers'
have, as far as it is possible, taken care to ensure that the
information given in this text is accurate and up to date.
However, readers are strongly advised to confirm that the
information, especially with regard to drug usage, complies
with the latest legislation and standards of practice.

The
publisher's
policy is to use
**paper manufactured
from sustainable forests**

Printed in China
NPCC

Contents

Contributors

Terry Bailey
Former special hospital patient. Now a mature student.
2. Care in context
A personal experience

Claire Barkley MBChB MRCPsych CertMHS
Consultant Forensic Psychiatrist, The Foundation NHS Trust, Stafford, UK
9. Seemingly intractable problems
Treatment resistance

Richard Bentall BSc(Hons)PhD MClinPsychol MA
Professor of Clinical Psychology, University of Liverpool, UK
4. Severe and enduring mental health problems
Cognitive–behaviour therapy for auditory hallucinations

Clancy Borastero RMN SRN RCNT CertAdEd
Lecturer Practitioner, Ashworth Hospital, Merseyside, UK
7. Firesetting
Group work with women who set fires

Clare Brabbins MBChB MRCPsych
Consultant Psychiatrist, Rathbone Hospital HDU, Liverpool, UK
8. Problematic substance use
Substance misuse complicating mental illness

Maureen Burke RGN RSCN RMN DipMS MA
Consultant Forensic Nurse, Ashworth Hospital, Merseyside, UK

5. Self-harming behaviours
Young people in forensic care

Hazel Chipchase BA(Hons) DipClinPsych
Clinical Psychologist, Stepping Hill Hospital, Stockport, UK
5. Self-harming behaviours
Women who self-harm in a high security hospital

Philip Clayton BSc(Hons) RNMH RMN ENB998
Senior Nurse Therapist, Calderstones Hospital, Lancashire, UK
7. Firesetting
Cognitive analytic therapy: learning disability and firesetting

J. Thomas Dalby PhD CPsych
Professor of Clinical Psychology, University of Calgary, and Psychology Coordinator, Peter Loughreed Centre, Calgary, Canada
3. Sexual offending
Adolescent sex offenders
7. Firesetting
Arson

Paula Ewers RMN DipHE PGDipCounselling MSc CBT
Clinical Nurse Specialist, The Scott Clinic, St Helens, Merseyside, UK
4. Severe and enduring mental health problems
Cognitive–behaviour therapy for delusions

Sara Finlayson BSc(Hons) MPhil DipClinPsychol
Clinical Psychologist, Rathbone Hospital HDU, Liverpool, UK

9. Seemingly intractable problems
Addressing institutionalisation

Joe Forster BA(Hons) RMN DipNurs
Nurse Team Leader, Rathbone Hospital HDU,
Liverpool, UK
9. Seemingly intractable problems
Addressing institutionalisation

Syd Fraser BSc(Hons) MSc PhD DipClinPsychol
CPsychol AFBPsS
Consultant Clinical Psychologist, Rampton
Hospital, Notts, UK
5. Self-harming behaviours
*A problem-solving approach to the treatment of
suicidal behaviour and self injury*

Ute Goldkuhle DrPH RN-ANP
Assistant Professor, University of Hawaii,
Monoa, School of Nursing, Honolulu, Hawaii,
USA
11. Community care
Inter-agency working in the USA

Jan Gregoire SRN RMN RGN PGDipCouns
CertSupervision ENB A74
Clinical Nurse Therapist, Ashworth Hospital,
Merseyside, UK
7. Firesetting
Group work with women who set fires

Gill Haddock BSc(Hons) MClinPsychol PhD
Clinical Psychologist and Lecturer in Clinical
Psychology, University of Manchester, UK
**4. Severe and enduring mental health
problems**
*Cognitive–behaviour therapy for auditory
hallucinations*

Dave Harper BA(Hons) MClinPsychol PhD
Clinical Psychologist and Clinical Tutor,
North Mersey Community NHS Trust and
Department of Clinical Psychology, University
of Liverpool, UK
8. Problematic substance use
Use and misuse of prescribed medication

Michael Howlett LLM(Hons)
Director, The Zito Trust, London, UK
2. Care in context
Victims and survivors

Clare Hughes
John Hughes
Parents of service user.
2. Care in context
Family and friends

Howard Jackson BSc(Hons) MClinPsychol PhD AFBPS
Clinical Director, The Transitional Rehabilitation
Unit, Haydock, Lancashire, UK
10. Personality disorders
*Relating neurological and neuropsychological deficits
to antisocial personality and offending behaviour*

Lawrence Jones BSc MSc CPsych
Clinical Psychologist, Rampton Hospital,
Notthinghamshire, UK
10. Personality disorders
Therapeutic community in a forensic setting

Simon Jones RMN DipMDO ENB770
Court Liaison Officer, Northallerton NHS Trust,
North Yorkshire, UK
11. Community care
Diversion from custody

Arlene Kent-Wilkinson RN BSN MN
Forensic Nurse Educator/Consultant, Alberta,
Calgary, Canada
12. Key issues in forensic care
*Practitioner training, future directions, and
challenges for practice*

Peter Kinderman MA MSc PhD
Senior Lecturer, Clinical Psychology, University
of Manchester, UK
4. Severe and enduring mental health problems
Cognitive–behaviour therapy for delusions

David Leadbetter MSc BA(Hons) CQSW DSW
CertSWED CertMTD
Director, CALM Training Services,
Clackmannanshire, UK
6. Violence and aggression
*Critical incident management: aggression and
violence*

Karen Leadley BSc(Hons) MPhil DipClinPsychol
Clinical Psychologist, The Socrates Project,
University of Liverpool, UK
4. Severe and enduring mental health problems
Cognitive–behaviour therapy for delusions

Helen Liebling BSc MPhil MSc RGN
Clinical Psychologist, Psycho-Legal Service,
High Royds Hospital, West Yorkshire, UK
5. Self-harming behaviours
Women who self-harm in a high security hospital

Joe Martin III BA(Hons)
Assistant Psychologist, The Transitional
Rehabilitation Unit, Billinge, Lancashire, UK
10. Personality disorders
*Relating neurological and neuropsychological deficits
to antisocial personality and offending behaviour*

Tom Mason BAc(Hons) PhD RGN RMN RNMH
Senior Lecturer, Department of Nursing,
University of Liverpool, Liverpool, UK
1. Introduction
8. Problematic substance use
Use and misuse of prescribed medication
9. Seemingly intractable problems
The silent resistance
12. Key issues in forensic care
*Practitioner training, future directions, and
challenges for practice*

Ged McCann BPhil MPH RMN DPSN
County Development Officer for Mentally
Disordered Offenders, North Yorkshire Health
Authority; Lecturer, University of York, York, UK
1. Introduction
4. Severe and enduring mental health problems
Family work
12. Key issues in forensic care
*Practitioner training, future directions, and
challenges for practice*

James McGuire MA MSc PhD AFBPsS
Senior Lecturer, Clinical Psychology, University
of Liverpool, UK
10. Personality disorders
*Problem-solving training: pilot work with secure
hospital patients*

Mick McKeown BP(Hons) RGN RMN DPSN
Lecturer, Department of Nursing, University of
Liverpool; Practitioner, North Merseyside
Community NHS Trust, Liverpool, UK
1. Introduction
4. Severe and enduring mental health problems
Family work

8. Problematic substance use
Relapse prevention for problematic alcohol use
12. Key issues in forensic care
*Practitioner training, future directions, and
challenges for practice*

Dave Mercer BA(Hons) MA RMN PGCE
Lecturer, Department of Nursing, University of
Liverpool, Liverpool, UK
1. Introduction
3. Sexual offending
Pornography and practice: the misfortunes of therapy
7. Firesetting
Group work with women who set fires
9. Seemingly intractable problems
The silent resistance
12. Key issues in forensic care
*Practitioner training, future directions, and
challenges for practice*

Christopher Minto MSc LLB(Hons) PGCE RGN RMN
RMNH
Senior Lecturer, Forensic Practice Research Unit,
University of Northumbria at Newcastle, UK
12. Key issues in forensic care
*Clinical supervision for nurses in a learning
disability forensic service*

Maureen Morrow BSc(Hons) PGCE DPSN FETC RMN
RGN
Senior Lecturer, Mental Health Division,
University of Northumbria at Newcastle, UK
12. Key issues in forensic care
*Clinical supervision for nurses in a learning
disability forensic service*

Aisling O'Kane BSc(Hons) MClinPsychol
Clinical Psychologist, Scott Clinic, Mersey
Forensic Psychiatry Service; Lecturer in Forensic
Behavioural Science, Department of Clinical
Psychology, University of Liverpool, Liverpool,
UK
3. Sexual offending
Assessment of mentally ill sex offenders

Brodie Paterson BA(Hons) Med RMN RNMH RNT
Lecturer, University of Stirling, Stirling, UK
6. Violence and aggression
*Critical incident management: aggression and
violence*

Michael Pavlovic BA(Hons) DipSW
North Yorkshire Probation Service, UK
11. Community care
Primary care, probation, and risk management

Cindy Peternelj-Taylor BScN MSc RN
Professor of Nursing, University of
Saskatchewan, Canada
6. Violence and aggression
Anger management

Rob Poole MB BS FRCPsych
Consultant Psychiatrist, Rathbone Hospital
HDU, Liverpool, UK
8. Problematic substance use
Substance misuse complicating mental illness

Sheila Rose RNLD
Lecturer in Nursing, Rampton Hospital, Notts,
UK
5. Self-harming behaviours
*A problem-solving approach to the treatment of
suicidal behaviour and self injury*

Penny Schafer RN BSN
Coordinator, McKenzie Unit, Regional
Psychiatric Centre, Saskatoon, Canada
6. Violence and aggression
Anger management

Howard Shimmin BA(Hons) DipCouns DipSW
Project Manager, The Wordsworth Project,
Ashworth Hospital, Merseyside, UK
10. Personality disorders
*Social therapy: a case study in developing a staffing
model for work with personality-disordered offenders*

Ged Smith BEd CQSW MSc
Family Therapist, Greenwich NHS Trust,
London, UK
3. Sexual offending
Working with survivors of sexual abuse

Tish Smyer DNSc MN BSN
Associate Professor, South Dakota State
University, USA
9. Seemingly intractable problems
The aged offender

Les Storey RGN MSc PG(Dip)HE
Lecturer, University of Central Lancashire,
Preston, UK

10. Personality disorders
*Social therapy: a case study in developing a staffing
model for work with personality-disordered offenders*

Mark Stowell-Smith BA(Hons) MSc PhD DipPSW
DipForPsych
Psychotherapist, Whiston Hospital, Merseyside,
UK
10. Personality disorders
*Psychodynamic psychotherapy, personality disorder
and offending*

Cheryl Tringham MPhil RNT RCNT RGN RNMH
Teaching Fellow, University of Stirling, UK
6. Violence and aggression
Critical incident management: aggression and violence

Peter Van Der Gucht BSc CQSW
Psychiatric Social Worker, North Yorkshire
Social Services, UK
11. Community care
Inter-agency working in the UK

Gregory Van Rybroek PhD JD
Deputy Director, Mendota Mental Health
Institute and University of Wisconsin – Madison
(Psychology, Psychiatry, Law), Wisconsin, USA
6. Violence and aggression
*Chronically dangerous patients: balancing staff
issues with treatment approaches*

Jack White BSc(Hons) PhD FAPS
Chair, College of Forensic Psychologists,
Australian Psychological Society, Australia
3. Sexual offending
Adolescent sex offenders
7. Firesetting
Arson

Richard Whittington BA(Hons) PhD RMN CPsychol
AFBPsS
Senior Lecturer, Department of Psychology,
University College of Chester, UK
6. Violence and aggression
*Changing the environment in the management of
aggression*

Phil Woods DipHC RMN EN(M) ENB870
Lecturer in Nursing, University of Manchester,
UK
12. Key issues in forensic care
Social assessment of risk: the Behavioural Status Index

Foreword

Mentally disordered offenders are in many respects little different from the clientele of the mental health services generally. They are predominantly distressed and disabled people, often showing multiple dysfunctions, who require the variety of therapeutic services expected in a modern mental health care system. However, mentally disordered offenders are not simply the mentally disordered who happen to offend, and two critical features distinguish forensic psychiatric services. First, the problems of mentally disordered offenders come to light because of the problems they cause for others. Second, these services are located at the shifting interface of the criminal justice and mental health systems, and their clinical functions are often compromised by the social and political roles they are expected to serve.

Providing treatment services under such conditions has never been easy. Violent patients are frequently unwilling participants in treatment, and can generate strong countertransference and stress in staff. Service priorities and the objectives of treatment for mentally disordered offenders are also frequently unclear. Secure hospitals that attempt to be more than 'benign warehouses' are liable to public criticism for being too liberal. More often, tension between the goals of public safety and individual treatment is resolved in favour of the former by a reliance on pharmacological treatment and containment as the mainstay of management and care. This dominance of the 'medical model' and the priorities accorded to security and institutional routines discourage attempts to understand and meet the complex needs of patients.

This books demonstrates that despite these obstacles to treatment innovation, many clinical staff in the forensic psychiatric services are actively engaged in treatment provision. It also illustrates the wide range of problems with which staff attempt to deal. These efforts to individualise treatment originated more than thirty years ago when psychodynamic and behavioural therapies were first introduced into the English special hospitals. Applications of these and other psychosocial treatment methods to the problems of mentally disordered offenders have subsequently been reported from forensic psychiatric services in a number of countries. However, descriptions of this work are often limited to research reports in specialist intradisciplinary journals and do not come to the attention of practitioners in different disciplines. Moreover, the development of community care for mentally disordered offenders has entailed the involvement of other disciplines and different contexts of treatment and management that remain unfamiliar to staff in more traditional secure settings.

The editors of this book have attempted to make these developments more accessible to practitioners by adopting a case study approach. This description is perhaps deceptive, because the chapters in this book go beyond mere anecdote or the description of 'interesting cases'. Instead many of the contributors set their therapeutic experiences in the context of the theory and research underpinning their procedures. They also describe the obstacles, frustrations and wider institutional and social constraints involved in attempting to achieve therapeutic change with mentally disordered offenders. As they amply demonstrate, success is rarely guaranteed and always hard won.

The book also emphasises that treatment services are being provided by a variety of disciplines. It is significant in this respect that the editors are experience forensic psychiatric nurses who have provided professional leadership in moving from a traditional custodial management role to a more active provision of therapeutic services. However, as many of these case studies illustrate, treatment practices are not only multidisciplinary but also interdisciplinary. Institutional treatments, for example, frequently involve the collaboration of psychologists, nurses and social workers, while interagency cooperation is crucial in community care. It will also be clear that the further development of services for mentally disordered offenders can profit from the interchange of the experiences and ideas of mental health professionals grappling with similar problems in other countries.

The editors are to be congratulated on bringing together a wealth of experience from a diversity of sources, including the often neglected recipients of services. They aim to illustrate what is being attempted with mentally disordered offenders rather than to demonstrate `what works' with this group. Despite significant progress in the development of interventions for offenders more generally, we actually know little about the effective ingredients of services for offenders who are disabled by mental disorder or about which treatment methods work best with which patients. Randomised controlled trials may eventually tell us something about the potential efficacy of particular procedures when applied to specific clinical problems. They are unlikely, however, to tell us which treatments are most effective in producing therapeutic change with patients who typically have multiple problems. Case studies of the kind reported by many of the contributors to this book are essential to inform us about the effectiveness of established or developing procedures when exported to complex clinical settings.

What case studies do not tell us is the extent to which mentally disordered offenders are receiving the therapeutic services illustrated. The number of patients provided with such services has always been small, and even a decade ago, surveys of forensic psychiatric services in Britain and America revealed that individualised treatment continued to be the exception rather than the rule. There may never be enough staff to meet the individual needs of mentally disordered offenders. However, if this book encourages greater recognition among mental health practitioners that many seemingly intractable clinical problems can be amenable to change, the editors' aims will be well satisfied.

Liverpool, 1999   Ron Blackburn

Preface

Few people today, professional or otherwise, could claim disinterest in the field of forensic mental health care, or dispassion about the disposal of disordered offenders. From tabloid headlines to Hollywood's box office billions, the criminal as madman (or woman) has achieved an almost unequalled media currency. If the haunting black-and-white imagery of *Psycho* captured the deranged killer as a collective fear of mass popular culture, then Hannibal Lecter must symbolise the depth of despair in psychiatric expertise. Yet these excessive and fictional examples are an important starting point for this text, in that they illustrate the enormous challenges facing those who work with a socially excluded and disadvantaged population. Here is the metaphor of violence and cruelty, the demand for retribution, the grail of rehabilitation, the stigma of otherness, the contagion of contact and the destruction of innocence. Most significantly, though, they situate forensic practice in relation to the larger political and moral debates which construct medicalised crime.

Despite the diverse assaults of conservative and liberal critics upon the ideal of treatment for offenders, the therapeutic enterprise has both survived and flourished. Sadly, this victory has been typically proclaimed in ways which are either rhetorical or remote from the practice domain. Individual 'clients' have been sacrificed to the statistics of recidivism, the science of the randomised controlled trial, and the silence of dominant discourses. None of this is to deny the relevance of research in establishing a solid foundation for the development of evidence-based intervention. Rather, it attests to the confusion and contradiction which characterise an, as yet, embryonic field. Between the disparate poles of 'nothing works' and asking 'what works?' are a growing number of allied groupings with a responsibility to manage and care for the perpetrators and survivors of interpersonal harm. This book is dedicated to hearing their stories, and learning from them.

If the aims of the book are modest, the challenges offered are more circumspect. Before we can talk to each other there needs to be a common language. Just as the disordered offender is homogenised in the literature, ideas about the role of the practitioner are often narrow and partisan. This is hardly desirable, yet no more does it reflect our own experience of clinical work in a forensic context. Contributors to the text represent both the providers and recipients of forensic care, and span a range of services, agencies and disciplines. This type of collaborative venture is fundamental to the promotion of good practice, premised upon reciprocity, respect and continuity. If these are laudable aspirations for success, their failure is the regrettable conclusion of too many official inquiry reports.

A further feature of the authors gathered in this text is their proximity to the point of practice or service delivery. In their candid accounts, using the medium of case studies, they restore a human face to the invisible players behind the headlines. And here is a second ambition of this book: to reflect upon what we do when things go wrong, just as much as when they go right. A notable adjunct to the professionalisation of forensic care has been the explosion of educational courses, affiliations, and product champions. While there is no shortage of gurus and mantras, critical narratives are less abundant. This is particularly problematic for forensic nursing in the UK, where in some senses a quasi-religious zeal has substituted blind faith for honest appraisal. This book may not set that world alight, but were it to do so there would be no shortage of 'fiddlers'.

If parochialism is a weakness, we have endeavoured to diminish its attrition by seeking an international perspective. Forensic practice is a global phenomenon and there is much to share with our colleagues around the world. Again, though, we need to be sensitive to the historical and cultural contexts which underpinned service development, and will continue to shape future directions. If the UK cannot claim a unified system of mental health legislation, there is a common emphasis upon offence-specific approaches, be they institutional or community orientated. Forensic practice in this sense embraces the Special Hospitals, regional secure units, prison medicine, policing and a range of diversion or liaison initiatives. The mentally disordered offender is a direct descendent of the 19th century 'dangerous individual', an embodiment of psychiatric power penetrating the criminal justice system. It is a progressive though not uncontested journey, which has taken over 150 years. Across the continent of North America, or in the antipodes, this 'correctional' focus would hardly begin to describe the scope of forensic practice.

Finally, the various interventions described in this collection of case studies is deliberately eclectic, with contributors selected on the basis of scholarly and clinical expertise in their respective fields of practice. The collective whole attempts to capture the actual diversity of provision for mentally disordered offenders across contemporary multi-agency services.

Liverpool, 1999

Dave Mercer
Tom Mason
Mick McKeown
Ged McCann

Abbreviations

AA	Alcoholics Anonymous
ABC	aggressive behaviour control
AID	apparent irrelevant decision-making
ASW	approved social worker
ATSA	Association for the Treatment of Sexual Abusers
BPD	borderline personality disorder
CAT	cognitive analytic therapy
CBT	cognitive-behaviour therapy
CHN	community health nurse
CICB	Criminal Injuries Compensation Board
CMHT	community mental health team
CPA	Care Programme Approach
CPN	community psychiatric nurse
CPS	Crown Prosecution Service
CSE	coping strategy enhancement
DAT	dementia of Alzheimer's type
DNR	do not resuscitate
DRAQ	Drug-related Attitude Questionnaire
DSM	Diagnostic and Statistical Manual
ECT	electro convulsive therapy
EE	expressed emotion
FCPN	forensic community psychiatric nurse
HAD scale	Hospital and Anxiety Depression scale

HDU	high dependency unit
IAFN	International Association of Forensic Nurses
HSPSCB	High Security Psychiatric Services Commissioning Board
MDT	multi-disciplinary team
MEPS	means end problem-solving
MHAC	Mental Health Act Commission
MHRT	Mental Health Review Tribunal
MMPI-2	Minnesota Multiphasic Personality Inventory-2
MSU	medium secure unit
PANSS	Positive and Negative Syndromes Scale
PCTM	patient care team meeting
PD	personality disorder
PDU	personality disorder unit
POA	Prison Officers' Association
PQRST	Personal Questionnaire Rapid Scaling Technique
PRN	pro re nata; as required
PSI	psychosocial intervention
RMO	responsible medical officer
SANE	sexual assault nurse examiner
SDR	sequential diagrammatic reformulation
SHSA	Special Hospitals Service Authority
TC	therapeutic community
TPP	target problems procedures
VRS	Violence Risk Scale
WISH	Women in Special Hospitals

Introduction

CONTENTS

Introduction

*Mick McKeown, Dave Mercer,
Tom Mason and Ged McCann*

This book draws together 39 case studies written to illustrate something of the diversity of experience and clinical practice which exemplifies the forensic practice arena. All excepting Michael Howlett's contribution in Chapter 2, which refers to a case already in the public domain because of the publication of an official inquiry report, have been anonymised to protect the identity of the subjects. The idea is to provide interested practitioners with a flavour of potentially useful issues and interventions, setting them in the context of real experience, as seen by key representatives of the various stakeholders in forensic care. It is hoped that the emphasis is on clinical utility rather than dry theory. In this way we hope to render an eclectic mix of therapies more easily accessible to line-level practitioners, and, ultimately, more likely to become employed in the course of routine practice and case management. This is not to say that this text should be read as a clinical handbook, directly inspiring and informing sophisticated therapies. Rather, it ought to be read as an introduction to these therapies, complete with reflections upon their use in practice, which could lead to them being taken up in practice given the possession of an appropriate level of competency and expertise, and adequate systems for clinical supervision.

Forensic care

In recent times forensic care has become the focus of much professional development and interest. This notion of forensic care usually refers to the treatment and rehabilitation of mentally disordered individuals who also exhibit a degree of criminality, with the context of this care more often than not involving placement in some sort of secure institution or close supervision within the community. However, what actually constitutes forensic care, or the work of forensic practitioners, has been subject to some flexibility of definition, especially with respect to international differences in the disposal of mentally disordered offenders and the organisation of appropriate services. Though the legal notion of diminished responsibility in relation to mental state is commonplace across mature criminal justice frameworks, sentencing patterns for offenders, whether to institutions which exist primarily as prisons or hospitals, vary widely amongst, or even within, nation states. Certain of these differences arise from the employment of distinct, or even divergent, legal or psychiatric taxonomies. Such definitional difficulties are exemplified in the controversy over the use of the medico-legal construct of psychopathy in England and Wales, yet not Scotland, with disposal decisions centring on the, often ambiguous, professional judgement of 'treatability'.

The recipients of forensic care are a diverse group, from whichever way they are regarded. They span the range of mental health problems and diagnoses, and the spectrum of criminal offences. It is also quite clear that, broadly speaking, the sort of stigma and public fear which surrounds mental illness generally is exaggerated, often in the extreme, in contemplation of this group. The media and politicians often exacerbate these matters by sensational over-identification with the highest profile and most extreme criminal acts of the minority of offenders. Notwithstanding such misrepresentation, the real focus on the management of dangerousness, of one form or other, is inescapable in the care of the majority. Given the strong association in the public consciousness of a relatively fixed and enduring attitude which links people with mental health problems to a fear of violence, it is not surprising that forensic patients receive a bad press. Wider issues of stigma and discrimination

against people with mental health problems have been challenged in mainstream psychiatry and among the general public by various initiatives, largely arising out of the politics of service-user involvement and empowerment.

Central to these efforts has been a challenge to the twin dynamics of oppressive power structures and the power of language itself in the construction of negative attitudes and personal responses to so-described individuals. A simple example of this would be the rejection of pejorative lay or medical labels, often applied to people who use services, especially where employed as a matter of routine by professionals. If we turn to forensic environments and institutions, it is clear that attempts to address such issues of progressive practice and civil liberties are both called for, but inherently problematic and complicated by the dual role of therapy and custody. A glaring example of this is the question of how to refer to the users of forensic services. Within mainstream services, the appellation of patient has largely been replaced by variants on the descriptor of client, reflecting historical and ideological movement towards a philosophy of consumerism in health. However, to refer to forensic 'patients' as 'clients' is palpably absurd given the absence of choice in the establishment of therapeutic relations for the majority of such people, especially those within the confines of secure hospital provision. Beyond this, however, there is ample room for improving professional discourse, attitudes and institutional practices, particularly with regard to the care of women and ethnic minority groups. Arguably, some of the negative effects of the psychiatric enterprise's engagement with issues of gender and ethnicity are seen in their most extreme form within the walls of forensic institutions. We have suggested elsewhere that attempts at staff education or consciousness raising, though laudable in themselves, are inadequate in addressing institutionalised discrimination without changes in the structures of administration and power.

The personnel who deliver forensic care are equally diverse, covering the range of professional health and criminal justice disciplines. Forensic psychiatry, and its related specialisms, represent a growing professional territory. Nurses comprise the largest section of the forensic workforce, with colleagues across a diverse range of allied professional and occupational groups including psychiatrists, clinical psychologists, social workers and probation officers, occupational therapists, prison health care staff, police officers and voluntary agencies. Typically, the professional literature has been dominated by medical perspectives, with a smaller, but growing, number of contributions from forensic psychology or forensic nursing. Yet, with the move towards multi-disciplinary and inter-agency practice the forensic mental health worker has assumed a more eclectic role, with interventions shaped by a collaborative framework rather than a narrow uni-disciplinary focus.

Bringing together practitioners, researchers and clinicians, the idea for this book grew out of the need to bridge a vaunted theory–practice gap, by explicating good practice and problem areas, within the clinical arena of forensic care. Such a focus will, it is hoped, provide a reference source for others and enhance quality standards in the field. The relevance of many of the issues covered here will not be restricted to forensic practitioners alone, having a broader value to mainstream arenas of care also. An obvious example of this cross-over would be the continuing importance of assessing and managing risk, regardless of the clinical setting. Though there is much work to be done in researching the effectiveness of interventions for mentally disordered offenders, and the systematic implementation of best practice is variable, this is not to say that the field is characterised by therapeutic pessimism. However, from the perspective of grass-roots practitioners, or students of forensic care, it can often be immensely difficult to glean practical information about key interventions from the research literature. Papers which evaluate certain interventions often given scant attention to detailed descriptions of the actual therapeutic techniques or strategy employed. The reliance on case study material here is aimed at making some of the practicalities of the interventions and relevant clinical issues much more accessible

to a wider readership. An important dimension of this task is the extent to which the authors attempt to honestly reflect upon the real-life difficulties of delivering some of these interventions in practice. Even if a particular intervention has not been wholly successful with a particular person (a rare event, possibly, in psychiatry, let alone forensic arenas, given the challenging and complex problems and needs presented), it is still possible to draw valuable learning experiences from contemplation of the factors which have contributed to the degree of success or failure which results.

Common themes, which reflect contemporary practice and policy, are drawn out in many of the case studies. The contributing authors describe relevant research and evidence upon which they base their practice, or call attention to gaps in the evidence base. Many of the case studies describe specific treatment modalities or therapeutic interventions applied to particular groups of mentally disordered offenders, either in terms of specific diagnoses or psychosocial problems, or with respect to different categories of offending.

Despite ambiguities of definition, there has been a rapid emergence and expansion of educational courses, curricula and, to a lesser degree, texts, aimed at satisfying increasing levels of demand for appropriately knowledgeable and skilled practitioners. This focus has attempted to draw out and delineate forensic practice as a discrete specialised field of working. Again, the wider relevance of matters central to forensic practice is evidenced within UK nursing education in the English National Board's (1995) recommendation for coverage of the care of mentally disordered offenders in all pre-registration level programmes. The growth of specific professional specialisms can be seen in the fact that degree and diploma courses with a forensic flavour are an increasingly marketable commodity in university and higher educational institutions, with the Internet providing opportunities for engagement with innovative distance learning materials. Most of these courses deal with therapeutic interventions and organisational care of mentally disordered offenders, but a wider definition of forensic practice brings in criminal investigative work, including the efforts of scene of crime personnel, offender profilers, and provision of victim support.

The philosophy of the International Association of Forensic Nurses (IAFN) is illustrative of an alternative dynamic in the relationship between health care, law enforcement and forensic science. This body, orchestrated largely by the efforts of a small number of sexual assault nurse examiners (SANE) in 1992, has resolved to include victims of violence no less than the perpetrators. Currently, it would be no surprise to find health care personnel working alongside police and agents of the criminal justice system. The scope of this practice will embrace such diverse activities as scene of crime investigation, collection of evidence, photo-documentation, trauma counselling and the whole range of mental health assessment.

There is an academic discourse concerning whether the 'forensic' component of any professional discipline constitutes a unique body of knowledge or merely represents traditional approaches targeted at a specific population. Aside from this theoretical debate, everyday practice continues. It is this pragmatic area of forensic operational practice that this book attempts to illuminate, through the use of case studies relating to a wide range of forensic settings, from institutional containment to community care.

Structure of the book

The book is constructed around 11 central, if difficult, areas of forensic care and management. Within each of these chapters, case studies will be used to present an assessment of problems, strategies of intervention and forms of outcome measure. Contributors are drawn from forensic practice in the UK, USA, Canada and Australia. International links are now evidenced in journal publications, conference presentations and exchange projects. To date, core texts dealing with forensic care have been overly theoretical, singularly focused and professionally parochial. This book, in contrast, is aimed at a wider readership united by practical and clinical difficulties

and dilemmas. All of the contributing authors are respected experts in their field of practice and representative of a multi-disciplinary approach over a diverse range of forensic settings. The case studies cover a number of different national contexts, in terms of legislation and service delivery, included to present an international perspective. Chapter headings have been selected as a structuring principle for the text and to reinforce the need for planned, and systematic, care provision. Overall themes of the volume include contextualising care relative to current policy, examination of risk management issues, ethical considerations and the identification of evidence-based practice. This illustrative device of the case study is intended to highlight not only instances of progressive practice but also engage with, rather than avoid, seemingly irresolvable problems.

In Chapter 2, *Care in Context*, the contributors have been selected to speak, authoritatively, from the perspective of key players in the career of mentally disordered offenders. Not untypically, the 'career' of the forensic patient commences in the wake of catastrophic events, which sadly are too often captured in sensationalist media reporting and attendant moral panics. The impact of offending behaviour is rarely understood in relation to the significant others, be they family and friends of the offender, or the victim/survivor and their intimates. If developments in the USA signal trends for the future of the forensic role, this inter-relationship is likely to be of much greater import. The case studies in this section address such an equation, from the support and involvement of family and friends to the experiences of those who become the recipients of forensic care. Against the contemporary professional lexicon of empowerment and human rights, public safety and risk management are explored from the perspectives of these primary informants to the debate. *Terry Bailey* offers a disturbing account of her life as a patient within a maximum security psychiatric hospital. In relating the inadequacies of such institutions to meet the needs of women, she poses some telling questions about their future. The impact of offending upon family life is powerfully described by *John* and *Clare Hughes*, whose son was admitted for a lengthy period to a secure hospital. This testimony details a wide range of difficulties and stresses which confront and challenge relatives who find themselves in similar circumstances, and points to means by which some of these can be resolved. Finally, *Michael Howlett*, Director of the Zito Trust, focuses on the direct and indirect consequences of mentally disordered offending. He draws upon the consistent recommendations of various inquiry reports, with a focus on one key case, to urge an improved response to victims of these specific crimes.

In Chapter 3, the vexed issue of the care and treatment of individuals who have engaged in *Sexual offending* is considered. The sex offender label in many ways exemplifies the dilemma between professional issues and public concerns. However, it would be a mistake to view perpetrators as a homogenous group or conceive of them as residing solely in maximum security psychiatric settings. The case studies in this section address the interaction between legal definitions, medical diagnoses and service delivery. *Aisling O'Kane* presents an argument for broad criminogenic factors to be taken into account when assessing mentally ill sex offenders, rather than a singular reliance upon psychopathological models. *Thomas Dalby* and *Jack White* tackle the issue of sexual offences committed by adolescents. They remain therapeutically optimistic with regard to this client group and make important observations for the clinical and judicial management of such cases. The issue of sexual offending is taken up from a different perspective by *Ged Smith*. He recounts the institutional failings in the care of a survivor of childhood abuse within a forensic context. Similarly, the confounding effects of institutional cultures are prominent in *Dave Mercer's* case study. Here, the challenge of enacting a therapeutic regime for perpetrators of serious sexual crime is in conflict with pervasive attitudes and practices regarding masculinity and pornography.

Interventions for people with *Severe and enduring mental health problems*, comprising the largest single group of mentally disordered offenders, with respect to diagnosis, are discussed in Chapter 4. Within mainstream psychiatry, there has been much critical concern and policy directives regarding perceived inadequacies in the care of this client group. The psychosocial intervention (PSI) approach has been suggested as most likely to address these concerns and secure hospitals have been in the vanguard of translating this community model of practice into in-patient settings. The case studies in this chapter illustrate alternate dimensions of this approach, focusing on different aspects of the psychotic experience. *Richard Bentall* and *Gill Haddock* describe the cognitive–behavioural treatment of a person with auditory hallucinations who has committed murder and highlight some of the problems in applying such an approach in forensic settings. *Paula Ewers*, *Karen Leadley* and *Peter Kinderman* outline attempts to modify persecutory delusions in a violent offender. They too rely on a cognitive–behavioural model of psychotic symptoms, basing their therapy on a systematic case formulation. The notion of psychosocial interventions is central to the work of *Ged McCann* and *Mick McKeown* with respect to involving and supporting the relatives of patients detained in a secure hospital. Attention is paid to the separate and joint needs of both groups.

Chapter 5 deals with a variety of *Self-harming behaviours*. British mental health legislation allows for the detention of the mentally disordered for reasons of risk to themselves or others. Regardless of offence status, the forensic practitioner will be confronted by a substantial number of patients for whom the target of harm is themselves and the primary care issue is one of vulnerability. Paradoxically, this scenario can be exacerbated by the institution in which people are ostensibly placed for their own safety. The case studies in this section illustrate interesting features of self-harm, most notably certain demarcations between types of behaviour, and how these may relate to gender issues. Through the collective experiences of a group of detained female patients, *Helen Liebling* and *Hazel Chipchase* reflect on the attempt to introduce a woman-centred approach to therapy into an environment dominated by masculinity.

The problems of resisting this historical legacy are noted, with recommendations for progressive and gender-sensitive services. If patterns of self-harming behaviour are typically compounded by institutional factors, their antecedents often reside in childhood traumas of neglect and abuse. In the context of a secure unit for adolescents, *Maureen Burke* illuminates the intrapsychic crises, and interpersonal dynamics, faced by one young woman struggling to rebuild her life. *Syd Fraser* and *Sheila Rose* consider the therapeutic options available to staff in secure settings when self-harm escalates into suicidal behaviour. Recognising the value of ongoing psychotherapeutic intervention, they focus on short-term problem-solving as a strategy of care and management. Significant results are documented and organisational issues elaborated.

Chapter 6 engages with *Violence and aggression*, an issue of central concern to many forensic practitioners. It is often a prominent feature of offending, and the archetypal forensic patient is typically constructed from an amalgam of professional and public fears. Although this may be an oversimplification, those working in a range of forensic services will undoubtedly need to be skilled in the management of aggression and violence. Given the prominence of these concerns, some of the most ubiquitous and well-researched initiatives have focused on effective risk assessment and a broad range of interventive techniques and strategies. The case studies in this section consider both long- and short-term measures, aimed at reducing individual violent behaviours or managing crisis situations. *Penny Schafer* and *Cindy Peternelj-Taylor* outline the content and process of the Aggressive Behaviour Control (ABC) programme operated by the Correctional Services of Canada. The project offers an intensive treatment package for federal inmates, targeted at behavioural changes related to violent and criminal offending. *Brodie Paterson, David Leadbetter* and *Cheryl Tringham* remind us of the legal and ethical implications in maintaining a safe environment for service users and staff. In working with a challenging population an awareness of internal and external 'triggers' to violence is central to the de-escalation of critical incidents. The theme of environmental factors influencing levels of aggression in either negative or positive ways is developed by *Richard Whittington*. His case study offers constructive suggestions for integrating the physical and psychological dimensions of care for inpatient settings where violence is an issue. *Greg Van Rybroek* takes up this theme, highlighting the role of staff and the institution rather than simply implying that chronic dangerousness is exclusively located in the patient

Chapter 7 addresses interventions with individuals who have been involved in *Fire setting*. The offence of arson is, arguably, one of the most serious facing forensic practitioners. The symbolism of fire as an element of destruction is reflected in the gravity by which the judicial system disposes of convicted individuals. *Jack White* and *Thomas Dalby* relay the case history of an individual convicted of arson to illustrate important themes which have emerged in the scientific literature. A novel application of cognitive analytic therapy (CAT) is described by *Philip Clayton* in the context of a forensic learning disabilities service. In contrast to the previous individualised approach, *Jan Gregoire, Clancy Borastero* and *Dave Mercer* reflect on a group intervention for women who set fires, detained in a high-security facility.

In Chapter 8 care and management issues relating to *Problematic substance use* are explored. Refraction through the judicial and psychiatric systems can lead to a high density of individuals with a history of substance misuse in secure facilities. Clinical management can be exacerbated by continued use, perhaps with attendant moral panic amongst staff. Attempts to implement progressive policy or interventions can raise tricky dilemmas with respect to the law on drug misuse. The following case studies highlight the diversity and difficulties of addressing both licit and illicit drug use. *Clare Brabbins* and *Rob Poole* describe the care of a person with severe mental health problems complicated by the use of various substances. Interestingly, they explore the dynamics within a care team which is split between operating a harm-reduction approach or a policy of prohibition in the context of a secure environment. The focus on drug misuse can act to obscure the fact that a commonly problematic substance in forensic care is alcohol, and *Mick McKeown* addresses this in discussing a group approach to relapse prevention. There is much anecdotal reporting of the misuse of prescribed medication within forensic institutions. This issue is explored by *Dave Harper* and *Tom Mason* in the context of wider concerns over the issue of treatment compliance and its implications.

Chapter 9 addresses typical barriers to therapeutic progress, either institutionally driven or idiosyncratic. The compulsory detention and forced treatment of psychiatric patients, generally against their wishes, may benefit public safety but compromise therapeutic relationships and intervention strategies. Practitioners in the forensic field will encounter those with *Seemingly intractable problems*. These might include individuals who actively resist treatment over prolonged periods, where silence itself is a powerful medium of communication, as described by *Tom Mason* and *Dave Mercer*. With more optimism, *Claire Barkley* discusses new medical interventions for treatment-resistant schizophrenia. Long-term secure care can result in its own problems, raising concerns around quality of life. There will always be a minority of patients for whom there may be very little therapeutic optimism and who are likely to spend the remainder of their lives in conditions of security. The last two case studies in this chapter address both the reasons for this scenario and the means by which the deleterious effects of long-term incarceration can be minimised or overcome. *Tish Smyer* deals with the issue of offenders ageing within the system, and *Sara Finlayson* and *Joe Forster* present a psychosocial approach to tackling the effects of institutionalisation.

The contributors to Chapter 10 explore the difficult issues which arise in the care of individuals deemed to suffer from *Personality disorders*. The whole issue of treatment for this group of patients is highly contested. However, forensic practitioners do not have the luxury of exclusively debating the constructed nature of this medico-legal category and are obliged to engage real people in effective interventions. A number of initiatives have been suggested as potentially useful which range from the intra-psychic to the interpersonal. *Mark Stowell-Smith* outlines a forensic psychodynamic approach to addressing offence-specific dangerousness in the context of individual therapy sessions. In contrast, *James McGuire* highlights the value of group therapy aimed at global problem-solving skills. The other two case studies in this section describe the potentially therapeutic influence of systems. *Lawrence Jones* details the impact upon an offender of a therapeutic community approach, whilst *Howard Shimmin* and *Les Storey* focus on the process of facilitating change amongst a whole team, grounded in a philosophy of social therapy. The extent to which organic factors may contribute to the aetiology of personality-disordered offenders is the theme of *Howard Jackson* and *Joe Martin III's* reflections on the case of a brain-injured individual.

Chapter 11 addresses *Community care*, a crucial and growing area of forensic intervention. Like no other client group, mentally disordered offenders highlight the inadequacies of care in the community and the gaps in current provision. Their complex needs require effective collaboration between health, social services and the criminal justice system; yet disparate agencies can be seen to work in isolation, drawing upon diverse theoretical or philosophical perspectives. The organisation of effective inter-agency working is addressed in the course of two separate case studies, offering a view from both sides of the Atlantic. *Ute Goldkuhle* describes the American experience of case management, whilst *Peter Van Der Gucht* draws on similar themes from a UK perspective. *Michael Pavlovic* and *Simon Jones*, respectively, explore the opposite ends of forensic practice's interface with the community. The former accounts for initiatives in primary care, probation and risk management consequential on the discharge of previously hospitalised offenders, whilst the latter exemplifies the process of diversion from custody, and hence the entry into forensic mental health care.

In Chapter 12, some *Key issues in forensic care* are taken up. *Phil Woods* offers a specific systematic approach to risk assessment, a perennial theme in forensic care. The final two contributions raise important issues in staff practice, welfare and professional development. *Chris Minto* and *Maureen Morrow* present a case for the introduction of clinical supervision for forensic practitioners, drawing on the narratives of participating nurses. The editors, together with *Arlene Kent-Wilkinson*, conclude the book with a look forward to future directions and challenges for practice. Innovative models of education are highlighted, with such training perceived as an important route to achieving lasting improvements in services and clinical practice.

REFERENCE

English National Board (1995) Response to the review of health and social services for mentally disordered offenders and others requiring similar services. English National Board, London

CHAPTER 2

Care in context

CHAPTER CONTENTS

A personal experience

Terry Bailey

I was born in England to Irish parents, the fifth oldest, fifth youngest of a family of nine. My father was a drunk who was away more often than he was at home, my mother a dutiful Catholic wife who never contemplated divorce or refusing her husband his conjugal rights. He would often beat her up and she in turn would beat us, her children. I bore the main brunt of her anger and frustration as I was the 'clever clogs' of the family and the most outspoken. I was 8 years old when we moved to Ireland. Where we had been bullied in England because of our Irish connection, we were now being bullied for having been born in England. I cannot remember when I first contemplated death and dying, but I was 12 years old when I first voiced the wish to die to my sisters. It was around this time that I began to drink heavily. It was easy to get hold of the alcohol because my family distilled 'poteen', an illegal spirit in Ireland. I felt I was different to others in that my intelligence singled me out for ridicule from my mother and special attention from the teachers. At the age of 15, following an attempted sexual assault by a neighbour, I left home. I was sent back by social workers, and remained in the family home until 1 year later, when I finally left for good.

I ended up on the streets of London. Already a seasoned drinker, I now discovered drugs and a world where nothing and no-one mattered. Over the next 3 years, I was in and out of prison on remand for larceny offences, mainly shoplifting. My only friends were other 'cons' or addicts and my sexual relationships were confined to one-night stands.

I was diagnosed as having a 'personality disorder' at the age of 19, following my first admission to a psychiatric hospital. This was just 4 months after I had given birth to twin boys. I was not told at the time that any diagnosis had been made and left the hospital 2 months later none the wiser about what had happened, or why. At no time was I asked why I felt so low, or why I had taken an overdose. I was given medication and asked to weave raffia seats onto stools. I recall seeing a psychologist once, but her only interest seemed to be in measuring my intelligence by asking me to perform a number of tests. After this I refused to work with her. The eldest of my twins died, aged just 7 months, from cot death.

Over the next 5 years, I was to spend time in and out of prison for theft, actual bodily harm (ABH) and criminal damage (I seemed to have acquired a taste for breaking windows). There were also several more admissions for drink and drug detox, plus depression, but never for more than 3 to 4 weeks. The only treatment consisted of medication and referrals to Alcoholics Anonymous (AA). Almost 5 years after the death of my son, my 9-month-old cousin died whilst in my care; again, the verdict was cot death. I joined a church and for the next few years remained clean and sober. I was elected onto the church board, became an adult student in the church school and helped teach the youth Sabbath school lessons. I left the church community after about 4 years and returned to the bottle. After a one-night stand with an old friend, I became pregnant again, returning to London where my family were then living. Just 2 months after I gave birth to a beautiful and healthy baby girl, she too succumbed to the phenomenon of cot death. This time I could not accept her loss and soon found myself caught up in the psychiatric system once more.

Prior to my index offence, I had set a small fire in the funeral parlour where my child had lain, for which I received a caution. Shortly after this, I set fire to the house which I was renting, but caused little damage. I was a voluntary patient on the 'open ward' of a psychiatric hospital when I set fire to a shop which catered for parents of newborn children. Following this

incident, I was transferred to a medium security unit. On arrival I was left alone in the day room with the other patients. There were no other females that I could see. One man was pacing endlessly around the room, in a circle, occasionally punching the air and shouting. Another sat in an armchair wearing only a dressing gown which was open (he often walked around naked). Someone came towards me with outspread arms, claiming that he was 'Jesus' and would take away my pain. It was a 'madhouse' and I was petrified. Anytime that I complained about harassment or intimidation by the male patients, I was told I needed to be more tolerant as these men were 'ill'. Therapy was offered, in groups, but once again I was the only female and 'Jesus' was a member of the group. I became quite aggressive and agitated and my mood hit a real low. Within 3 months, my psychiatrist had decided to refer me to a high-security hospital, or 'Special' as they are more commonly known.

Confirmation of the realisation that I no longer had any rights under the law, and of my invisibility as a person, came when entering my plea of guilty and again during sentencing. The psychiatrist had written a summary of my life, parts of which I disagreed with and other parts which I felt had been misinterpreted. Though I was not asked to contribute to my own biography, my family were, although we had enjoyed little or no contact for 10 years. My sister informed the doctor that I had set fires in Ireland and this was presented as a fact to the judge. In reality, I have never been charged, let alone convicted, of arson in Ireland. Contrary to instructions, my barrister did not challenge any of the psychiatric findings. Although I was adamant that I would not accept treatment, I was sentenced to the Special for an indefinite term: a section 37/41 of the Mental Health Act 1983.

I was a child in this system. Once I was sent to bed early for giggling, which was interpreted as my being 'high', with a named nurse who insisted I refer to her as 'nanny'. We were 'their girls' (the staff's), though we were also considered dangerous and evil women when it suited their purposes. I spent 2 years on the admission ward which held women who had already been there 5 years or more, some having spent 15 to 20 years in the system. Many had entered the system as 18- or 20-year-old women. The majority of women of my own age, 30 when admitted, had already been in the hospital several years and were tired of trying to figure the system out. They would tell me I was naive when I insisted change could happen, had to happen.

There was nothing to do on the ward apart from sewing or knitting, the table tennis making only an occasional appearance (usually when there were visitors on the ward). I used to walk up and down the corridor and was medicated in an attempt to make me sit quietly like the others. Out of boredom, frustration and anger, I began causing as much disruption to the ward routine as I could. It was incredibly easy to cause a security alert and I used their paranoia to be as annoying as possible. I mostly hid spoons or stole the crockery and distributed it amongst the other women. Because I was considered intelligent I was also considered to be highly dangerous. I was placed on close observations with severe restrictions including limited communication with my peers on the ward and no contact with other patients in the hospital.

The majority of patients in the Special were men and the majority of them were sex offenders, with whom even their own gender would refuse to mix if they were in prison. Although they had their own separate wards, we were expected to integrate with them in the Education Centre or at social events. There was a 'women only' workshop but that tended to concentrate on arts and crafts, rather than work or learning a skill. I complained to my solicitor, who advised me to comply with the system. WISH (Women in Special Hospitals) were assured that attending socials was not compulsory, yet my refusal to do so was raised as a concern at my Tribunal (MHRT). It left me feeling dirty, worthless and unimportant. Imagine the outcry if female prisoners were forced to mix with their male counterparts? The behaviour of the men also impacted upon our lives on the ward. We were often prevented access to the garden area because one or other of the men was feeling hostile towards women that day and had been allowed to 'walk it

off' outside the ward. On another occasion, a male patient threw hot water over someone on his ward and so we were no longer allowed to make our own tea or coffee. At the same time, though, these restrictions were not brought to bear on him. Making my own coffee had been the only thing I had been allowed to do for myself and the taking away of even the most basic of tasks was completely disempowering. When we heard of men escaping over the wall, we had trouble comprehending how that was possible. We never had space where staff were not four or five paces behind, let alone the opportunity to plan and make an escape. Similarly, women had their videos and computer equipment confiscated when the story broke about the pornography which male patients had access to, although no female patient had been involved. The knowledge that men were having unsupervised visits with their children, although their crimes should have dictated otherwise, was painful to all the mothers who had no access to theirs; or who, like me, always had a staff member present at visits.

The staff who worked in the Special were nearly all local people whose parents and grandparents had worked there. Approximately half the staff had no qualifications at all and were known as nursing assistants. The female assistants were used as 'stand-ins' for qualified staff who did not have time to talk or listen to us. The male staff were there to intimidate and keep us quiet. Once, after one of the male assistants had threatened a female patient, we all signed a complaint against him. The independent investigator concentrated more on the fact that she had used a swear word than on the physical size of the man, or his threat, which had caused considerable fear and distress to all the women and not just the individual concerned.

Probably the hardest part was that this treatment and lack of understanding were encouraged and often participated in by female staff, some of whom were qualified in mental health and called themselves 'nurses'. At times they would deny us clean sanitary towels or toilet paper and when placed on constant observation, they would take your panties off leaving you with nothing with which to hold your pad on by. I cannot begin to express how humiliating and degrading that experience can be, or why I was often filled with a bitter self-loathing when I saw or was subjected to those practices. Since emotion had to be suppressed, distress or attempts to regain some form of control over our lives was often exhibited through self-harm or by an eating disorder.

Initially, the prevalence of self-harm and other disorders was dismissed as 'attention seeking' until the Mental Health Act Commission (MHAC) and other groups began to express real concern. Following a training day on understanding eating disorders, our staff decided it would be easier to simply restrict our food intake and applied this rule even to women who had no history of abusing their food. For guidance about self-harm, staff were dispatched to America and returned with medical terms and American slang that the women patients were unable to identify with; but at least now the hospital could show they were taking these issues seriously. One woman who had a history of self-harm prior to admission, and was again feeling the urge to cut herself, approached staff about joining the programme. She was told that she was not eligible, having refrained from that kind of behaviour for some time. She felt she had been told to 'cut up or shut up'.

When '24-hour opening' (access to own room) was introduced to the Special that I was imprisoned in, there was a lot of resentment from staff and scaremongering by the Prison Officers Association (POA). Again, the men fared better than us women in the deal. While men could get up at night to make tea, have a 'cuppa', etc., we were simply given a few extra hours before 'compulsory' bedtime. Though our cells were no longer locked at night, we were made aware that they would be if we refused to stay in them once sent to bed, as our psychiatrist would simply prescribe 'locked doors' which would also mean an earlier bedtime. I did get up once to ask for a drink as I was anxious about my MHRT the following day. I was refused the drink, but offered PRN (as required) medication. When the nurse realised I was not prescribed any medication, she panicked and I had to assure her I would be fine and returned voluntarily to my cell. Their fear of having to deal with us without the aid of medication and/or seclusion would be comic if our lives were not being ruined by them.

There are several incidents which haunt me still. One involves a woman who warned me that a member of staff was planning to have me beaten up by other patients (to 'bring me down a peg or two'). She was later goaded into attacking the said staff member and sentenced to a prison term. The hospital gave her leave of absence to do her time and then recalled her to another of the Specials. Another shocking incident I witnessed involved a young black woman who would scrape at her skin, or cover herself in talc, in an attempt to make herself white. Staff openly made fun of what they termed her 'antics'.

I only ever met one black staff member in the Special Hospital. She was a female social worker, yet had been assigned to work with male patients. I saw no black nursing staff in my 3 years there, or since. I still visit the Special to see a friend, or when WISH hold a conference there, and little has changed. During one of these visits, on my way to the female villa, I passed male patients out enjoying the sun, while the women were locked away inside for their own protection. Though the POA members constantly highlight a need for tightened security and tougher measures to be introduced, citing staff vulnerability to attack, to my knowledge of all the inquiries into the three Special Hospitals none has been convened as a result of injury and/or death of a staff member.

People say the Special Hospitals can reform. I say 'Dream on'. We have had inquiry after inquiry and nothing has changed. The system is totally resistant: there are too many vested interests in keeping things the same. These are prisons first and foremost and it is predominantly a prison culture … And women, there are about 220 women in these hospitals, and most of them do not need to be there at all. They experience a culture that is abusive and infantilising beyond belief … People are being kept in what amounts to prison for years on end simply because the system is not capable of providing the care they need. In a modern, democratic society, that is obscene.

These words were written by Ray Rowden (1998), Director of the High Secure Psychiatric

Services Commissioning Board (HSPSCB), for the journal *Mental Health Care*.

Ray Rowden left the HSPSCB after 2 years because he felt he would not be allowed to make the changes in the system that he believed to be necessary. Unfortunately, that is usually what happens when any staff member attempts to bring about change in the system. The new post of Advisor to Women was vacated after just 6 months and the title changed to Manager of Women's Services, but she too gave up in 1997 after less than 2 years. They, and all the others who have left, are testimony to the fact that things are not changing regardless of what the hospitals' glossy annual reports would have us believe. The only psychotherapist employed by the hospital has also since left, making access to any real or beneficial treatment even more unlikely.

The MHAC, WISH and other advocacy organisations have no power to change anything and can merely express concerns regarding treatment, or the lack of it. They tend to give an air of respectability to the Specials and create the illusion that women are being heard and represented. Having once been a member of the Patients Council, I am also aware of how the institution uses such mechanisms to prove that they are listening, when in fact the Council is merely another stepping stone toward the good practice the Specials would have everyone believe they embrace.

Simply opening Women Only units, yet employing the same staff with the same views and attitudes that currently prevail, is not the answer. To start with, the time you can legally be held should have a limit which corresponds with a prison sentence for the same type of crime. Psychiatrists should be legally required to specify what type of treatment they are offering and what alternatives are available should the patient not respond to one particular type of therapy/medication. All staff should have training in 'women's studies', with a core staff equipped to help ethnic minorities whose behaviours and fears are ignored or misunderstood because their culture was not considered.

Those of us taken to court and held to be responsible for our crimes should also be given the responsibility of choosing between treatment or punishment. The Specials were established for the criminally insane, but are now used by lazy doctors as the dumping grounds for patients who need more than a tot of Largactil and a pat on the head. I was discharged in 1996 but many of the women, without whose support I would never have survived, remain stuck in a system that offers little treatment, no understanding, and even less hope. In the words of Ray Rowden (1998): 'In a modern democratic society, that is obscene.'

REFERENCE

Rowden R 1998 Special treatment: inside outside. Mental Health Care 1 (9): 295

CONTENTS

Family and friends

John and Clare Hughes

You must not allow yourself to become victims of this terrible tragedy.

These words from a close friend were the best advice we were given in the aftermath of our 18-year-old son James's index offence, which led to his detention in Ashworth high-security hospital 15 years ago. He is still there and we have been supporting him in whatever ways we could during all those years.

James always had great difficulty in adjusting to new experiences and situations outside the immediate family environment, unlike our other three children, who grew up well able to express themselves and to cope with the usual 'ups and downs' of family life. Whenever he was subjected to competitive pressures, for example school exams, or situations where he was required to talk about himself, James always found great difficulty in communicating with others and chose to retreat into silence. Increasing failure to achieve or progress in such areas only served to deepen his lack of confidence and distress, manifesting themselves in various ways, for instance, he would become tense, listless and deeply withdrawn. Often, with help and encouragement, he would be able to adjust and there would be a return of confidence with him becoming cheerful and more able to cope. The crisis would be over, until the next one was precipitated by another sudden pressure on him.

At other times he was unable to adjust and he would have to be removed from the distressful situation temporarily, perhaps a week or two at

19

home away from school, or even a transfer to a special school environment for a period. Such changes were always impatiently welcomed by James, so anxious was he to escape from the current predicament, but then the novelty of the new regime would wear thin and he would eventually become restless and unhappy and want to be back in the former environment again.

Eventually, at the age of 12, he suddenly announced his desire to leave his special school, where he had been making some progress in learning and socialisation, and transfer to a 'normal' secondary school. He did in fact complete the basic period of secondary education, but during these 4 years there were many crises in the classroom or playground and, on occasion, we felt it necessary to keep him at home until the current problem had passed and James felt more or less able to face up to school life once again.

Though James himself wanted to stay on into the 6th Form, the school felt he would not be able to undertake 'A'-level work and his educational psychologist found him a 2 year course instead at a local Further Education College. This offered young people with learning and other disabilities opportunities to learn from a wide range of subjects, without the pressure of examinations. James settled in quite well at first, but soon started to complain at the presence of various physically disabled people on the course. He felt he was himself being classed as 'handicapped'. The course tutor reported that he was often very tense in class 'like a volcano about to erupt'.

From this point until the index offence was committed only 6 months later, things went downhill very rapidly for James. He quit college, had several stormy sessions with a psychiatrist and was prescribed various tranquillisers. After further violent family scenes, he was admitted, as a reluctant voluntary patient, to an open ward in the local psychiatric hospital. A period followed where he revolved between hospital and home, started drinking and generally showed various kinds of incongruous behaviours which left us bewildered and apprehensive. All of this culminated in the final horror of his fatally attacking an elderly fellow-patient in the hospital grounds with a single blow of a kitchen knife.

At the time of his offence, it seemed hard for us, bewildered and traumatised by the rapid succession of arrest, police interrogation, court appearances, remand prison and so forth, to feel we were anything else but victims of a horrendous chain of events. These eventually resulted in his transfer to Ashworth Special Hospital after a court plea of manslaughter with diminished responsibility was finally accepted 6 months later.

During all this time we had our other three younger children to care for and protect from the stigma of having a member of the family in such a shameful predicament. All three were attending the same school that James had so recently left. We had to make sure that they would not be subjected to any publicity, either at school or elsewhere. Unfortunately, the local commercial radio station announced our son's name in connection with the incident in the hospital grounds, while we were at the police station trying to find out the details. We had not even been told what had happened, only that he was in custody. Our children were listening to the radio and were devastated, angry and very frightened. How were they going to face everyone in school the next day? Would their friends desert them? In the event, their close friends, and ours, 'came up trumps' and were very supportive. However, there are always the prurient, the scandal-mongers and nosy newspaper reporters to contend with. Up until the final court hearing 6 months later, it was a time fraught with unbearable tensions.

Nor does the fear of stigma ever fade away completely. Having a close family relative in a high-security hospital is actually worse than having a relative in prison. It has been very difficult for James's sisters and brother to explain, when they started to have new and serious relationships of their own, the whereabouts of their elder brother. As for ourselves, we have often had to field innocent questions from new acquaintances, enquiring after our 'other' son, with evasive answers. We have learnt over the years to be circumspect on these occasions, and when we have to mention, albeit reluctantly, the name of the hospital, we are by now well accustomed to hearing that sharp intake of breath and the embarrassed, 'Oh … isn't that where so-and-so is?' All of this reflected the regrettable notoriety of the institution at that time.

Nevertheless, our first reaction after his transfer from the barbaric prison system was a feeling of great relief that at last James was in the safe professional hands of medical and nursing staff, who would work with him therapeutically towards his eventual rehabilitation and resettlement in the outside world. But we very soon came to realise how little we knew about the aetiology or pathology of James's illness, or the long-term treatment methods used in such institutions.

The worst of it was that nobody within the hospital seemed at all anxious to enlighten us on these matters. For instance, the first official communication we received from the hospital, some weeks after James's admission, was a 'Handbook for Visitors' which was literally quite forbidding. It forbade much more than it permitted or encouraged in terms of patient–visitor contacts. We eventually got to find out who James's responsible medical officer (RMO) was and we were allowed a brief and non-committal interview with him. This was the first of a series of interviews with a succession of RMOs which, until more recent times, left us more frustrated and bewildered than enlightened. As for the ward staff, there seemed to be a similar reluctance to impart any information regarding our son's care plan, or even to help or advise us in coping with James's often disturbed behaviour during those early visits with him while he was still on the admission ward. If we asked for specific information about his treatment or progress, we were simply told to write to his RMO (which we would dutifully do, although replies were not always forthcoming).

On reflection, the first weeks and months after admission of a relative into such a closed and forbidding environment are obviously times of the greatest anxiety and stress for the family, who will have already been through traumatic upheavals during the periods of their relative's deteriorating mental health, culminating in many cases in an index offence and detention. It is particularly crucial, therefore, for the caring relatives to receive as much helpful information and support as possible from the ward nursing staff, as this is a period of conflicting emotions for families, and often includes a burden of guilt and social stigma for the relative's criminal offence or antisocial behaviour. To quote from the Blom Cooper Inquiry Report (Committee of Inquiry 1992):

…regrettably, the regime at Ashworth … seems to have been designed to deter rather than encourage relatives to participate in their relatives' care. (p 233)

This was some 9 years after we, ourselves, first recognised similar staff attitudes. In the same chapter of the Report, social workers Susan Machin and Jonathan Best point out that:

…relatives often perceive themselves as powerless, and only through kind-hearted compliance can they contribute to the care of the patient. (p 233)

The Support Group

During these early years, there were many occasions when we felt the lack of any mutual support network among relatives and friends of patients at Ashworth. A network which could have explored matters of common interest concerning not only patients' welfare but the well-being of us relatives as well. Sharing the concerns and experiences of people in similar predicaments can often help in the process of alleviating one's sense of powerlessness and isolation in the face of what can seem an impersonal and impenetrable system. It was only in the aftermath of the scandals that led to the Blom Cooper Inquiry that Ashworth very belatedly began the process of creating a forum for relatives and friends (or 'significant others') to meet regularly. At first, this pilot project was restricted to one ward and was indeed largely initiated and developed through the sterling efforts of some members of the Hazlitt Ward nursing team.

Hazlitt happened to be our son's ward at this time (autumn 1991) and so we were very pleased to be invited, along with other relatives, to be involved in the creation of a ward-based

Relatives and Friends Support Group. From its inception, the staff members involved encouraged us to take responsibility for the structure and agenda of the Group into our own hands, with nursing or ward management presence as, and when, invited. After some initial wariness, with prospective Group members finding it hard to realise that they were actually being given a voice in their relatives' care and that their concerns might actually be heard by the 'professionals', the Group stabilised and flourished, with constant background support. We drew up a simple constitution, appointed a chair on a rotating basis and arranged a programme of monthly meetings in the ward library. We mainly discussed matters of mutual concern regarding our relatives' care and welfare, but we also invited appropriate professionals within the hospital to discuss topics such as the effects and management of schizophrenia within the family, medication, diet, the provisions of the Mental Health Act 1983 and Mental Health Review Tribunal procedures. In all such matters we relatives were involved in a steep learning curve!

A detailed account of the Group's setting-up and development is contained in McCann's (1993) evaluation study. Here, we can only mention some of the major benefits and spin-offs of the Support Group initiative as we and our fellow Group members came to experience them:

- Our physical presence on the ward during meetings was valued, not only by ourselves and our respective relatives but also by the other patients, many of whom seemed never to receive visits themselves. They began to feel that the Group members, by their very presence, were giving them all an extra voice in the ward's affairs, and some asked to sit in on our meetings from time to time, adding their own comments and insights to the agenda.
- We now enjoyed a face-to-face communication link to ward staff, who were no longer disembodied voices on a telephone line. There was less of a sense of 'them and us' in our dealings with them, and more of a growing feeling of partnership in the therapeutic process of our son's care and rehabilitation. We relatives were able to meet with primary nurses and discuss problems and concerns, and in particular to amplify, in more human detail than through phone calls or gleaned from clinical notes, our own versions of the patients' histories that had led to their present detention.

- From our own son's perspective, there was a marked improvement in his relations with his primary nurse as we all met together, after Group meetings on the ward, to talk over James's current care plan and to make arrangements for such special events as his first day visit home after 9 years' incarceration. Formerly, he had been suspicious of the nursing regime generally and, at times, even non-co-operative in matters such as keeping up his personal hygiene or his attendance at social or work activities. Now, as he joined us in openly sharing our concerns with him and his nurses face-to-face on the ward, he seemed less inclined to split, to keep up his 'me and them' attitude, and more inclined to negotiate and be reasonable in his reactions to the daily routines of the ward.
- As the Group grew in cohesion and confidence, a valuable sense of camaraderie developed among the members, united as we were in our common concerns. We compared notes and shared stresses and strains both inside and outside the hospital walls, and we involved ourselves in occasional social events on the ward which brought together patients, staff and visitors in an informal setting.
- Above all, we experienced a growing feeling of empowerment, being able to make a contribution and a difference, which in turn engendered hope and even optimism for our son's eventual recovery where there had been little or none before. These positive feelings came to be reflected in our meetings with our relatives and friends in Ashworth, which made visiting times more pleasurable experiences all round.

It would be gratifying to report that the achievements of the Hazlitt Ward Support Group had spread through other wards and inspired them to similar ventures, but in spite of our proselytising zeal, and the Clinical Rehabilitation Department staff's best efforts, this did not happen. One or two other wards did initiate Support Groups of their own, but for various reasons they did not survive.

However, about this time, members of our Support Group became closely involved in the planning of a new initiative launched by the hospital. This was the building of a Visitors' Centre designed to offer social and support facilities, as well as overnight accommodation to those visitors who hitherto would have had to make a very long return journey in one day or stay in hotels. The Centre eventually opened its doors in March 1993 and has since proved its value many times over. The Centre offers a welcoming reception point for visiting relatives and friends in a neutral setting, just outside the hospital walls. It also provides the venue for the ongoing monthly meetings of the Visitors Action and Support Group, the present successor of our original Hazlitt Ward Support Group. This Centre group at last provides a hospital-wide forum for the relatives' collective voice to be heard at senior management level on a wide range of issues and concerns. This is particularly relevant now as Ashworth experiences another judicial inquiry and yet more organisational and personnel changes, which are making life within its walls more restrictive for patients, staff and visitors alike.

A Relatives' Charter?

As far back as 1992, the Blom Cooper Inquiry Report recommended that:

…The Special Health Services Authority should develop a clear policy about the values, principles and practices which govern relationships between hospital staff and patients' close relatives, recognising relatives' rights to information; practical involvement in care and treatment plans; and their need for emotional support and help. We received written evidence that the SHSA [Special Hospitals Service

Authority] intended to develop such a policy during 1992/3. (p 235)

Even before then, we and our colleagues in the Hazlitt Ward Support Group had come to realise the stark fact that only a small proportion of relatives and friends had, or indeed still have, any clear idea of their rights and responsibilities when visiting and supporting patients. We talked with many who had no knowledge of the formal patients' complaints procedure or the extent of their right to be involved in their relatives' care plans or case conferences.

What we saw that was needed was just such a 'clear' policy as recommended by Blom Cooper: a 'Relatives' Charter', to be given to each patient's nearest relative upon admission. This would clearly set out their rights and responsibilities in all aspects of visiting and supporting their relatives in Ashworth, and on similar lines to the SHSA 'Patients' Charters' (SHSA 1994). Thus, we became involved with a small working group of relatives and hospital officials in drafting such a document, but unfortunately it remains in draft form to this day, a victim of the ongoing management upheavals during the recent crisis and subsequent Fallon Inquiry.

Below are just one or two examples of the main entitlements to be guaranteed by the hospital in the Charter, as and when it eventually sees the light of day:

- Whilst your relative is being treated at Ashworth Hospital, you will have access to advice, support and counselling at the Visitors Centre, as well as facilities for overnight accommodation.
- Confidential information about your relative will only be available to the nearest relative/significant other following consent from the patient.
- You have the right to have any complaint investigated thoroughly, quickly and impartially in accordance with the complaints procedure. If required, you can have access to translation services.

Many of the draft Charter's provisions emphasise rights to information on hospital procedures and legal matters likely to affect their relative's welfare and treatment; other sections are devoted to corresponding responsibilities whilst visiting. Matters such as attitudes to staff and other patients and the adherence to the hospital's policy on visiting, covering such points as appropriate dress and the prohibition of supplying forbidden substances to patients, are included.

In spite of the current delays and uncertainties at a hospital management level, we feel confident that the Charter, once adopted and circulated, will provide a comprehensive and user-friendly guide for relatives making their first apprehensive visits to the hospital – such a guide we ourselves would have greatly valued 15 years ago.

Conclusion

In retrospect, we see that the good relationship we now enjoy with our son's care team (including his RMO) owes much to the mutual support and encouragement we shared with the other members of the original ward Support Group. We now feel ourselves able to contribute usefully to reviewing James's care and treatment on formal occasions such as his periodical case conferences or Mental Health Review Tribunals (where the presiding Chairman has clearly welcomed our presence and input to the proceedings). And outside the hospital, his home visits are looked forward to as successful and enjoyable occasions for the family, but equally for his primary nurse, who works with us in advance planning for the best use of James's precious hours at home.

There is no doubt that knowledge empowers. This has become evident to us in our long, and at times very stressful, experience as caring parents of a patient in a high-security hospital. But it can also de-victimise, conferring respect and a measure of responsibility on the relatives in such a situation, making them feel less isolated and helpless as they become more actively involved with patients, staff and other relatives in a network of mutual therapeutic aims.

REFERENCES

Committee of Inquiry into Complaints about Ashworth Hospital 1992 Report of the committee of inquiry into complaints about Ashworth Hospital (Blom Cooper Report) Cmnd 2028. HMSO, London
McCann G 1993 Relatives support groups in a special hospital: an evaluation study. Journal of Advanced Nursing 18: 1883–1888
Special Hospitals Service Authority (SHSA) 1994 Special hospitals service authority: patients' charter. SHSA, London

CONTENTS

Victims and survivors

Michael Howlett

Introduction

This case study begins by taking a brief look at the way independent inquiries into homicide by people with a mental illness have become established since 1994, following the publication of the inquiry into the care and treatment of Christopher Clunis, before focusing in more depth on the relationship between informal primary carers and the severely mentally ill. Attention will be given, in particular, to a case study of a patient in receipt of in-patient and out-patient mental health services over a period of years, who eventually committed homicide and attempted homicide, and whose care and treatment are described in a published independent inquiry report.

The purpose of the case study is to highlight two separate but inter-related themes. First, the very serious difficulties faced by informal carers as they attempt to engage services for family members who are generally regarded by those services as 'difficult to treat', which usually means their mental illness is compounded by a number of other risk indicators, such as a history of violence, alcohol and substance abuse, non-compliance with treatment, homelessness and unemployment. Second, the case study moves on to look at the place of 'secondary' victims in these community care tragedies and how they are treated by the process following the homicide.

Background: independent inquiries and community care – the Clunis case

The Zito Trust, a registered mental health charity, was set up in 1994 in response to the inquiry into the care and treatment of Christopher Clunis (Ritchie et al 1994), which examined the circumstances leading to the homicide, in December 1992, of Jonathan Zito. The Trust's objectives are to campaign for improvements in the way community care services are organised and delivered to the severely mentally ill, and to provide support and advice to those who are affected by a broad range of failures in community care services.

The Clunis inquiry has quickly established itself as seminal in the currently expanding field of independent inquiries into homicides committed by people with mental illness. The breakdown of care in this case, described in intricate detail by the inquiry report, represents something of a marker in the implementation of community care policy and, with the incident involving Ben Silcock in the lions' den at London Zoo on New Year's Eve 1992, began the process of raising concerns, both lay and official, which has gained in momentum ever since.

Between July 1994 and April 1999, there were 50 independent homicide inquiry reports published under guidance issued by the NHS Executive in 1994 (Department of Health 1994b). A further 30 inquiries are currently under way. As these inquiries are commissioned on a local basis, there is no central initiative for ensuring that their many recommendations are implemented nationally. Bringing the central recommendations together (Sheppard 1996), or analysing particular themes (Howlett 1998), may provide a focus for all services responsible for community mental health, but there is currently no requirement for purchasers and providers of services either to disseminate their inquiry reports widely or to avail themselves of reports published outside their locality. Indeed, one of the issues raised about implementing mental health policy by NHS Guidance, rather than by primary legislation, concerns the actual status of

the measures once they are in place. This is certainly the case with the introduction of supervision registers (Department of Health 1994a), which have been criticised as vague and open to legal challenge (Baker 1997).

A recurring theme in the majority of published inquiry reports is communication. It is evident that the fragmentation of services in many cases of patients who are deemed 'difficult to treat' leads to a breakdown in communication within and between agencies, so that full information is never in the hands of one service, agency or individual at any one time. Cases like Clunis are exacerbated by a reluctance, conscious or otherwise, on the part of professionals to engage with patients who have a history of violence. As Coid (1994) put it, 'Many psychiatrists currently practising in the Greater London Area will personally know a colleague who was directly involved in the care of Christopher Clunis.' Coid goes on to describe Clunis's movements during the 4-year period of his care in London:

He … lived in one bail hostel, two rehabilitation hostels, two hostels for the homeless and six separate bed and breakfast accommodations. The geographical pattern of his movements are of considerable interest. He crossed the River Thames from one side of the city to the other on four separate occasions, either by chance or deliberate placement, and with additional sideways moves between different in-patient and aftercare services. He meanwhile passed through three out of the four former Thames Regional Health Authorities.

In retrospect it was to become evident that, despite the protracted involvement of different professionals, any systematic or co-ordinated approach to care planning had broken down. During his last hospital admission Christopher Clunis had been considered fit for discharge by the responsible psychiatrists, but supervisory relationships and ongoing assessments of risk were disorganised and disparate. He stopped taking his medication, missed appointments and lost regular contact with health and social service agents. Local residents had expressed concern about Christopher's bizarre and, at times, threatening behaviour, but police had failed to consider the serious risk suggested by his previous history. Subsequently, Christopher Clunis stabbed Jonathan Zito, a complete stranger, to death in an underground railway station in London. The case was to receive widespread, and often sensationalised, reportage in the media, precipitating scrutiny and action at senior levels of government.

CASE STUDY: MARTIN MURSELL

Context: when things go wrong, informal carers and victims

Martin Mursell was born in 1967. He began suffering from mental illness at about the age of 17, but was not formally diagnosed until his first hospital admission some 4 years later. In May 1988, he seriously assaulted his girlfriend. He was remanded in custody for 4 months and then sentenced to 2 months' imprisonment, suspended for 1 year, for actual bodily harm (ABH). His mother had wanted this opportunity to be used to get proper treatment for her son so, accordingly, sought legal advice. Her solicitor's response was, 'You don't want him locked up for life in a mental institution, do you?'

In February 1989, Martin was admitted to hospital under section 2 of the Mental Health Act 1983 and was subsequently detained under section 3. He was given section 17 leave at the end of March, which continued until his discharge in July. He was subsequently admitted to hospital on four further occasions between 1990 and 1993 under section 3. In 1994, he was admitted as an informal patient in July and discharged in August. He had a history of non-compliance with medication, including non-attendance at out-patient appointments. He also misused alcohol and other substances.

In October 1994, Martin killed his stepfather Joseph Collins and attempted to kill his mother. Both were stabbed in the family home. In January 1996, he insisted on pleading guilty to murder and attempted murder, notwithstanding the availability to him of a plea of manslaughter on the grounds of diminished responsibility. He was sentenced to imprisonment for life, and 10 years, for the two offences. He is now a detained patient in one of the Special Hospitals, having been transferred from prison under section 48 of the Mental Health Act 1983. An independent inquiry into the care and treatment of Martin Mursell was commissioned by Camden and Islington Health Authority in 1996 and it published its report in 1997 (Crawford et al 1997).

Identified problems

It is evident from the inquiry report that the bare facts of the case as they are set out here give no indication of the extent to which Martin's mother suffered as her son's primary carer since the first symptoms of mental illness manifested themselves in the family home in 1984, continuing until the fatal and near-fatal attacks in 1994. During this 10-year period, every attempt was made by her to engage the appropriate services on behalf of her son. Her efforts, which exacted a heavy and unacceptable emotional and physical toll, and which ultimately devastated her life, drew in all possible sources of help and intervention, to no avail, including health, social services, housing, the voluntary sector, her MP, the prison service and her solicitor. In her many attempts to have her son assessed for community care services under the National Health Service Community Care Act 1990, she was consistently advised by the statutory authorities to call the police if she became unduly concerned.

Interventions

The following synopsis of the ways in which fundamental interventions by health, housing and social services respectively might have prevented the breakdown of care in Martin's case, a breakdown which ultimately led to tragedy, focuses principally on the period leading up to the fateful events in October 1994. In compressing analysis in this way, however, it should not be forgotten how Martin's mother had fought tenaciously for many years to get adequate care for her son and how, towards the end, she was clearly putting her own well-being and safety at risk.

Health

Martin had received treatment from the health service for a number of years before the attacks on his mother and stepfather. As he had been detained compulsorily on five of the six hospital admissions between 1989 and 1994, he was legally entitled to aftercare services under section 117 of the Mental Health Act 1983. The appropriate level of care under section 117 is assessed according to local implementation of the Care Programme Approach (CPA), introduced nationally in 1991 (Department of Health 1990). The inquiry report notes (Crawford et al 1997:64) that Martin Mursell should have been entitled to level 3 CPA, the highest level, intended for severely mentally ill patients who present a serious risk to themselves or others and who are eligible for inclusion on the supervision register (Department of Health 1994a). As already noted, Martin had a history of non-compliance with medication.

Initially, Martin had good contact from the community psychiatric nurse (CPN) allocated to his care. The absence of an effective, co-ordinated care plan, however, led to a progressive deterioration in CPN care. This was not helped by a reluctance on the part of the CPN in question to follow a single care plan, to implement the multi-disciplinary process inherent in section 117 aftercare or to write a formal care plan for Martin. The CPN stated to the inquiry that he was 'of a generation of [nurses] who were brought up not writing care plans', and that they were 'a formalisation of a way of thinking' (Crawford et al 1997:68).

At the time of Martin's final discharge from hospital in August 1994 to bed and breakfast accommodation, it was assumed that a CPN would provide support to him and his mother. This did not happen. Little notice was taken by the responsible medical officer (RMO) of Martin's history of violence and the risk he posed. The CPA had not been fully implemented by the health authority and no formal care plan was prepared for Martin. It was assumed by the RMO, however, that Martin's mother would be happy with the discharge arrangements.

The inquiry report notes that she was, in fact, 'thoroughly displeased' with the arrangements (Crawford et al 1997:78).

Housing

The failures to support Martin and his mother in the community were described by the inquiry's chairman as 'fundamental and depressing' (Lee 1997). The admission of Martin as a voluntary patient to hospital in July 1994 was at his own request, but he was discharged against his and his mother's will 2 weeks later. All the agencies involved at this stage disagree about the manner in which the discharge took place (Crawford et al 1997:46). The RMO felt that 'housing' would offer Martin accommodation; social services declared that Martin was being discharged at the insistence of the hospital; the housing officer felt 'dumped on' because the hospital simply rang up and told him Martin was on his way over in a cab. At this point he was officially homeless, having been advised by housing in 1992 to give up the tenancy on his flat as 'the logical and uncontroversial thing to do' (Crawford et al 1997:43). He was therefore given bed and breakfast accommodation.

Social services

The inquiry report makes it clear that Martin's needs were complex and that he required an allocated social worker. Yet, in March 1994, he was transferred from his allocated worker to the duty system because of pressures arising elsewhere within child protection. Neither Martin nor his mother were informed that he had been 'de-allocated'. Following discharge from hospital in August 1994 into bed and breakfast accommodation, his mother telephoned social services to express her concerns and asked for the name of the allocated social worker. Social services would not tell her. A week before the tragedy, she wrote to social services and received a curt and unhelpful response which stated that appropriate services would be offered to her son in the event of a crisis.

Outcomes: the carer as victim

The mother of Martin Mursell is in a unique position. She was her son's primary carer during the years of his illness. She became a primary victim when she was left for dead by her son following multiple stab wounds. She is a secondary victim as the bereaved widow of her husband, Joseph.

Discussion

Without the formal inquiry process, to which she was able to give extensive evidence, Martin's mother would have found it difficult to begin to come to terms with her loss, including the loss of her son to the high-security psychiatric services. The process itself, culminating in the public launch of the report, allowed her, as with many secondary victims, to channel some of her energies into an attempt to understand how the services could have failed so fundamentally in her case. The treatment of victims by the criminal justice system is well documented (Zedner 1997) and increasingly their needs beyond the role officially required of them as witnesses are now being recognised (Rock 1996).

As yet, however, there is no place for secondary victims in the civil courts. The case of Clunis is instructive on this point. In December 1997, the Court of Appeal decided that Clunis had no right to claim damages against the health authority he alleged had breached its duty of care towards him. The Court took the view that as Clunis pleaded guilty to manslaughter on the grounds of diminished responsibility, and was not therefore 'insane' at the time of the offence, he should not be permitted to benefit financially from having committed an illegal act. It was also held that Parliament could not have intended there to be a common law duty of care arising from a statutory breach of section 117 of the Mental Health Act 1983.

It is clear in this, and other cases like it (Horsnell 1998), that primary and secondary victims are in an even weaker position than patients nominally in receipt of services at the time of the alleged breach, insofar as they need to meet the three basic criteria established by precedent in the law of negligence: a legal duty of care, breach of that duty and consequent damage arising from the breach.

There is, furthermore, no requirement on the part of Mental Health Review Tribunals to inform or advise secondary victims of the imminent discharge of the mentally disordered offender in question from hospital. There is no place for victims to give evidence to the Tribunals. This closed system, whose decisions can have serious consequences for individuals and their families, differs from the criminal justice system which encourages the probation service to communicate with victims of crime.

In the case of Martin's mother, it was as if nothing whatsoever had been learned from what had happened to her when, in 1997, she received a letter from the social work department of the Special Hospital in which her son is a patient, asking for her response to the possibility of his returning to live with her in the family home on discharge from hospital (Jackson 1997). Having taken immediate advice, Martin's mother contacted the hospital on the day she received the letter and was told that the social worker who had written it had gone on holiday and would not be back for 2 weeks. It was eventually explained that the letter would have been automatically triggered by the need for a 'home report' following her son's application to a Mental Health Review Tribunal, an application which he subsequently withdrew.

Conclusions

This case study highlights the 'before and after' of community care failure. Failed attempts to engage services which do not communicate with each other and which are fundamentally in disarray and ineffectually managed place unrealistic burdens on so-called 'informal' carers. Familial bonds are often manipulated, consciously or otherwise, until they reach breaking point. Feelings after the tragedy has taken place are not mitigated by a disturbing tendency to keep victims at arm's length, most probably out of a primitive fear of other people's grief, rather than engage them in a comprehensive and informative process which is both meaningful, constructive and potentially therapeutic.

REFERENCES

Baker E 1997 The introduction of supervision registers in England and Wales: a risk communications analysis. Journal of Forensic Psychiatry 8(1): 15–35

Coid J 1994 The Christopher Clunis Inquiry. Psychiatric Bulletin 18: 449–452

Crawford L, Devaux M, Ferris R, Hayward P 1997 The report into the care and treatment of Martin Mursell. Camden and Islington Health Authority, London

Department of Health 1990 Caring for people: the care programme approach for people with a mental illness referred to the special psychiatric services: HC(90)23/LASSL(90)11. Department of Health, London

Department of Health 1994a Introduction of supervision registers for mentally ill people from 1 April 1994: HSG(94)5. Department of Health, London

Department of Health 1994b Guidance on the discharge of mentally disordered people and their continuing care in the community: HSG(94)27/LASSL(94)4. Department of Health, London

National Health Service Community Care Act 1990. HMSO, London

Howlett M 1998 Medication, non-compliance and mentally disordered offenders. The Zito Trust, London

Horsnell M 1998 Mother of murdered girl loses cash claim. The Times 19 February

Jackson L 1997 Widow asked if killer son can come home. The Sunday Telegraph 23 March

Lee A 1997 Schizophrenic who killed was let down by system. The Times 8 March

National Health Service Community Care Act 1990

Ritchie J, Dick D, Lingham R 1994 Report of the inquiry into the care and treatment of Christopher Clunis. HMSO, London

Rock P 1996 The inquiry and victims' families. In: Peay J (ed) Inquiries after homicide. Gerald Duckworth, London, ch 8

Sheppard D 1996 Learning the lessons: mental health inquiry reports published in England and Wales between 1969 and 1996 and their recommendations for improving practice, 2nd edn. The Zito Trust, London

Zedner L 1997 Victims. In: Maguire M, Morgan R, Reiner R (eds) The Oxford handbook of criminology. Clarendon Press, Oxford, ch 17

Sexual offending

CHAPTER CONTENTS

CONTENTS

Assessment of mentally ill sex offenders

Aisling O'Kane

Introduction

The relationship between mental illness and violence has stimulated much debate among both researchers and the public alike. There is undoubtedly considerable tension between public perception of the mentally ill person representing a high risk of violence and the reality of statistics that demonstrate relatively low levels of violence among this group. Given the steady increase in the proportion of sex offenders relative to the total offender population in recent years (Motiuk & Belcourt 1996), it is perhaps not surprising that current public opinion is that individuals with a mental illness are primarily responsible for sexual offences, particularly those perpetrated against children (Murray et al 1992). Given that the majority of those who commit sexual offences are not in fact suffering from a mental disorder (Chiswick 1983), such fears are largely unfounded. Nonetheless, a small number of sex offenders are present in criminal mental health services who are suffering from a mental illness and who pose considerable challenges to forensic practitioners in relation to risk assessment and future planning.

The particular difficulties associated with working with this group of offenders will be highlighted by outlining briefly some of the work which has been carried out on the links between mental disorder and violence. This leads into a review of the small body of literature addressed specifically at sexual violence and psychosis. Discussion of a particular case illustrates the need for broad-based assessments which do not focus exclusively on psychopathology but also include consideration of relevant criminogenic factors.

Mental disorder and violence

Much of the empirical work which has attempted to explore the complex relationship between violence and mental disorder has focused on a general category of violence rather than specific offence categories such as sexual offending. Some of these studies have attempted to address this area by focusing on the occurrence of violent behaviour among psychiatric patients in institutions (Crichton 1995; Hiday 1988) and also rates of mental disorder among prisoners (Swank & Winer 1976, Taylor & Gunn 1994). More recently, a comprehensive review has been provided by Bonta et al (1998) who carried out a meta-anlysis to establish whether predictors of recidivism among mentally disordered offenders differed from other offenders. Drawing from the literature on non-disordered offenders, they explored the relative contribution of both sociology, criminology and social psychology perspectives, in addition to psychopathology models. The authors suggest that this approach serves to assist in improving our understanding and explanation of the antisocial conduct of mentally disordered offenders. They conclude that in order to understand the behaviour of this group, the application of what have previously been identified as the predictors of violence among general offending populations should be utilised.

Their work highlighted the fact that the strongest predictor of adult offender recidivism in mentally disordered offenders was criminal history, a finding consistent with earlier work carried out by Monaghan (1993). Similarly, variables including juvenile delinquency, family problems, poor living arrangements and substance misuse were also shown to play an important role in respect of risk prediction. This is identified by the authors as providing substantial support for adopting a social psychological approach to understanding the

anti-social conduct of mentally disordered offenders. Interestingly, the clinical variables which were included in the meta-analysis yielded little in relation to predictive validity. Indeed, the more severe mental disorders such as psychosis and schizophrenia were in fact inversely related to both general and violent recidivism, a finding that is in contrast to work by other authors in the field such as Robins & Regier (1991) and Swanson (1994). The authors note that one explanation for the variability across some of the studies may be due to the way mental disorder is defined in the country where the research is being carried out.

Research to date, which has looked at particular psychotic symptoms and their relative contribution to future violence, has yielded some interesting findings. Recent research has certainly indicated that the presence of specific symptoms may increase the likelihood of violence taking place. For example, organised delusions (Nestor et al 1995, Taylor 1993), thought disorder (Gardner et al 1996), and command hallucinations (Bartels et al 1991)

The apparent lack of consensus regarding the role and relative influence of psychotic symptoms in relation to violent behaviour may in part be attributable to the paucity of literature which looks at specific categories of violence, thus failing to account for relevant criminogenic factors. This poses particular challenges for the forensic practitioner who is faced with the task of carrying out individual risk assessments on mentally disordered offenders. According to Bonta et al (1998), theories which have been identified as providing explanation for the behaviour of so-called rational offenders are likely to have significance for understanding mentally disordered offenders. What appears to be central to this field is clarification regarding which specific symptoms may, in conjunction with other risk factors, result in an increase in the likelihood of violent behaviour or, specifically, sexual violence occurring. The behaviour of mentally ill sex offenders might, therefore, be better understood in the context of criminological theory in addition to psychopathological frameworks.

Sexual offending and psychosis

Chiswick (1983), in his review of psychiatric aspects of serious sexual offences, concludes that only a small number of sex offenders are suffering from a mental illness. Research on adolescent sex offenders also indicates that conduct disorder is more commonly diagnosed in this group than mental illness (Kavoussi et al 1988). Chiswick (1983) goes on to suggest that understanding offences in this group requires a comprehensive understanding of the offender, the victim and the environment, warning against adhering to rigid psychiatric nosology. Given the small numbers of sex offenders who have a mental illness, together with some of the methodological and conceptual complexities briefly alluded to, it is perhaps not surprising that research in this area has been sparse and has tended to report on surveys (Henn et al 1976, Gibbens & Robertson 1983, Murray et al 1992), or case studies (Craissati & Hodes 1992, Huckle & Jones 1993, Meloy & Gacono 1992).

Surveys in this area have generally comprised mentally ill sex offenders as a sub-sample. Henn et al (1976) examined records of 239 individuals charged with sexual offences and found that major mental illness was very rare among both those who had been charged with rape and those who had offended against children. The subjects in Gibbens & Robertson's (1983) survey of all men receiving hospital orders in the UK in the year 1963–64, excluding those given restriction orders, were followed up over 15 years with regard to subsequent offences and convictions and hospital admissions. The authors noted that out of a sample of 378 patients with a mental illness, 17 had committed a sexual assault, of which five were described as 'serious assaulters' defined as having three or four convictions.

In what is the largest published review of sex offenders in the Special Hospital system, Murray et al (1992) identified 32 patients with a mental illness out of a group of 106 sex offenders, with five subjects being excluded from the study because of a dual diagnosis of psychopathic disorder and mental illness. Of interest here are the apparent similarities and differences between this group and the other Special Hospital sex offenders. Significantly, choice of victim was noted to be different among the mentally ill group with only 6% targeting victims under 11 years of age, compared to 28% and 33% in a psychopathic disordered group and mentally handicapped group respectively. Further, 94% of the mentally ill group had offended against females compared with 72% and 43% in the other groups. Interestingly, the range of sexual offences committed by the three groups was consistent with a high percentage of subjects engaging in at least one offence in the 'sexual touching', 'exhibitionism' and 'other including sexual threats' categories. The authors concluded that in light of their findings overall, there may be a case for including mentally ill sex offenders in treatment programmes for other sex offenders. Such an assertion would indicate that factors other than those associated with the offenders' illness may also be an important target for treatment.

In addition to Special Hospitals, sex offenders with a mental illness are also located in medium secure provision. Craissati & Hodes (1992) described a sample of 11 male sex offenders suffering from a psychotic illness resident in a medium secure unit, with 10 of the patients reported to have a diagnosis of schizophrenia. Interviews with nine of the patients revealed that the offences involved minimal violence, leading the authors to conclude that sociopathic traits were not a feature of this group. This work provides an interesting contrast with Kalichman's (1990) findings, which suggest that rapists have traits in common with other offenders in general. These include poor impulse control and, significantly, sociopathic traits. Somewhat surprisingly, in light of work described above, Craissati & Hodes also reported that a history of delinquency or family history of criminality was not a feature of this group. Rather, they concluded that the primary causal factor in their offending was sexual disinhibition. While phallometric assessment was not employed in this particular study, it might be useful for future research to delineate further the nature of this sexual disinhibition.

Huckle & Jones (1993) provided a commentary on the above study suggesting that there may be an alternative explanation for the mentally ill sex offenders' behaviour. They stress the importance of carrying out a full mental state examination as soon as possible after the commission of the offence to ensure that the practitioner does not miss the presence of command hallucinations at the material time. However, they also suggest that patients may actively hide their symptoms at the time of the assessment. In an attempt to provide some empirical support for this position, Jones et al (1992) explored the possible links between the role of command hallucinations and sexually assaultative behaviour by examining four case studies in which the two were reported to co-exist. The four men aged between 22 and 28 had all committed sexual assaults on adult women. In each case, third person auditory hallucinations were described by the individuals as instructing them to carry out a sexual attack. These included 'he should rape a girl to cure him of all his ills', 'have sex with young women as part of the master-plan', 'he must have sex by midnight or he would be killed' and 'go on, she wants it'. In addition to auditory hallucinations, the authors noted that family background was characterised by a dominant mother and absent or emotionally distant father, which they suggest may have contributed to the later development of psychopathology. Further, they noted that the men were lacking in social skills and had limited heterosexual experience. Treatment involved neuroleptic medication combined with ECT for two patients and lithium for one patient. Social skills training was offered to one of the patients focusing on his approach to women. The authors suggest that a package of treatment should be considered including social skills training, problem-solving training and cognitive therapy.

A number of other studies have emphasised the role of hallucinations in the prediction of hostility, such as that of Bartels et al (1991). However, the complexities inherent in this relationship are undoubtedly considerable, not least of which being that in the context of risk assessment, it is not merely the presence of hallucinations which is of importance but also the response made by an individual to those hallucinations. Honig (1991) suggests that most patients who experience command hallucinations are able to ignore them but that repetitive commands which occur over an extended period can increase the likelihood that the patient will respond to the command. A study by Junginger (1990) looking at how we might predict who might comply with command hallucinations indicated that those subjects who reported hallucination-related delusions and who were also able to identify the voices were more likely to respond to them. It would also seem that the content of command hallucinations may differ from other hallucinations with the former being characterised more often by themes of aggression, dependency and self-punishment (Rogers et al 1990).

In attempting to explain the link between command hallucinations and sexual violence, it may be that it is the presence of what Link & Steuve (1994) refer to as the 'threat/control override' (TCO) quality of some psychotic phenomena which increases the likelihood of violence being carried out. They suggest that those individuals who report that they felt threatened by others and were unable to exercise control over their own thoughts were more likely to engage in acts of violence. To date it is not known what specific role TCO may play in relation to the commission of sexual offences.

In reviewing the evidence in this area, it seems that researchers have varied in respect of the relative emphasis which they have placed on the contribution of specific psychotic symptoms in the commission of sexual offences. Nonetheless, in the absence of large-scale research, there is an inherent danger that assumptions regarding causality will be made such that motivation for sexual offending in a mentally ill sample will always be regarded as inextricably linked to the individual's illness despite the lack of strong empirical evidence for this position. A study carried out by Hafner & Boker (1982) indicated that among a sample of 533 mentally disordered offenders only 20% appeared to be what they described as apparently motiveless. Given the retrospective nature of this study, it is likely that this percentage may include individuals whose motive was unknown at the time of assessment rather than non-existent.

In conclusion, it would seem crucial to explore the criminogenic features of this group, including those associated with violence in general such as procriminal attitudes and lifestyle variables (Gendreau et al 1997) and also those which are known correlates of sexual offending.

CASE STUDY: GEORGE

The case study here describes a sex offender with a psychotic illness who was referred for a risk assessment to a clinical psychology department. An account of the assessment which was carried out is briefly described and the findings are considered in the overall context of risk assessment with this group.

George, a 35-year-old man, classified as mentally ill under the Mental Health Act 1983, was resident in a high-security hospital at the time of referral. A transfer to conditions of lesser security was proposed and an assessment of his potential risk for future sexual offending was therefore requested. During his 9 years at the hospital, he had been compliant with medication and a reduction in his symptoms had been noted. George had also engaged in anger management work and had attended a social skills group. Reports of his motivation and commitment in relation to these therapies had been positive and his clinical team were largely supportive of his transfer.

Background details

At the age of 26, George had been found guilty of committing two sexual offences against adult women and following psychiatric recommendation was transferred from prison to Special Hospital. Neither victim was known to him, and the offences took place 4 months apart. At the time of the offences, he had been attending a day centre for adults with mental health problems and had been prescribed neuroleptic medication, although his compliance with the regime had

been somewhat questionable, and his illness was not reported to be well controlled. Specifically, he had been described as experiencing delusions of grandiosity, which included the belief that he was something of a 'Don Juan' with women. This was in contrast with the fact that he had only ever had one sexual relationship with a woman which had lasted 3 months. In addition, George was also described as exhibiting paranoid ideation, characterised by his feeling that people he did not know were looking at him and laughing at him behind his back. George himself attributed his offences to the disinhibiting effect of his illness, asserting that he no longer posed a threat to women since his medication had been altered. George did not use either drugs or alcohol, stating that he did not like to feel out of control.

The assessment

Three clinical interviews were carried out and, in line with recommendations from Beckett et al (1994), covered information relating to George's family and personal history, his sexual history, including details about his sexual interests, current and previous fantasies, the details of his offence history including antecedents and consequences of his offence behaviour, victim empathy, and cognitive distortions together with his perception of his own risk and future treatment needs.

In addition to the interviews, the following psychometric tests were administered:

1. The Minnesota Multiphasic Personality Inventory-2 (MMPI-2) (Hathaway & McKinley 1989). This is a broad band test comprising 567 items which assesses a number of the major patterns of personality and emotional disorders.
2. The Rust Inventory of Schizotypal Cognitions (RISC). This is a 26-item, self-report scale for assessing the schizotypal cognitions associated with the positive symptoms of schizophrenia and schizotypal personality.
3. The Multiphasic Sex Inventory (MSI) (Nicholls & Molinder 1984). This is a

300-item, self-report questionnaire comprising 20 scales which assess sexual deviance, treatment attitudes, social sexual desirability, sexual obsessions, lie scale, cognitive distortions, immaturity, justifications, paraphilias, sexual dysfunction, sexual knowledge and beliefs and sexual history.

4. The Hypermasculinity Scale (HIS) (Mosher & Sirkin 1984). This is a 30-item, forced choice questionnaire which measures macho personality constellation consisting of three components: violence as manly; danger as exciting; and callous sexual attitudes towards women.

5. The Rape Myth Acceptance Scale (RMAS) (Burt 1980). This is a 19-item, self-report questionnaire which measures adherence to common myths about rape.

6. Attitudes to Women Scale (AWS) (Spence et al 1973). This is a 45-item, self-report scale which measures stereotyped and traditional attitudes to male/female roles.

This list is not meant to be definitive for this type of assessment but merely serves to illustrate some of the available measures appropriate for this area.

Results

The full details of George's risk assessment will not be reiterated here but rather some of the important issues which it raises will be considered. George's scores on the MMPI-2 fell mostly within the normal range apart from two scales which were moderately elevated. These included the masculinity/femininity scale and one of the validity scales, specifically the lie scale. The latter while not invalidating his performance on the inventory may indicate an individual who is over-controlled and lacks insight into his behaviour and also has considerable difficulty admitting to personal weakness. Such characteristics have important implications in relation to the prognosis for future psychological intervention. This was further compounded by his lack of awareness of the likely impact

the offences may have had on his victims. Interestingly, George did not score highly on either the schizophrenia scale of the MMPI nor were his scores marked on the RISC. This was consistent with reports from staff, and also George's own account of his mental state.

George's performance on the MSI again highlighted his apparent wish to present himself in a positive light. His performance on the validity scales indicates that he was unwilling to admit to normal sexual interests and desires. Significantly, a low score on social/sexual desirability may be indicative of someone wishing to portray themselves as asexual and may also provide evidence that the individual is 'faking good'. Interestingly, he also asserted that he masturbated once a week to consenting adult fantasies denying ever having non-consenting or coercive sexual fantasies. Further significant findings were available from George's performance on the masculinity femininity scale on the MMPI-2 and the AWS. Taken in conjunction with his elevated score on the RMAS and the HIS this would suggest that George holds stereotyped attitudes towards women which are characterised by hostility and this in turn influences his perception of rape as justifiable.

In conclusion, the assessment highlighted a number of issues relevant to the prediction of George's dangerousness. His reported attitudes towards women and rape, the suppression of his sexual feelings and the associated denial of his own risk, together with his impaired ability to perspective-take, particularly in relation to his own victims, are of considerable concern. The nature and content of George's psychotic symptoms are indicative of a man whose self-image appears fragile and this, taken in context of the above findings, may suggest that future deterioration in his mental state might have a disinhibiting and destabilising effect on his behaviour in relation to women. The fact that he was unable to acknowledge this risk or indeed identify any other factors which would increase his risk of future offending is perhaps further evidence that for George even thinking about these issues was too personally threatening.

Issues highlighted by George's assessment

It is important to stress here that George is not being cited as typifying other sex offenders with a mental illness. Indeed in the absence of empirical evidence regarding the aetiology of offending in this offender group, the importance of individualised risk assessment is paramount. Attention to those factors which have previously been shown to correlate with sexually assaultive behaviour must be paid before assumptions about causality of offending can be made. Examples of such correlates include poor empathy (Hudson et al 1995), attitudes towards victims (Quinsey 1986), opinions about their sexual behaviour (Marshall & Eccles 1991) and criminal responsibility (Segal & Stermac 1990).

The integration of information from such a complex and not always consistent body of knowledge is a challenging task. An example of this can be found in considering typologies in relation to sexual offending and individuals with a mental illness. Certainly, Grubin & Kennedy (1991) conclude that while many of the existing typologies have a certain logic and a degree of face validity, a meaningful and reliable classification system for sex offenders is still in an early stage of development. Grubin & Wingate (1996) suggest that much of the research in relation to sexual offending does little more than offer circular explanations for things. They suggest that more dynamic variables need to be explored and explained if the prediction of re-offending by individuals is to be improved. Such a move would increase the clinical relevance of actuarial studies in individual risk assessment. Clearly, the effective reduction of recidivism has been the major goal of many researchers working in the field of sexual offending. Implicit in much of this work is the assumption that targeting pro-criminal beliefs will reduce offending behaviours, and treatment programmes have reflected this.

Considerable strides have been made in understanding pro-criminal thinking and the role played by cognitive distortions in the acquisition and maintenance of sexual offending. Of particular interest are the attributions made by offenders themselves for their sexually deviant behaviour and the variance according to victim type. Individuals who have been convicted of child sex offences tend to attribute their offending to internal, stable and uncontrollable causes. Rapists, on the other hand, appear to attribute their offending to external, stable and uncontrollable causes. In contrast to child sex offenders, the other offending groups, including property and violence, generally attribute their sexual behaviour and sexual arousal to external, unstable and controllable causes (McKay et al 1996). It is perhaps not surprising that mentally ill sex offenders such as George will wish to attribute their offending behaviour to their mental state as this is consistent with the notion that sex offenders tend to make external attributions for their behaviour. In this context, illness may be construed as beyond their control and therefore their responsibility.

If this hypothesis is correct and mentally disordered offenders do make such attributions for self-serving reasons, this may have implications for those studies which have relied on mentally disordered offenders' self-report in assessing the link between violence and mental illness. However, such attributions also have implications for the motivation of offenders in relation to treatment. Adherence to medication, despite unwelcome side effects, may appear a more attractive choice to the mentally ill sex offender than participating in a lengthy and challenging therapy group, if such an option were available. At the time of writing, there was no identified programme of treatment specifically designed to target the needs of the mentally ill sex offender in the Special Hospital system, a major service provider for this group in the UK. The implications of this are perhaps reflected in the findings of a study carried out by Grounds (1991) which looked at the length of time spent by prisoners transferred to Special Hospital between 1960 and 1983 and reported that sex offenders stayed significantly longer than other categories of offenders.

Finally, a further factor relevant to all forms of criminal behaviour and, arguably, particularly so in relation to sexual offending, is the cultural context in which the behaviour takes place. Anthropological evidence would suggest that there are so-called rape-prone societies which are characterised by high levels of interpersonal violence, sexual repression and male dominance (Sanday & Reeves 1981). Similarly, other identified factors include the prevalence of pornography and its effects on attitudes to sexual violence. Recognising which aspects of the social context are most influential in the development of sexual offending, while extremely complex, must also be considered in any equivalent exploration of sexual violence in the mentally disordered offender.

Conclusions

Given the relatively small numbers of sex offenders with a mental illness, it can be argued that pertinent, reliable and sensitive assessment instruments are essential. This may, in part, be due to the reliance on models of change which are underpinned by medical models of psychopathology. According to Bonta et al (1998), given the presence of co-existing criminogenic variables, treatment programmes which do not address these are unlikely to succeed. Similarly, the issue of co-morbidity is one which researchers have not taken full account of in considering risk assessment in this area.

Perhaps, as Hiday (1995) suggests, the most realistic conclusion to be drawn from a literature which is characterised by conflicting findings is that a number of different explanations exist which may go some way towards explaining the behaviour of mentally disordered offenders and importantly, their sexually deviant behaviour. The first of these relates to the presence of antisocial personality disorder in this group and/or co-occurring substance misuse. Second, the role of active psychosis where the symptoms directly lead the individual into violence. Finally, psychotic symptoms where an individual's experience of suspicion or mistrust results in what have been termed TCO symptoms which can themselves result in violence. It is suggested here that testing these postulations can only take place if account is taken of the co-occurring criminogenic features which are associated with violence as a whole, and also those factors which have been shown to correlate with particular offence categories, in this instance sexual offending behaviour. This in no way overlooks the important role that psychopathology plays in this context. Rather, it serves to elaborate more fully the nature of any offending behaviour, identifying how effective risk management and appropriate treatment can be designed such that simplistic assumptions about causality are avoided.

REFERENCES

Bartels J, Drake R, Wallach M, Freeman D 1991 Characteristic hostility in schizophrenic outpatients. Schizophrenic Bulletin 17: 763–771

Beckett R, Beech A, Fisher D, Fordham A 1994 Community-based treatment for sex offenders: an evaluation of seven treatment programmes. Crown, London

Bonta J, Law M, Hanson K 1998 The prediction of criminal and violent recidivism among mentally disordered offenders. Psychological Bulletin 123: 123–142

Burt M 1980 Cultural myths and support for rape. Journal of Personality and Social Psychology 38: 217–230

Chiswick D 1983 Sex crimes. British Journal of Psychiatry 143: 236–242

Craissati J, Hodes P 1992 Mentally ill sex offenders. British Journal of Psychiatry 161: 846–849

Crichton J 1995 Psychiatric inpatient violence. In: Walker N (ed) Dangerous people. Blackstone, London

Gardner W, Lidz C, Mulvey E, Shaw E 1996 Clinical versus actuarial predictions of violence in patients with mental illness. Journal of Consulting and Clinical Psychology 64: 602–609

Gendreau P, Goggin C, Law M 1997 Predicting prison misconducts. Criminal Justice and Behaviour 24: 414–431

Gibbens T, Robertson G 1983 A survey of the criminal careers of restriction order patients. British Journal of Psychiatry 143: 370–375

Grounds A 1991 The transfer of sentenced prisoners to hospital 1960–1983: a study in one special hospital. British Journal of Criminology 31(1): 54–71

Grubin D, Kennedy H 1991 The classification of sexual offenders. Criminal Behaviour and Mental Health 1: 123–129

Grubin D, Wingate S 1996 Sexual offence recidivism. Criminal Behaviour and Mental Health 6: 349–359

Hafner H, Boker W 1982 Crimes of violence by mentally abnormal offenders: a psychiatric and epidemiological study in the Federal German Republic. Cambridge University Press, Cambridge.

Hathaway S, McKinley J 1989 MMPI-2: Manual for administration and scoring. The University of Minnesota Press, Minneapolis

Henn F, Herjanc M, Vanderpearl R 1976 Forensic psychiatry: profiles of two types of sex offenders. American Journal of Psychiatry 133: 694–696

Hiday V 1988 Civil commitment: a review of empirical research. Behavioral Sciences and the Law 6: 15–44

Hiday V 1995 The social context of mental illness and violence. Journal of Health and Social Behaviour 36: 122–137

Honig A 1991 Psychotherapy with command hallucinations in chronic schizophrenia: the use of action techniques within a surrogate family setting. Journal of Group Psychotherapy, Psychodrama and Sociometry 44: (1) 3–18

Huckle P, Jones G 1993 Mentally ill sex offenders. British Journal of Psychiatry 162: 568

Hudson S, Marshall W, Ward T, Johnsten P 1995 Kia Marama: a cognitive–behavioural program for incarcerated child molesters. Behaviour Change 12(2): 69–80

Jones G, Huckle P, Tanaghow A 1992 Command hallucinations, schizophrenia and sexual assaults. Irish Journal of Psychological Medicine 9: (1) 47–49

Junginger J 1990 Predicting compliance with command hallucinations. American Journal of Psychiatry 147: 245–247

Kalichman S 1990 Affective and personality characteristics of MMPI profile subgroups of incarcerated rapists. Archives of Sexual Behaviour 19: 443–459

Kavoussi R, Kaplan M, Becker J 1988 Psychiatric diagnosis in adolescent sex offenders. Journal of the American Academy of Child and Adolescent Psychiatry 27: 241–243

Link B, Steuve A 1994 Psychotic symptoms and the violent/illegal behavior of mental patients compared to community controls. In: Monaghan J, Steadman H (eds) Violence and mental disorder: developments in risk assessment. University of Chicago Press, Chicago, p 137–159

McKay M, Chapman J, Long N 1996 Causal attributions for criminal offending and sexual arousal: comparison of child sex offenders with other offenders. British Journal of Clinical Psychology 35(1): 63–75

Marshall W, Eccles A 1991 Issues in clinical practice with sex offenders. Journal of Interpersonal Violence, 6(1): 68–93

Meloy J, Gacono C 1992 A psychotic (sexual) psychopath: 'I just had a violent thought …' Journal of Personality Assessment 58: 480–493

Monaghan J 1993 Mental disorder and violence: another look. In: Hodgins S (ed) Mental disorder and crime. Sage, Newbury Park, CA, p 287–302

Mosher D, Sirkin M 1984 Measuring a macho personality constellation. Journal of Research in Personality 20: 77–94

Motiuk L, Belcourt R 1996 Profiling the Canadian Federal sex offender population. Forum Corrections Research 8(2): 3–7

Murray G, Briggs D, Davis C 1992 Psychopathic disordered, mentally ill and mentally handicapped sex offenders: a comparative study. Medicine, Science and Law 32(4): 331–336

Nestor P, Haycock J, Doiron S, Kelly J, Kelly D 1995 Lethal violence and psychosis. Bulletin of American Academic Psychiatry and Law 23: 331–341

Nichols H, Molinder M 1984 Manual for the Multiphasic Sex Inventory. Tacoma, WA, USA

Quinsey V 1986 Men who have sex with children. In: Weisstub D (ed) Law and mental health: international perspectives, vol 2. Pergamon, New York

Robins L, Regier D 1991 Psychiatric disorders in America: the Epidemiological Catchment Area study. Free Press, New York

Rogers R, Gillis J, Turner E, Frise-Smith T 1990 The clinical presentation of command hallucinations in a forensic population. American Journal of Psychiatry 147: 1304–1307

Sanday P, Reevesüit 1981 The socio-cultural context of rape: a cross-cultural study. Journal of Social Issues 37(4): 5–27

Segal Z, Stermac L 1990 The role of cognition in sexual assault. In: Marshall W, Laws D, Barbaree H (eds) Handbook of sexual assault: issues, theories and treatment of the offender. Plenum, New York

Spence J, Helmreich R, Stapp J 1973 A short version of the Attitudes towards Women Scale. Bulletin of the Psychonomic Society 2: 219–220

Swank G, Winer D 1976 Occurrence of psychiatric disorder in a county jail population. American Journal of Psychiatry 133: 1331–1333

Swanson J 1994 Mental disorder, substance abuse and community violence: an epidemiological approach. In Monaghan J, Steadman H (eds) Violence and mental disorder: developments in risk assessment. University of Chicago Press, Chicago, p 101–136

Taylor P 1993 Schizophrenia and crime: distinctive patterns in association. In: Hodgins S (ed) Crime and mental disorder. Sage, Newbury Park, CA, p 63–85

Taylor P, Gunn J 1994 Violence and psychosis – risk of violence among psychiatric men. British Medical Journal 228: 1945–1949

CONTENTS

Adolescent sex offenders

J. Thomas Dalby and Jack White

Introduction

Sex offences committed by adolescents are a rising problem, accounting for 20 to 30% of rapes and 30 to 60% of child molestation cases. Half of all adult offenders began their aberrant pattern of sex offending while juveniles. It is of vital importance to identify the type of offending pattern in juvenile sex offenders, as outcome research has shown an excellent response to specialised treatment and supervision in this population of offenders. We illustrate the spectrum of juvenile sex offenders with two brief vignettes. Research on this population shows that although each case adjudicated must be individually scrutinised, the vast majority are best left in the juvenile justice system rather than raised to adult court, and that relapse prevention and follow-up are vital components of any intervention with this younger age group.

Theoretical background

When over 50% of adult sex offenders begin their offending careers as juveniles, it becomes important to focus resources on rehabilitation in this population. In the past, juvenile sex offending has been minimised and many mental health workers looked upon these crimes as adolescent experimentation (Barbaree et al 1993, Groth & Loredo 1981, Longo 1982). Most adolescent sexual offenders, when detected, have already committed multiple offences. However, they carry treatment advantages over adult offenders as their atypical arousal patterns are less entrenched and they may not have developed an array of sexual aberrations seen in their adult counterparts.

Perry & Orchard (1992) counter many of the myths that are held regarding adolescent sex offenders with the following summary of facts:

- Their offending behaviours are not simply attempts to learn about sex.
- Not all offenders are male (*see* Mathews et al 1997).
- They derive from all races, socio-economic classes and levels of intellect.
- The victims are often known to the perpetrator.
- Adolescent sexually deviant conduct will not go away with simple maturity.
- The label of sex offender will not predispose the youth to re-offend.
- Sexual assaults are not primarily sexually motivated behaviours.
- Sexual offences are largely planned actions.
- The trauma to victims does not vary with the age of the offender.
- Adolescent offenders typically have committed more than one offence when apprehended.
- Adolescent sex offenders require sex-offender-specific treatment.
- Not all adolescent sex offenders have been victims of sexual abuse.

Like their adult counterparts, adolescent sex offenders must be considered as a heterogeneous group. Again, this becomes obvious when we contemplate the genesis of adult patterns of offending. Knight & Prentky (1993) have reviewed the classification schemes for juvenile sex offenders and the taxonomy presented borrows from a body of research with adult categorisations. Some of the most important classification dimensions reviewed include family environment (physical abuse was correlated with increased sexual violence in adolescence); sexual history and adjustment (sexual abuse was found to be higher in adolescent sex offenders than the general population); social competence (up to 65% of adolescent sex offenders showed serious social isolation); behavioural problems (adolescent sex offenders frequently have histories of other criminal activity); neurological and cognitive problems (cognitive weaknesses are not uniformly found in adolescent sex offenders but may be linked to those showing more violent conduct); school achievement (many adolescent sex offenders show learning difficulties); level of force and physical injury to victims (adolescents are less likely than adults to use weapons or injure their victims physically in their assaults); and race (in the US studies, blacks are over-represented, especially in cases of forcible rape, although arrest rates are biased against blacks).

The primary taxonomic division in sex offences is between rapists and child molesters. For the rapists, dimensions such as anger, opportunism, vindictiveness, sadism and social competence are used to structure different types. With child molesters, the offenders are usually divided into high or low fixation (paedophilia vs situational offending), then issues of meaning of contact (sexual or interpersonal), sadism and aggression are analysed. Awad & Saunders (1989) have contributed to our understanding of adolescent child molesters by reviewing demographic and clinical variables, further noting that unlike many adult sex offenders alcohol and drug abuse rarely played a role in the commission of the offences. Other classification schemes for sexually abusive adolescents have focused on victim-age selection or preference and relationship to the victim (Richardson et al 1997). This work in classification becomes important in structuring a specific treatment programme for the individual in need. A programme designed to facilitate social competence will not impact on sexual offending if this underlying variable is not important in the particular offender.

CASE STUDY 1: OLIVER

History

Oliver was just 11 years old when he first sexually abused the 3-year-old niece whom he was baby-sitting. The young girl reported to her mother that Oliver had molested her by manipulating her genitals. She was taken to the family physician, but the mother did not want police involvement as it was deemed to be a 'family matter'. 'Counselling' was to have been arranged with the family physician, but this never occurred. 3 years later, while Oliver was at a cousin's home playing, he went upstairs and removed the clothing of another 4-year-old niece and performed cunnilingus. The police were notified and Oliver was arrested and then released into the custody of his parents. After an assessment was conducted, the Crown Prosecutor agreed to a diversionary arrangement of active treatment for 1 year.

Identified problems and needs

Oliver was an only child, born with a cleft palate which required surgery and subsequent speech therapy. He had failed a year in school and was deemed to have low average intelligence. Much of his time was spent in the company of his mother, as his father was often away from home on business. Oliver had no exposure to alcohol or drug use and had no prior criminal history. Personality testing (MMPI-A and High School Personality Questionnaire) showed valid profiles with no evidence of psychopathic qualities but mild depression and anxiety with a strongly introverted character. He was a concrete thinker, was serious minded and timid and was rather lax of social rules. He had a profoundly poor self-esteem, rarely expressed negative emotions and was concerned with demonstrating his sexual identity through exceptional endorsement of stereotypic masculine interests. Additionally, he displayed poor knowledge of human sexual functioning and had no experience with age peers in sexual behaviour. He reported not being the subject of any form of abuse. Oliver reported few fantasies that were related to his offending and was at times overwhelmed with guilt for his behaviour.

Interventions

Oliver participated in an individualised treatment programme that emphasised gaining knowledge of human sexual hygiene, behaviour and psychology and developing appropriate heterosexual social skills. Assertiveness training, modelling and relationship-building skills were targets for change. He was then referred for participation in a group 'relapse prevention' programme, which was provided to boys who had already completed a course of treatment.

Outcomes

2 years after the completion of treatment, Oliver has developed increased relationships with peers, joined several social clubs through his school and has had several positive dating experiences. He has shown no further aberrant sexual behaviour or other antisocial actions.

CASE STUDY 2: CHRISTOPHER

History

Christopher was arrested at the age of 16, after following a 22-year-old woman off the public transportation system and raping her at knifepoint. He had been using marijuana that evening. He had a prior conviction for the forcible sexual assault of a girlfriend 2 years earlier, but had received a probationary sentence on the basis of his intoxication at the time. He left a group treatment service for adolescent sex offenders after two sessions and was seen in individual treatment for his substance abuse. Christopher's mother was a single parent and alcohol abuse was frequent in the home setting. He showed criminal versatility, with offences spanning property and assault crimes.

Identified problems and needs

Christopher, on formal testing, showed average intelligence with age-appropriate academic achievement. His MMPI-A profile revealed strong antisocial characteristics, including family discord and resentment for parental and societal authority. His profile suggested that he was comfortable and confident in social situations, but felt that he was getting a 'raw deal' from life. He was often bored and restless and tended to have unrealistic evaluations of his own abilities and self-worth. Concurrent substance abuse was seen as a secondary concern. In interview, he lacked empathy for his victim, noting that she was not a virgin. This was expressed in a callous, cocky and glib response to any suggestion that others' rights were important. At the same time, he was well spoken and friendly during contacts. He had good knowledge of human sexual functioning and described a high sexual drive and range of experiences. He has had frequent sexual contact with female peers and casually described situations akin to 'date-rape'. He volunteered that it was common knowledge that in the female vocabulary 'no' meant 'yes'. In his background, Christopher had been subjected to physical and emotional hurt, but said that he had not been sexually abused. He acknowledged frequent sexual fantasy, of a wide range, including aggressive sexual contacts.

Interventions

Christopher was identified as having a conduct disorder, with strong elements of a developing psychopathic nature. He received a 2-year sentence of incarceration for the instant offence, but little treatment was provided during this time. He did, however, attend school sessions offered in the juvenile detention system as well as a course on substance abuse. Upon release to the community, he presented a treatment challenge, as he was unmotivated and had experienced previous treatment failure. At this point, he was paired with a senior, and well-experienced, male therapist whose interventive style was direct and confrontive. The therapeutic focus was on anger and frustration management and empathy training. The development of an offence cycle was jointly constructed with the aim of allowing Christopher strategies to break the pattern at different points in the cycle. He was placed in a work setting as a carpenter's helper and maintained this employment with few complaints by the employer.

Outcomes

After 3 years of his release from jail for sexual assault, Christopher has served several short sentences of incarceration on drug charges, but has not repeated a sexual assault. He was identified as a high-risk offender and participated in relapse-prevention group treatment, but his participation was interrupted by a short period of incarceration. He continued to have contact with female peers and several of those interviewed did not indicate aggressive actions on Christopher's part.

Discussion

The Association for the Treatment of Sexual Abusers (ATSA) in a position paper (1997) noted that current data suggest juveniles account for an alarmingly high percentage of rape and child molestation cases in the USA. Further, they cite recent prospective and clinical outcome studies which indicate that most juveniles who sexually abuse will cease this behaviour by the time they reach adulthood, especially if they are provided with specialised treatment and supervision. Their position is that adult sentences (and appearances in adult courts) for the majority of juvenile sexual offenders are inappropriate, and that most offenders can be safely and effectively managed in the community with specialised treatment and court supervision. Notification of the community, if imposed at all for juveniles, should be done conscientiously, cautiously and selectively. While some jurisdictions (and countries) prohibit the release of information on young offenders, there is a strong push to rescind these civil protections. Research in linking classification and risk assessment was given priority by ATSA.

Oliver illustrates one of the more common examples seen in juvenile sex offenders. Poor social competence and an avoidant personality often underlie these reports. It should not be intimated that juvenile sex offending is simply curiosity or experimentation, as this would involve consensual peer exploration. He showed little mental pathology outside of his sexual behaviour, which may have developed over time into strongly paedophilic tendencies. His prognosis appears promising.

Christopher represents a less common, and more difficult, long-term rehabilitative challenge. His sexual aggression was but one expression of antisocial tendencies and his psychopathic demeanour would be more difficult to alter than single offences. He was able to maintain employment and was only involved in minor, non-violent offences during follow-up, but his risk would remain elevated requiring long-term monitoring. When treating adolescent sex offenders, the therapist should examine his or her own attitudes toward the offender. In an excellent position paper, Marshall (1996) reminds us that sexual offenders are neither 'monsters' nor 'victims' and should therefore be treated like all other clients. He suggests that we shift from a preoccupation with procedures and instead give attention to process features of treatment. A therapeutic style which enhances the offender's self-esteem may be best.

REFERENCES

Association for The Treatment of Sexual Abusers 1997 Position on the effective legal management of juvenile sexual offenders. ATSA, Oregon

Awad G A, Saunders E B 1989 Adolescent child molesters: clinical observations. Child Psychiatry and Human Development 19: 195–206

Barbaree H E, Hudson S M, Seto M C 1993 Sexual assault in society: the role of the juvenile offender. In: Barbaree H E, Marshall W L, Hudson S M (eds) The juvenile sex offender. Guilford Press, New York

Groth A N, Loredo C M 1981 Juvenile sexual offenders: guidelines for assessment. International Journal of Offender Therapy and Comparative Criminology 25: 31–39

Knight R A, Prentky R A 1993 Exploring characteristics for classifying juvenile sex offenders. In: Barbaree H E, Marshall W L, Hudson S M (eds) The juvenile sex offender. Guilford Press, New York

Longo R E 1982 Sexual learning and experience among adolescent sexual offenders. International Journal of Offender Therapy and Comparative Criminology 26: 235–241

Marshall W L 1996 The sexual offender: monster, victim, or everyman? Sexual Abuse: A Journal of Research and Treatment 8: 317–335

Mathews R, Hunter J A, Vuz J 1997 Juvenile female sexual offenders: clinical characteristics and treatment issues. Sexual Abuse: A Journal of Research and Treatment 9: 187–199

Perry G P, Orchard J 1992 Assessment and treatment of adolescent sex offenders. Professional Resource Press, Sarasota, FL

Richardson G, Kelly T, Graham F, Bhate S 1997 Group differences in abuser and abuse characteristics in a British sample of sexually abusive adolescents. Sexual Abuse: A Journal of Research and Treatment 9: 239–257

CONTENTS

Working with survivors of sexual abuse

Ged Smith

Introduction

This is an account of therapeutic work, with a female survivor of sexual abuse, in a secure psychiatric unit. It is presented within the context of the power dynamics which exist both within the institution and in social structures generally. It is proposed that those who hold power can abuse it unwittingly, that abuses in 'benign' form can be just as damaging as any other kind and that the disempowering regimes of most psychiatric institutions cannot possibly be helpful to those whose major suffering was having power taken away from them. Examples of the therapeutic approach are included and a proposal to distinguish between the problem behaviours and the person.

Theoretical background

Mental health services are discriminatory, particularly on the grounds of gender (Allen 1987, Gelsthorpe 1989, Morris 1989), race (Fernando 1991, Kareem & Littlewood 1992) and class (Richards 1995). As with prisons, psychiatric institutions are full of people marginalised from the power bases in society. The social construction of gender, just like race and class, contributes to both misdiagnoses and to psychological distress. Women are more likely to be seen as appropriate subjects for psychiatric intervention simply because they are women and, in turn, this dynamic causes psychological distress in itself. Women make up 4% of the general prison population, yet account for 20% of Special Hospital patients (Herman 1992). Furthermore, the desire for 'feminised' behaviour often means that certain of women's behaviours (e.g. drunkenness, promiscuity, drug abuse, violence) will alert psychiatric services, while the same actions in men are seen as 'normal' (Morris 1989).

Psychiatric institutions, like prisons, were designed by men for men and of course the loci of real power – from the hospital director and psychiatrist to the local MP – are highly likely to be with men. Women patients have to fit in. This is the case even if they are survivors of sexual abuse and violence sharing a ward with male perpetrators of abuse and violence, which is not an uncommon occurrence. Those professionals with less power (nurses and other ward staff) are, again, more likely to be women. A combination of directives from above, pressures of work and insufficient training will often make them, despite best intentions, agents of further abusive practices upon patients.

Psychiatric care can be very good. However, it is my contention, and clinical experience, that the single most important factor – power – is a neglected concept amongst most staff. For those who already belong to a traditionally marginalised group in society, this negligence has a more damaging effect. Crucially, if you have also been severely abused in childhood, then these abuses of professional power in 'benign' form will do nothing to aid recovery. Any intervention which takes power away from such people cannot possibly be helpful.

A parallel process

Currently, there are several police investigations around Britain into the institutional abuse of children in care (sic), ranging over the past 30 years. Many of these survivors, now adults, are seeking counselling for the effects of this abuse and most are also seeking financial compensation from the Criminal Injuries Compensation Board (CICB). After years of being disbelieved, these people are now assisting the authorities as witnesses, although the experience of making a statement to the police and giving

evidence in court often leads to the opening up of old wounds and memories which leaves them in unbearable pain. The counselling services offered to them are woefully inadequate, the waiting lists are months long and the intensity of support usually needed is just not available.

Many men, abused as children, are left feeling that they have been used again and left abandoned, with their well-repressed anger and hurt resurfaced against their will, to get on with it. To top it all, the CICB often rejects their claims on the grounds that many of them have criminal records. Another interpretation is that they have hit back at the authority and establishment figures who incarcerated and abused them, embarking upon lives of crime, drug use and other self-destructive behaviours.

The kinds of abuse suffered by these people while in 'care' are of a different order from the main subject of this case study, but, as noted, some of the abuses perpetrated in 'benign' form can have effects which are just as damaging. Social constructionist theory has led many to question the relationship between the individual and wider social systems. Grand theories which proclaim universal truths are viewed with suspicion as we come to recognise that our view of the world is culturally conditioned; we see the world not as it is, but as we are. Through the influence of thinkers like Foucault (1973) and Kristeva (1980), the voices of the most powerful, and their practices, have come to be critically questioned. Psychiatric theory, just like history, could be said to be no more than agreed upon fable, where power is having one particular version of reality accepted. Schizophrenia may one day be viewed much as hysteria (Showalter 1987) or drapetomania (Fernando 1992) are today. Each was a culturally constructed diagnostic label where medical science embraced the dominant, and derisory, 19th century ideologies about women and people of colour.

CASE STUDY: KIM

There is a clear link between all of the above and the experiences of a woman I worked with on a secure unit for psychiatrically ill 'patients' who were considered to be dangerous. Kim was a 33-year-old woman, whose risk to society was based on the fact that she had twice set fire to houses causing considerable damage. Arson is, indeed, a very serious and worrying offence. The psychiatric assessments which followed these offences led to her being diagnosed as suffering from paranoid schizophrenia at the age of 18. Since that time, Kim had been resident in a number of secure establishments. Kim had recently disclosed to ward staff that she had been sexually abused as a girl and wanted some help with the effects that this was having on her life. As I had recently been involved in some teaching to ward staff on this topic, I was asked to see Kim. She had asked for help in dealing with the effects of her recently disclosed sexual abuse and staff agreed that this was an important focus for therapeutic intervention.

I recalled that during the teaching I had spent considerable time with the ward staff looking at the question: 'Within the context of a secure unit, where does the idea of empowerment fit when working with survivors of child sexual abuse?' A thorny question, given the disempowering regime of this and most psychiatric secure units, and one which the staff really struggled with. Interestingly, I had also been invited in response to the recent suicide of a former patient who, after years of self-harm through cutting, had fatally slashed her wrists. The woman had been physically restrained from cutting herself a month before her suicide because of senior staff alarm. When she finally got the space, after 1 month, she took the opportunity to finally end the torture. One could not wish for a better example of the dangers of taking away a person's freedom to act, but I remained unconvinced of what lessons had been learned.

Kim had been brutally sexually abused by her father, her brothers and various associates of her father during her early teen years. At a point where she could take it no more, she decided to set fire to the bed where all the abuse had occurred. The fire raged out of control and, while the rest of the family escaped, it took the fire brigade to rescue Kim. Though her recollection was hazy she thinks she wanted to see if her father would save her from the flames, but he only acted to save his sons. The cause of the fire was quickly established and Kim was detained while assessments were conducted. She recalls that the manner of those carrying out the assessments was such that she could never tell them the reasons behind starting the fire. Soon after this, she absconded from detention and was picked up by the police outside the house of one of her father's associates who had sexually abused her. She was carrying petrol and matches, but again found it impossible to give any explanation to people who she found accusatory, intimidating and verbally and physically abusive. Of course, she was also silenced by the threats issued by her abusers about what would happen if she should ever tell. Ironically, one of these threats was that she would not be believed, but would be called 'mad'. She was diagnosed as suffering from paranoid schizophrenia and admitted into Ashworth Special Hospital at just 18 years of age.

For 15 years Kim lived through the regimes of Ashworth and later the local secure unit for psychiatrically ill patients who are deemed a danger to the public. She developed eating disorders, started cutting her arms and cut off her hair, and was seen as 'troublesome' by staff. She was heavily drugged and felt that years had gone by while in a 'zombie state'. It took these 15 years before she found anybody who she felt able, or ready, to share her story with. This was a ward nurse who had acted very sympathetically to Kim's story and befriended her. The nurse, though, felt that she had done as much as she could at the point when she contacted myself.

Therapeutic considerations

A lot of preliminary work followed before I met with Kim, particularly concerning the issues of sex and gender. Staff reassured me that she was happy to undertake therapy with a man, and I later found this to be the case.

Because of the risks associated with arson it was decided that a member of the hospital staff must always be present during our sessions, in case Kim should become agitated and more of a risk. It is a truism that, after embarking upon therapy, people often do feel worse before they feel better. This is particularly so for people with a history of abuse, where hidden wounds may be reopened and buried memories revived. Precaution with a convicted arsonist makes sense, but the balance between this and the necessary empowerment to aid progress must also be considered. Owing to resource implications, and the absence of the anticipated agitation, hospital staff decided after 10 meetings to stop providing a nurse to observe our sessions. Instead, they relied on myself to contact them if I had any concerns regarding Kim's increased levels of risk. I never did have any fears, but, in keeping with my own practice, I arranged to send Kim a letter after each session, outlining what we had talked about and presenting her with further questions to ponder prior to our next session. We agreed that a copy of this letter would also go to ward staff.

Many interesting sessions followed during which Kim made good progress, as reported by herself and staff. In one session she confronted me with a question which had been bothering her for a while. Her key-worker had encouraged her to spend 10 minutes in the gym every day, kicking a football and screaming to let her anger out. She could easily 'kick fuck out of the ball' she told me, but could not scream and wanted to know why. Initially, I had no idea, but within an hour of exploration and questioning, an answer had emerged from Kim. It was one which she found satisfactory. As a child she was often told she was 'mad' (especially by her abusers and the mother she had tried to tell but who could not afford to believe her) and that she would end up in the very hospital she was now in. Kim had also picked up the message that mad people scream in a deranged and senseless way. These messages had been 'forgotten' by Kim, but remained with her at an unconscious level, and were strong enough to stop her screaming while kicking the football. This awareness helped her to let go of the injunction, the more she realised and believed that it was those abusive people who were bad and guilty, not her.

This revisioning of her own story is consistent with my approach to working with survivors of sexual abuse, who are often blind to their own strengths and resources while privileging their perceived weaknesses. Kim was very articulate with an hilarious sense of humour, but she had never been told this by anybody. When I referred to it, she was surprised, and responded that it was not at all how she saw herself. I asked Kim what she thought that I saw in her to give me this impression, whereupon she rattled off a list of examples of her humour and intelligence. Hearing herself do this, so readily, had a marked impression on Kim. It was as if she had unearthed aspects of herself hitherto visible only to others. One of the main effects of sexual abuse is the assault it makes on the person's self-perception, and I see challenging this, with gentleness and humour, as one of my fundamental tasks.

The other fundamental area of our work together involved the examination of what I call 'obstacles to resolution'. This moved away from notions of causation, history and pathology (though there is a place for these things at other times in therapy) towards examining what kept the problems alive in Kim's life. There is a subtle, but crucial, difference between the questions 'What caused this problem?' and 'What keeps it alive?' The former invites an historical account of things already known to the client, and is therefore of limited use, while the latter offers a reflexivity which is more likely to provide insights.

Endings

After more than 30 sessions, Kim was progressing well on her journey away from self-hate, self-blame and self-destructive behaviours. She had told me a lot about the effects of the abuse that she suffered, but never talked in depth about the abuse itself. I had always made it clear to her that I was available to hear this detail if she wanted to disclose it, but the timing and decision were always with her. Being alone in a room with a more powerful man was resonant enough with the abuse, without me telling her what was good for her. Now she was getting near to being willing, and able, to talk of the abuse, but needing more control over the circumstances. She now wanted no more copies of my post-session letters to her to be forwarded to ward staff and asked that no details be shared at ward rounds or anywhere else. Despite my appeals, senior staff were not agreeable to this. As a consequence, Kim refused to continue and our work came to an end. Kim hit out against having power and control taken away from her again – a common feature in her life. Further crises followed and Kim tried to stop eating, but was force fed. She cut herself more and was placed under constant surveillance. She could not sleep at night and was prevented from sleeping during the day. At this point, she had less power over her own life than she had had for a long time.

The last meeting I had with the staff was during a ward round, where I sat through detailed discussion of people I did not know. Kim's case was discussed in the presence of several people who did not know her. This was exactly the situation Kim had tried to protest about – the objectifying 'gaze' of those in positions of power over those they label, judge, diagnose, drug and incarcerate. The last time I saw Kim she looked drawn and thin. She had lost her sparkle and her sense of humour. Her last words to me were: 'You can't do anything in this place.'

This downward spiral does not all stem from Kim's lack of power to choose or her lack of choice over who knew what about her. Some staff say she thought she was on the verge of release and found the prospect terrifying, so acted against it (so-called 'gate fever'). Some doubt that she was ever abused at all (she continues to be disbelieved) and was 'spinning me along' with great manipulative skill. In a sense, though, the 'truth' is irrelevant. For although I believe all that Kim told me, her distress was beyond doubt and that is what we can try to help with. The fundamental principle, yet to be grasped by many schooled in a medical model, is that taking power and control away from people who have suffered powerlessness at the hands of family and institution cannot aid recovery. In incestuous abuse, the whole dynamic is power and we should focus our efforts, in collaboration with our clients, on having power and control over certain behaviours, not over the person.

REFERENCES

Allen H 1987 Justice unbalanced: gender, psychiatry and judicial decisions. Open University Press, Milton Keynes

Fernando S 1991 Mental health, race and culture. Macmillan, London

Fernando S 1992 Roots of racism. Open Mind 59: 10–11

Foucault M 1973 The birth of the clinic: an archaeology of medical perception. Tavistock, London

Gelsthorpe L 1989 Sexism and the female offender. Gower, Aldershot

Herman J 1992 Trauma and recovery. Harper Collins, London

Kareem J, Littlewood R 1992 Intercultural therapy. Blackwell, Oxford

Kristeva J (1980) Powers of horror. An essay on abjection. Columbia University Press, New York

Morris A 1989 Women, crime and criminal justice. Blackwell, Oxford

Richards B 1995 Psycotherapy and the injuries of class. BPS Newsletter 17: 21–35

Showalter E 1987 The female malady: women, madness and English culture, 1830–1980. Virago, London

CONTENTS

Pornography and practice: the misfortunes of therapy

Dave Mercer

Introduction

This case study looks at the introduction of a group treatment approach for sexual offenders in a maximum secure psychiatric hospital. Institutional impediments to a therapeutic model are illustrated, with a specific focus on pornography as an important clinical concern for forensic staff. It suggests that therapy cannot be enacted in an ideological vacuum and argues for the incorporation of a sexual–political agenda within the development of progressive practice.

Theoretical background

Trends in the treatment of sexual offenders reflect wider theoretical and political debates about sexualised violence and gender relations (Vogelman 1990). The shift away from a medical model which explained sexual crime in terms of genetic defect, mental disease and brain damage is in large part attributable to the impact of the Women's Movement in the 1970s (Watts & Courtois 1981). Social science research which demonstrated that most rapists did not fit a psychiatric profile (Amir 1971) supported the pioneering work of feminist critics who reconfigured rape as an expression of male power within patriarchal society (Brownmiller 1975, Millett 1971). Yet, if such recognition has challenged those popular mythologies, which blame and stigmatise victims, the discourses of law and psychiatry have been more resistant to change (Scott & Dickens 1989). Ironically, as sexual violence has assumed a central position in theorising about patriarchal power, the gaze has remained firmly fixed on the experiences of women. The neglect of inquiry into the social reality of men, the 'real experts' on sexual violence, has left dominant pathological explanations unchallenged: 'Such insight is acquired only through invading and critically examining the social constructions of men who rape' (Scully 1990).

The emergence of the 'dangerous individual' in mid-19th century Europe (Foucault 1978) provided a foundation for medico-legal decision-making about criminal responsibility. Nowhere is this more clearly evidenced than in 'the diagnosis and treatment of psychosexual abnormality as manifested by violent sexual criminals' (Cameron & Frazer 1987). It is suggested that, despite internal differences, diverse disciplines such as psychoanalysis and sexology share the traditional pathologising process of medicine. The clinical categories of 'psychopathy' and 'personality disorder', so often conflated with the cultural category of 'sex murderer', noticeably fail to problematise gender. Little critical commentary is devoted to explaining why most psychopaths are male, or that the focus of their characteristic impulsivity is seldom random in its expression: 'They often have a sexual component and are systematically misogynistic' (Cameron & Frazer 1987:91).

If most of the serious sexual offenders in the UK still receive a penal sentence (Gunn 1991), those deemed to be suffering from a mental disorder are likely to be detained under the Mental Health Act 1983 in one of the Special Hospitals. Though sexual deviancy itself does not fall within the legislative criteria, underlying problems such as psychopathic disorder serve to qualify as suitable grounds for treatment (Fitzgerald 1991). Thus, whilst this system of disposal contains dangerous and high-risk offenders, such individuals are not strictly designated as 'sex offenders' (Houston et al 1994). If the hospital setting is seen as more advantageous than prison for a treatment approach (Perkins 1991), secure psychiatric institutions are not without their own set of contextual and cultural barriers. Currently, a range of interventive modalities

co-exist, but the cognitive–behavioural 'relapse-prevention' philosophy (Laws 1989) has been particularly important in moving practice from a biological to a psychological framework. This model of working, furthermore, permits ideological arguments about sexual offending to be incorporated within an anti-oppressive value base for treatment (Cowburn & Wilson 1992).

Pornography: a clinical concern

It has been suggested that individual nurses, and the profession collectively, should actively embrace the manifesto of the anti-pornography lobby (Orr 1988). Such claims are grounded in a set of concerns, at a series of levels, about pornography in relation to health care services: thematic content of sexualised violence, the objectification of women, representations of the nursing role, workplace harassment and gendered inequities in career advancement. Despite important implications, these issues are inversely addressed in the professional arena. Psychiatric nursing literature, particularly, shows a lack of reference regarding the health risks associated with pornography consumption or perceptions of educators about possible effects (Drake 1994).

The emergence of specialist forensic practice further crystallises pornography as a clinical dilemma; access to legally available materials by detained patients is an area of growing concern, though few effective policy statements have been formulated (Duff 1995). The dual role, of care and custody, is beset by tensions around empowerment, citizenship and human rights (Burrow 1991), yet individual choice and self-determination have increasingly become the benchmarks of progress. To suggest that limitations, or restrictions, might need to be placed upon materials such as pornography conflicts sharply with this philosophy (McKeown & Mercer 1995).

In relation to specific therapeutic work with sexual offenders, pornography manifests concerns that are both clinical and contextual. Commercially available books, magazines and films can be understood as a mechanism for maintaining the masculine power characteristic of high-security settings (Mercer & McKeown 1997). In addition to this, a spectrum of media images, which sexualise women and children (Kelly 1992), can be manipulated and manufactured as masturbatory materials akin to offence behaviours, thus complicating a simplistic, censorial response to the sexually explicit. At the same time, the massive expansion in communications technology has created a network of 'deviant technicways' through cyberspace, severely testing traditional means of regulating and controlling pornography (Durkin & Bryant 1995). Recent events in high-security services, captured in tabloid headlines (Harding 1997), echo the urgency of critically exploring the place of pornography in relation to rehabilitative ideals.

Pornography and sexual offending

Evidence of a relationship between pornography and sexual crime is based upon diverse forms of data, from macro-level analyses of crime rates (Court 1976) to the testimonies of individual victims (Lovelace 1982). Experimental research into the harmful effects of pornography focus on two discrete categories of sexually explicit materials, the violent and non-violent (Check & Guloien 1989). Consistently, academic and social science studies have linked the use of these kinds of pornography to sexual aggression and negative attitudes toward women. A third grouping, the erotic, depicting consensual and pleasurable relations cannot be shown to produce similar results.

Sexual offenders are known to be heavy users of pornography (Blackburn 1993), but compared with 'normal' populations the evidence of pornography as a criminogenic factor remains equivocal (Langevin et al 1988). Thus, despite being the research focus of innumerable studies, scientific links between pornography and harm are a contested territory, which is, in part, attributed to methodological problems and emotive interpretations (Fukui & Westmore 1994). Aside from debates about the validity of experimental designs, significant findings emerge from the

clinical practice of sex offender therapists (Lee 1988). Similarly, it has been noted that pornography can be implicated at each of the key phases in a cyclical model of offending: predisposition, fantasy, grooming, planning and the commission of sexual crime (Wyre 1992). In moving away from a uni-directional search for 'cause and effect', pornography can be seen as one component of a multi-factorial explanation of sexual violence (Russell 1988).

One major contribution of feminism as a political force has been to redefine pornography as an issue of harm rather than obscenity; where evidence of a correlation between negative representations of women and sexual violence is sufficient to justify legislative action (Itzin 1992). This recognition that the production and consumption of pornography, eroticising power relations and gender hatred, *is itself* violence against women (Dworkin 1981, Russell 1993) cannot be ignored in the treatment setting. Much of the behavioural literature has emphasised arousal toward the sexually explicit as a purely biological imperative, failing to account for the process by which any image is interpreted as arousing. Thus, sexuality can be seen as 'meaningfully scripted behaviour', facilitated by the 'symbolic scripts' of pornography and learned in a social context (Ashley & Ashley 1984). This perspective has resonance for any understanding of the actions of those who move beyond words and symbols, as evidenced in the narrative accounts of convicted rapists (Kellett 1995). Heterosexual pornography becomes part of a discourse which not only perpetuates physical–sexual domination, but constructs defensive strategies for those who engage in abusive behaviours (Cameron & Frazer 1992). Beyond the pictorial and written content of pornography, then, are a series of discourses that texture the therapeutic space of forensic practice. In what follows, it will be suggested that 'treatment' needs to be deconstructed and politically driven.

CASE STUDY: VERNON

In a material sense, at least, the childhood and later life experiences of Vernon contrast sharply with that stereotypical image of the offender as a product of deprivation and hardship. With his two elder brothers, he shared the privilege, security and status of a wealthy family, whose name dominated the rural community in which he grew up. His father, a prominent landowner, exerted considerable influence in the area, both as employer and local dignitary.

Retrospectively, one can identify a pattern of factors which contributed, collectively, to the construction of a predatory and abusive young man. Sadly, at each stage of development, the increasingly excessive cruelty of his behaviour was emasculated by the ideological blindness of social class and gender relations. Unlike his two siblings, who would follow a predictable route of private education and professional standing, Vernon adhered to a reckless and unruly pursuit of personal gratification.

His frequent temper tantrums at primary school would lead to the profile of an aggressive and arrogant adolescent. Vernon was a tall and physically strong boy, who believed that any opposition could be bullied or bought. Despite the social embarrassment caused, there were few parental restraints to curb his growing sense of self-importance. Indeed, it was the indulgence of unending financial support which made possible the purchase of his hedonistic tokens; the ownership of 'objects' which signified his being would, with tragic consequences, come to include those women who were drawn into his world.

By the time he had reached his late teens, Vernon cast a prescient shadow across his peers. He owned an impressive sports car, paraded in the latest fashions and purveyed alcohol and drugs in a form of colonial comradeship. Vernon was to become a familiar figure in the Magistrates' court and derived notoriety from the charges of 'fast driving' and 'fast living'. Fines would always be paid and adverse publicity kept to a minimum. This family patronage extended to his sexual relations. Brief and cavalier affairs with young women, two of whom became pregnant, were reduced to the substance of small town gossip.

Though an assertive and articulate individual, Vernon's academic performance was poor. As a result, employment opportunities were limited and could never equal the fantasy version of his life which was becoming more deeply entrenched. A series of low paid and routine jobs failed to deliver the excitement that he craved.

When, at 23, Vernon married, naive assumptions that he would settle down were short lived. Rather than changing, his exploitative behaviour shifted from the public domain into the privacy of his new home. At a young age, Vernon had discovered, and purloined, the pornographic magazines secreted by his elder brothers. Now, his obsessive interest in sexually explicit materials entered a new realm, where his wife was to become a reluctant participant. Vernon accumulated a diverse collection of books, magazines and films with a specific theme of sex and violence. Acting out the sadistic scenarios became the defining feature of his marriage, where attempts at resistance met with savage and brutal episodes of domestic assault.

Outside the home, Vernon continued to pursue and solicit the attentions of other women, always younger than himself. His capacity to be charming and persuasive was equalled by a growing hatred for the 'objects' of his desire. If women submitted to his badgering persistence, they were unworthy of respect; if they repelled him, it fuelled his burgeoning anger. It was precisely these circumstances which precipitated the horrific death of a young woman and marked Vernon's entry into the arena of medicalised criminality. After meeting in a public house, the 17-year-old had accepted a lift home from Vernon. Instead, she was abducted and taken to a remote farm building where she was systematically raped and tortured over several days. Finally, the young woman was killed and her body concealed in a disused woodshed.

Hospital

Psychiatric assessment found Vernon to be suffering from a psychopathic disorder. He was admitted, without limit of time, to a maximum secure Special Hospital. At the time that he was referred to a 'sex offender therapy group', Vernon had already spent over 15 years reconstructing his life within the confines of an isolated and oppressive institution. The perversity of his survival in this environment is worth, briefly, sketching out in terms of this case study. It illustrates how the collusive elements of a closed system are counterproductive to their espoused aims and signal the challenges facing those who attempt to intervene at either interpersonal or structural levels.

Despite the public and policy messages about psychiatric disposal, admission into the Special Hospitals, until recently, paralleled a penal career for offenders. Harsh custodial regimes promoted the 'otherness' of inmates, maintaining a spatial and moral distance between the keepers and the kept. But, for Vernon, the enclosed world he now inhabited was a microcosm of his universe outside. The Public Inquiry at Ashworth (Committee of Inquiry 1992), shortly followed by a judicial inquiry, are the most recent expressions of concern about the sinister and secretive world of secure psychiatry. They force us to consider the context of any treatment and dispel the lingering myth of 'milieu therapy'. Let us now consider some of these institutional factors in relation to any kind of therapeutic engagement with Vernon during the early years of his incarceration.

- *Densely macho cultures*. For both patients and staff this represents a 'survival of the fittest' mentality. Status is rooted in power and conflated in a tradition of toughness and masculinity.
- *Dangerousness as currency*. An elitism has developed around the concept of forensic nursing which is based upon the risk, and 'glamour', of managing a proportionally small number of notorious offenders. This is expressed in a folk-loric language where expertise is a family tradition.
- *Custody and containment*. The role of nursing is reduced to a function of security. Incidents (typically defined by violent encounters) become 'perks' of the job.
- *Therapeutic pessimism*. Alternative approaches to practice, which move beyond surveillance and policing, are derided and feminised.

- *Role of women*. Historically, the ratio of female staff has signalled a powerful message about their status within such organisations and reflected sexual divisions in society. Women have been seen as 'decorative' features of the ward, with an innate calming influence in an all-male enclave. Their lesser numbers in the workforce are a totem of weakness and vulnerability, compounded by the allocation of domestic duties.

Treatment in context

The introduction of an offence-specific treatment group into the environment outlined above presented a range of organisational and operational difficulties, requiring much discussion, negotiation and careful planning. Clinical matters such as the assessment and selection of patients, or recruitment of facilitators, had to be managed alongside much more mundane issues that were no less important to the survival of the project. Concerns included:

- *The 'name' of the group*. This was significant because, given the fundamental problem of denial with sexual offenders, symbolically the group needed to represent the offenders' recognition and ownership of their abusive behaviours, with a desire to stop offending. In contrast, the hospital propagated a climate of institutional collusion. Sexual offenders had an interest in concealing the nature of their crimes and manufacturing fictional biographies to enhance peer status and ensure physical safety. Attending a group with the designation of 'sex offender therapy' introduced the possibility of identification and visibility, with the risk of reprisal.
- *The location of the group*. It was decided that the sessions should take place in a purpose-built suite in the Psychology Department. The room was equipped with observation facilities and audio-visual recording systems. Being away from the ward environment reduced the chances of exposure and maintained a clear boundary between therapeutic work and the interactions of

day-to-day living. However, information exchange, and collaboration, between group facilitators and those involved in the primary care of patients was a major focus.

• *Movement of patients.* Within the confines of perimeter security, escorting arrangements for group members challenged the bureaucratic policies of the institution. In terms of transporting patients from their respective wards to the treatment venue, existing procedures compromised anonymity and restricted available time. An alternative strategy was devised, the execution of which hinged upon the agreement of clinical, security and hospital managers.

• *Recruitment and preparation of facilitators.* Given the complex demands of interventive work in this area, the selection of motivated and appropriately skilled personnel is a critical factor. With limited resources, no official training budget and an unpopular patient group, the commitment of individual practitioners was a driving force. Still, the urgency to address prurient interest, or punitive attitudes in disguise, was an early obstacle.

In line with progressive developments in the UK penal system (Grubin & Thornton 1994) and treatment programmes documented in the literature (Nelson et al 1989), a cognitive–behavioural (relapse-prevention) framework was adopted. Vernon was one of nine men who volunteered to be in the first cohort of the group. The sessions, lasting 2 hours, took place one afternoon per week for a proposed 12-month period; given the patient population and treatment context this was later extended to 18 months. Staff representing a range of disciplines (psychology, nursing, psychiatry, and social work) and gender balance, rotated between facilitator and supportive observer roles.

The content of the programme, with some adaptation, followed a modularised formula and in this sense was unremarkable. The nature of the work included, for example, challenging cognitive distortion and denial; the construction of individual offence cycles; apparent irrelevant decision (AID) making; identification of high-risk situations and stressors, and triggers to relapse; victim empathy. More noteworthy here, is an account of how the therapeutic process interfaced with the wider organisational culture and the dilemma of bridging this distance. Here, the debate about pornography-related violence will be used as a vehicle to explore the political dimensions of sexual offending and the implications for harm-reduction strategies.

Reflections on therapy

For the first time since admission into hospital, Vernon was in a situation where he had to openly confront his offending behaviour. It was tacitly acknowledged that his main motivation to participate was instrumental, seeking transfer to a less secure setting, and that any change process would be difficult and slow. Vernon had constructed the identity of a 'political prisoner' for himself. Contemptuous of, and litigious towards, a system that continued to detain him, Vernon's claims for justice failed to consider past actions or future risks. He had been rewarded for 'good behaviour': parole status to move freely around the hospital site; a trusted position of work in the patient library; residence on a ward with a relaxed regime and minimal security. During his time in the group, each of these traditional measures of progress was to emerge as grounds for serious concern.

In the early stages of group work, Vernon professed that his religious faith betokened a redemption beyond the purview of peers or facilitators. Regular church attendance, he claimed, signified a new-found spirituality. Rather than revisit his index offence, the young woman's destruction became a catalyst for salvation and attonement. Strategies of denial are not untypical, and information exchange with personnel in the wider organisation proved valuable in formulating a therapeutic challenge. Fragments of Vernon's behaviour, collectively, afforded a larger picture. He was corresponding with a young woman who attended the hospital services as a member of the Christian Fellowship. In art classes, Vernon had been described as producing talented and creative work, but aesthetic judgement had submerged any clinical concerns; one of his paintings depicted the crucifixion, where the body of Christ had been replaced with that of a young woman.

With little prompting, Vernon's conservative ideas about the role of women evidenced a much more fundamental distinction of the 'Madonna/whore' type; rigid categories of good and bad, deserving and undeserving women. At ward level, reports and nursing notes singled out Vernon's 'personal hygiene' and 'tidy room' as positive features in his care. Less attention, however, was given to the content or context of his possessions. Unlike many other patient rooms in the hospital, covered with sexually explicit pictures torn from pornographic magazines, Vernon had decorated his walls with framed photographs. Without exception, the selected subjects were women, singers, actresses or fashion models, who merged into a single stereotype defined by age, physical appearance and hair colour. Alone, these representational images may indicate little more than the societal manufacture of an idealised femininity. Other items, though, directly connected his views about women to the violent expression of sexuality. A collection of video-tapes, disguised with bland titles, contained a personal library of sadistic-sexual recordings; some were part of an organised trade in illicit pornography, others were carefully edited from films broadcast on television. All of the technical equipment required for the construction, and consumption, of these materials formed part of Vernon's legitimate property.

To the casual observer, Vernon's reading materials might have appeared as an innocuous assortment of 'contemporary classics'. Closer inspection, though, again revealed a choice of titles distinct from literary merit; two examples, *Last Exit to Brooklyn* (1990) and *American Psycho* (1991), are notable for their graphic depictions of rape and sexual torture. A locker full of commercial pornography magazines, in the absence of any official policy, had never been considered in relation to Vernon's offending history.

The dynamics of the treatment group were noticeably influenced by the gender of the facilitators. Vernon's attempts to avoid discussion with the women became angry and hostile if confronted. These collusive, and abusive, responses were paralleled by interactions on the ward. Vernon's size and power, enhanced by daily gym sessions, exerted an intimidating presence without the use of force. With male staff, this was expressed in a 'mock combat with the enemy' (*see* Richman 1998); with females, it took the form of invading personal space and sexualising routine exchanges, particularly with those perceived as less powerful in the organisation such as domestic and auxilliary grades.

The topic of pornography, fantasy and offending was explored as a specific issue within the group programme. The subject generated intense emotion and a defensive commentary, where claims of 'normality' and 'freedom' contrasted with evidence of harm. Survivor testimonies and research evidence were used to explore the pattern of Vernon's use of pornography from an early age, later domestic violence and escalation to sexual murder. Unlike other sexual offences (Osanka & Johann 1989), pornography was not directly implicated at the scene of Vernon's crime. Explorations in the context of therapeutic work, though, revealed a more pernicious role in contributing to sexual violence, and constructing the sexual offender.

Conclusions and recommendations for practice

Along with other members of the group, Vernon contributed to a narrative discourse about the use of pornography in relation to sexually abusive behaviour. These accounts compared closely with the research findings of Jensen (1998), derived from interviews with sexual offenders in treatment, and supported similar conclusions. That is, pornography emerged as an important 'actor' in the construction of a male-dominated version of sexuality. Distinct from a simplistic 'cause–effect' relationship, pornography was implicated in the commission of sexual violence in specific and thematic ways: it provided early instructional information about the content and expression of sexual activity; presented sexualised images of male power and control as exciting and arousing; fostered a denigratory and stereotypical objectification of women; trivialised crimes such as rape and incestuous abuse, desensitising feelings toward the survivors of those offences; and, as a masturbatory aid, reinforced the eroticisation of sexual inequality and suffering.

Some treatment settings, or programmes, operate an inflexible policy of prohibition in relation to pornography (Jensen 1998), with its destruction signifying commitment to change. In large institutional settings, where sexual offenders comprise only a section of the total population, rigid restrictions become more difficult to justify and implement. In working with offenders such as Vernon, exposure to sexually explicit images is an issue that needs careful attention. As Schimmer (1993) notes, clear answers are needed if action is to be taken, but clear answers in this domain are elusive. In the formulation of policy statements, or the construction of guidelines for practice, a number of points need to be given prominence:

- Traditional attempts to define pornography in moral terms, such as 'obscene', are of limited value in the treatment setting.
- Progressive definitions of pornography focus on evidence of harm.
- Commercially produced pornography, marketed as 'entertainment', promotes sexual objectification generally and features specific themes of control and domination.
- Pornography contributes to a climate of institutional sexism, exploitation and intimidation.
- The use of sexually explicit materials in a clinical environment needs to be understood in relation to offence-specific interests.
- The introduction of restrictions on sexual materials needs to be linked to individual care planning.
- Policies have to be embraced, and taken seriously, by staff at all levels of the organisation.
- Ownership of a policy should be promoted, and supported, through education and training initiatives.
- Patients/clients should be informed of the reasons for restrictions as a therapeutic rather than punitive measure.
- Involvement of personnel skilled in information technology in monitoring patient/client use of computer equipment.

REFERENCES

Amir M 1971 Patterns in forcible rape. University of Chicago Press, Chicago

Ashley B, Ashley D 1984 Sex as violence: the body against intimacy. International Journal of Women's Studies 7(4): 352–371

Blackburn R 1993 The psychology of criminal conduct. Wiley, London

Brownmiller S 1975 Against our will: men, women and rape. Simon and Schuster, New York

Burrow S 1991 The special hospital nurse and the dilemma of therapeutic custody. Journal of Advances in Health and Nursing Care 1(3): 21–38

Cameron D, Frazer E 1987 The lust to kill: a feminist investigation of sexual murder. Polity Press, Cambridge

Cameron D, Frazer E 1992 On the question of pornography and sexual violence: moving beyond cause and effect. In: Itzin C (ed) Pornography: women, violence and civil liberties. Oxford University Press, Oxford

Check J, Guloien T 1989 Reported proclivity for coercive sex following repeated exposure to sexually violent pornography, non-violent dehumanising pornography and erotica. In: Zillman D, Bryant J (eds) Pornography: research advances and policy considerations. Erlbaun, Hillsdale NJ

Committee of Inquiry into Complaints about Ashworth Hospital 1992 Report of the committee of inquiry into complaints at Ashworth Hospital (Blom Cooper Report) Cmnd 2028. HMSO, London

Court J 1976 Pornography and sex crimes: a re-evaluation in the light of recent trends around the world. International Journal of Criminology and Penology 5: 129–157

Cowburn M, Wilson C (1992) The underlying framework: research, theory and values. In: Loewenstein P (ed)

Changing men: a practice guide to working with adult male sex offenders. Nottinghamshire Probation Service, Nottingham, England

Drake R 1994 Potential health hazards of pornography consumption as viewed by psychiatric nurses. Archives of Psychiatric Nursing 8(2): 101–106

Duff A 1995 Pornography and censorship: the problems of policy formation in a psychiatric setting. Psychiatric Care 2(4): 137–140

Durkin K, Bryant C 1995 'Log onto sex': some notes on the carnal computer and erotic cyberspace as an emerging research frontier. Deviant Behaviour: An Interdisciplinary Journal 16(3): 179–200

Dworkin A 1981 Pornography: men possessing women. Women's Press, London

Easton Ellis B 1991 American psycho. Pan, London

Fitzgerald E (1991) 'Back to therapy': sentencing of sexual offenders. Criminal Behaviour and Mental Health 1: 175–180

Foucault M 1978 About the concept of the dangerous individual in nineteenth century legal psychiatry. International Journal of Law and Psychiatry 1: 1–18

Fukui A, Westmore B 1994 To see or not to see: the debate over pornography and its relationship to sexual aggression. Australian and New Zealand Journal of Psychiatry 28(4): 600–606

Grubin D, Thornton D 1994 A national programme for the assessment and treatment of sexual offenders in the English prison system. Criminal Justice and Behaviour 21(1): 55–71

Gunn J 1991 The role of the psychiatrist. Criminal Behaviour and Mental Health 1(2): 109–113.

Harding L 1997 Within these walls: abuse, racketeering – what's going on inside Ashworth Hospital? The Guardian 17 February (2): 1–3

Houston J, Thomson P, Wragg J 1994 A survey of forensic psychologists' work with sex offenders in England and Wales. Criminal Behaviour and Mental Health 4: 118–129

Itzin C 1992 A briefing for MPs and MEPs on evidence of pornography related harm and a progressive new approach to legislating against pornography without censorship. Violence, Abuse and Gender Relations Research Unit, Bradford University, England

Jensen R 1998 Using pornography. In: Dines G, Jensen R, Russo A (eds) Pornography: the production and consumption of inequality. Routledge, London

Kellett P 1995 Acts of power, control and resistance: narrative accounts of convicted rapists. In: Whilcock R, Slayden D (eds) Hate speech. Sage, London

Kelly L 1992 Pornography and child sexual abuse. In: Itzin C (ed) Pornography: Women, violence and civil liberties. Oxford University Press, Oxford

Langevin R, Lang R, Wright P, Handy L, Frenzel R, Black E 1988 Pornography and sexual offences. Annals of Sex Research 1: 335–362

Laws R (ed) (1989) Relapse prevention with sex offenders. Guilford Press, New York

Lee R 1988 Attitudes of sex offenders. In: Minneapolis City Council Government Operations Committee. Pornography and sexual violence: evidence of the links. Everywoman, London

Lovelace L 1982 Ordeal: an autobiography. WH Allen, London

McKeown M, Mercer D 1995 Is a written charter really the answer? Human rights in secure mental health settings. Psychiatric Care 1(6): 219–223

Mercer D, McKeown M 1997 Pornography: some implications for nursing. Health Care Analysis 5(1): 56–61

Millett K 1971 Sexual politics. Rupert Hart-Davis, London

Nelson C, Miner M, Marques J, Russell K, Achterkirchen J 1989 Relapse prevention: a cognitive–behavioral model for treatment of the rapist and child molester. Journal of Social Work and Human Sexuality 7(2): 125–143

Orr J 1988 The porn brokers. Nursing Times 84(20): 22

Osanka F, Johann S 1989 Sourcebook on pornography. Lexington Books, Massachusetts, Toronto

Perkins D 1991 Treatment in hospital. Criminal Behaviour and Mental Health 1: 152–168

Richman J 1998 The ceremonial and moral order of a ward for psychopaths. In: Mason T, Mercer D (eds) Critical perspectives in forensic care: inside out. Macmillan, London

Russell D 1988 Pornography and rape: a causal model. Political Psychology 9(1): 41–73

Russell D 1993 Against pornography: the evidence of harm. Russell Publications, Berkeley, California

Schimmer R 1993 The impact of sexually stimulating materials on group care residents: a question of harm. Residential Treatment for Children and Youth 11(2): 37–55

Scott S, Dickens A 1989 Police and the professionalisation of rape. In: Dunhill C (ed) The boys in blue: women's challenge to the police. Virago, London

Scully D 1990 Understanding sexual violence: a study of convicted rapists. Unwin Hyman, London

Selby H Jr 1990 Last exit to Brooklyn. Paladin, London

Vogelman L 1990 The sexual face of violence: rapists on rape. Ravan Press, Johannesburg

Watts A, Courtois C 1981 Trends in the treatment of men who commit violence against women. The Personnel and Guidance Journal 60(4): 245–249

Wyre R 1992 Pornography and sexual violence: working with sex offenders. In: Itzin C (ed) Pornography: women, violence and civil liberties. Oxford University Press, Oxford

Severe and enduring mental health problems

CONTENTS

Cognitive–behaviour therapy for auditory hallucinations

Richard Bentall and Gill Haddock

Introduction

In this case study we will describe the attempted cognitive–behavioural treatment of a patient suffering from a psychotic illness, who had been detained in a Special Hospital following the murder of his girlfriend. The principal complaint of the patient, Albert, was auditory hallucinations and this symptom was the focus of his treatment. The therapy was not delivered in a conventional manner, as Albert had been recruited to a clinical trial designed to assess the efficacy of cognitive–behaviour therapy (CBT) for the treatment of hallucinations. For this reason, the treatment was time-limited and was not well-integrated with other treatments that Albert was receiving, and the treatment-protocol was determined in advance of any knowledge of Albert's history or difficulties. The case study therefore illustrates some of the limitations of clinical trials of psychological therapies, which do not allow the flexibility in treatment often desirable in routine practice. The study also provides an opportunity to consider the current status of cognitive–behavioural treatments for hallucinations. Finally, as the events leading to Albert's detention in hospital became an important issue during the progress of therapy, the case study illustrates some of the difficulties encountered when applying CBT in forensic settings.

Theoretical background

Until recently, hallucinations have been the subject of comparatively little psychological research

(Slade & Bentall 1988). This is partly because they have long been considered pathognomic symptoms of schizophrenia rather than worthy of investigation in their own right. Auditory–verbal hallucinations were included in Schneider's (1959) list of first-rank symptoms of the disorder. Consistent with Schneider's account, they are one of the commonest symptoms encountered in patients who meet conventional criteria for schizophrenia (Sartorius et al 1974). However, they are also reported by patients diagnosed as suffering from many other psychiatric and neurological conditions and for this reason their special status with respect to schizophrenia has been questioned by some commentators (Asaad & Shapiro 1986).

Although various definitions of hallucination have been proposed, Slade & Bentall (1988) have suggested that they are best described as percept-like experiences that: (a) occur in the absence of appropriate stimuli; (b) have the full force or impact of real perceptions; and (c) are not amenable to the direct voluntary control of the experiencer. In Western psychiatric practice, the most common type of hallucination reported by patients is auditory–verbal and may take the form of one or more voices talking to the patient, or commenting on his or her intentions or actions (Sims 1995). They may be experienced as external to the self (and therefore perceived through the ears) or as originating within the head (in which case they are still perceived as entirely alien to the self). The term 'pseudo-hallucination' has sometimes been used for the latter phenomenon, although the official diagnostic manual of the American Psychiatric Association notes that no significance should be attributed to the distinction between this type of experience and voices that appear to originate from an external source (American Psychiatric Association 1994). Although voices are often described by patients as critical or abusive, this is not invariably the case. In an interview study of chronically-ill schizophrenia patients in the USA, Miller et al (1993) found that a large proportion reported positive voices, which the patients felt some attachment towards,

and which had therefore been integrated into the patients' otherwise impoverished social networks.

Conventional psychiatric theory notwithstanding, it has become evident that by far the majority of people who experience hallucinations do not seek or require psychiatric treatment. Surveys of apparently 'normal' individuals consistently reveal a sizeable minority who experience voices (Bentall 1990). In the most comprehensive study of this sort (of over 18 000 randomly-selected US citizens) it was estimated that the lifetime prevalence of hallucinations was approximately 10% (Tien 1991), which exceeds the lifetime risk of a diagnosis of schizophrenia by at least a factor of 10. In Holland, the social psychiatrist Marius Romme has formed a national society for people who hear voices and many of its members have had little or no contact with psychiatric services (Romme & Escher 1993).

The severity of hallucinations may fluctuate over time. Studies with psychiatric patients show that voices are most likely to be experienced during periods of intense but unpatterned auditory stimulation (Gallagher et al 1994, Margo et al 1981). On the other hand, ongoing cognitive activity such as reading, thinking or concentrating on complex stimuli tends to reduce the experience of hallucinations (Erickson & Gustafson 1968, Gallagher et al 1995, James 1983). Both case study and psychophysiological data indicate that patients are most likely to experience hallucinations during periods of stress (Cooklin et al 1983), a finding which is consistent with more general observations of the negative impact of stress on psychotic patients.

In recent years, a number of authors have proposed psychological models of hallucinations (Bentall 1990, Frith 1992, Heilbrun 1996, Hoffman 1986). As these models are very similar, a consensus account has emerged, in which hallucinations are hypothesised to be mental events which the individual misattributes to a source which is external or alien to the self. In the case of auditory hallucinations, the individual mistakes the source of his or her own 'inner speech' (covert self-talk or verbal thought).

Evidence in favour of this hypothesis is available from electrophysiological studies, which have revealed increased activity in the speech muscles during periods of hallucination (Gould 1948, Gould 1950, Green & Kinsbourne 1990, Inouye & Shimizu 1970); muscular activity of this sort accompanies normal verbal thought. This account explains the influence on hallucinations of the various factors described above. During periods of unpatterned stimulation, less stimulus information is available to the individual to allow external and self-generated stimuli to be distinguished. As ongoing cognitive activity will tend to inhibit unintended inner speech (you cannot talk idly to yourself while concentrating on a difficult task), it will also tend to inhibit hallucinations. Stress, on the other hand, is likely to facilitate hallucinations because it adversely affects the accuracy of higher-level cognitive judgements.

The emergence of this consensus account has raised the possibility of psychological interventions for people who experience troublesome hallucinations. In a review of the literature conducted 10 years ago, Slade & Bentall (1988) found that a wide range of treatments had been reported in case studies, but that these could be grouped into three main types: anxiety-reduction treatments, interventions in which patients were encouraged to distract themselves from their voices (e.g. by engaging in cognitive tasks) and interventions in which the individual was encouraged to focus on their voices. Although Slade & Bentall argued that therapeutic benefits were likely from all three approaches, they suggested that only the last approach would lead to a lasting re-integration of voices with the self. It was in order to test this prediction that they planned the clinical trial which included Albert as a patient.

Treatment protocol

The clinical trial to which Albert was recruited has been described in detail elsewhere (Bentall et al 1994, Haddock et al 1993, Haddock et al 1998). Briefly, it was decided to compare two treatment strategies. The first, which was anticipated to be most effective, involved encouraging patients to focus on their voices and consider their meaning and significance, in the hope that this would lead them to recognise that they were self-generated. This strategy was called 'focusing'. The second, which was predicted to be less effective, involved encouraging patients to employ various kinds of cognitive activities (such as listening to music, performing simple mental tasks) which we hoped would inhibit their hallucinations. This second strategy was called 'distraction'. In order to be entered into the trial, potential patients had to meet the DSM-III-R criteria for schizophrenia (American Psychiatric Association 1987) and had to be suffering from severe hallucinations at least three times a week and unresponsive to neuroleptic medication. When these criteria were given to local consultant psychiatrists, the referrals that ensued were generally long-term patients who had enjoyed little benefit from conventional psychiatric treatment. (The mean length of illness of those completing the trial was 15 years.)

A total of 63 patients were referred and, of these, 33 were judged suitable: 14 patients were assigned to focusing therapy, 11 to distraction and 8 to a treatment-as-usual control group. Because of drop outs at various stages, at 2-year follow-up only 11 remained in the focusing group, 8 in the distraction group and 5 in the control group. These small numbers made interpretation of the long-term outcome difficult. However, it is fair to say that the overall results were disappointing for reasons which will be discussed below.

Albert was a 42-year-old man referred by a consultant at a nearby Special (secure) Hospital and assigned to the 'focusing' condition. He was seen by the first author (RB). Initial assessment consisted of a battery of measures which had been selected for the study, and which therefore did not yield a great deal of information about his history. These included the 9th edition of the Present State Examination (Wing et al 1974), an interview schedule designed to provide a comprehensive overview of patients' symptoms, a detailed interview assessment of hallucinations specifically designed for the study and various questionnaire and psychometric measures including the Hospital Anxiety and Depression (HAD) Scale.

Progress during treatment was assessed using the Personal Questionnaire Rapid Scaling Technique (PQRST) (Mulhall 1978). This involves repeatedly presenting the same questionnaire items (e.g. 'During the last week, the amount of time I have spent experiencing hallucinations has been …') along with different pairs of adjectives (e.g. 'moderate' vs 'very considerable'). Patients respond by choosing the most appropriate adjective from each pair and a final score, together with an indication of the reliability of the patients' responses, can be determined by examining the pattern of choices. Although this technique has been recommended for use with psychotic patients because of its in-built reliability measure, we found it tedious in practice and just as meaningful results were achieved using simple daily diary sheets, which included three visual analogue scales.

CASE STUDY: ALBERT

Albert was a large, jovial man of Afro-Caribbean origin. Throughout the assessment and treatment he was highly cooperative. A brief IQ assessment conducted at the initial assessment revealed that he was of average intelligence. He had grown up in Wolverhampton in a family of six. His father had worked for an engineering firm and his mother had stayed at home. No other members of his family had a psychiatric history and, when interviewed, he had not had any contact with his parents, brothers or sisters for a period of more than 2 years.

At the age of 16 he had left school, run away from home and embarked on a career of petty offences, mainly burglary. This had led to a period in borstal, where he had acquired skills as a painter and decorator. Psychiatric records indicated that Albert had first begun to experience psychotic symptoms during his early 20s. However, his admission to Special Hospital in the early 1980s had occurred after he had stabbed his girlfriend to death.

Albert complained of auditory and visual hallucinations, both of which were sometimes bizarre in content and often concerned sexual themes. For example, his voices might comment about the attractiveness of one of the female staff and this would lead him to construct 'a story' in his mind about himself kissing her and then having sex with her. Albert denied that these experiences were ordinary sexual fantasies because they seemed to happen all the time without his bidding. Similarly, he described visual experiences of women taking their clothes off and stated that these could not be fantasies because, 'You can only imagine someone you've met, and I've never met these women.' Other hallucinatory experiences were less prosaic. For example, Albert complained that he could sometimes see flying, disembodied penises. He also attempted to describe, in a slightly incoherent manner, his experience that the hospital he was in was in some way a copy of the real hospital, which existed alongside the real hospital, perhaps in a separate location or even on a separate plane of existence. The therapist found this experience particularly difficult to understand and it was not addressed in the course of treatment. However, the experience may have been similar to the 'delusion of inanimate doubles' described by Anderson (1988).

During early treatment sessions, Albert was asked to consider the similarity between his hallucinatory experiences and his normal mental processes. He found this difficult because he said that he had no thoughts and, indeed, that his lack of thoughts was more troubling to him than his voices. However, with encouragement he was able to consider five possible (and not necessarily mutually exclusive) explanations for his experiences:

1. He was 'picking up vibes from somewhere else'.
2. He had a brain disorder.
3. They were caused by his imagination.
4. They were his thoughts.
5. They were normal.

In order to assist Albert to consider the merits of these different accounts, he was encouraged to perform focusing exercises, in which he systematically listened to his voices for short periods of time. In the first exercise, carried out in the second session and repeated in later sessions, he was asked to note the physical characteristics of the voices. He reported that they appeared to vary in location, but typically originated from his head, eyes, throat or neck (as the subvocalisation hypothesis implies). He also became aware that he could sometimes ignore the voices, but that this was most difficult if they had a sexual content, if he was bored, or during periods of disharmony with the nursing staff.

After practising these focusing exercises between sessions, Albert reported a reduction of the frequency of his voices, which was reflected in changing scores on the PQRST (see Fig. 4.1, sessions 1–10). During this period, he reported that he felt a considerable degree of depression, which was reflected in his scores on the HAD. Consistent with the treatment protocol, little effort was made to address wider issues, such as his offence and his feelings towards his family. However, Albert brought these issues to the fore in the sixth session, which marked a fairly dramatic change in his attitude towards the treatment, and which occurred after a short break in therapy caused by a bank holiday.

Albert began the session by complaining about his persisting depression, which he felt had worsened in the 2 weeks since the therapist had last seen him. However, he acknowledged that his voices had been much less bothersome. Suddenly, he stated that the therapist's absence had contributed to his feeling of 'being low' and that, otherwise, he had begun to feel much more optimistic about his future. He reported that, since the therapy had begun, he had felt much more able to talk to the staff in the hospital, and especially to the therapist. He then stated that he would like to talk about his offence. There followed a lengthy discussion of his feelings of confusion running up to the murder of his girlfriend, which had occurred following an angry argument. Albert attributed his violent actions to his voices, but at the same time acknowledged that the content of his voices at the time had reflected his own

extreme emotions. For the rest of the session, the therapist attempted to assist Albert in reaching a formulation of his problems at the time of the offence which: (a) allowed him to acknowledge that his voices were his own thoughts; (b) allowed him to recognise the role of anger in the offence; and (c) moderated his very considerable guilt about what he had done. This approach led Albert to acknowledge that, not only had he been mentally ill at the time of the offence, but that he had remained mentally ill ever since.

Exercises in subsequent sessions began to focus on the content and meaning of Albert's voices. For example, in session 7, Albert monitored his voices by speaking them out aloud. In this way, he reported that his voices were saying, 'You're not worth a fuck', which the therapist interpreted as reflecting Albert's low self-esteem. In this way, the idea that Albert's voices were related to his feelings was reinforced. Later on in the session, Albert reported that his voice said, 'You don't seem to understand what Richard wants you to see', which was interpreted as reflecting Albert's anxiety about making progress.

A major setback in the progress of therapy appeared to occur in session 11, which again followed a break, this time occasioned by the therapist going on holiday for 2 weeks. In stark contrast to many of the preceding sessions, Albert started by stating that he felt very well. He then immediately stated that he had decided that his voices did not belong to himself. The therapist experienced great difficulty in challenging this idea without being confrontative and without damaging the therapeutic relationship. At about this time, Albert's PQRST ratings recorded an increase in the frequency of his voices, which fortunately was not maintained in the later sessions.

Throughout the following sessions, Albert never fully embraced the possibility that his voices were self-generated and the therapist decided that it would be unhelpful to focus further on this issue as doing so seemed to make Albert anxious. During this time, the content of Albert's voices often seemed to reflect

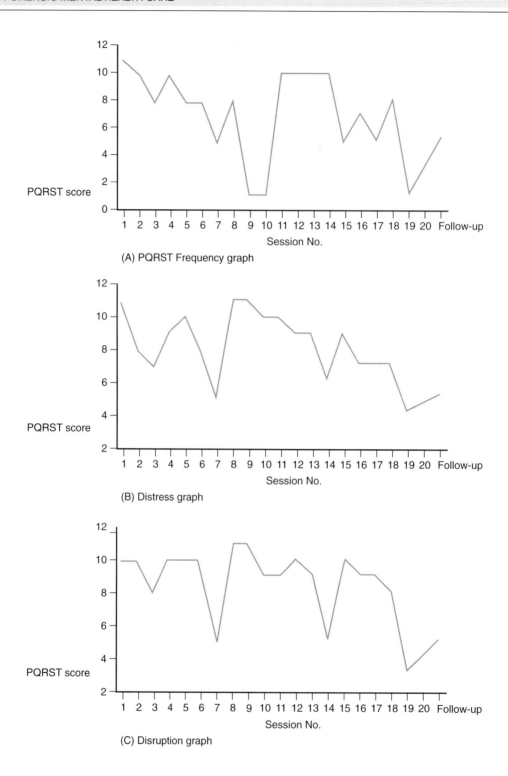

Fig. 4.1 PQRST ratings of the frequency of voices, and the disruption to life and distress.

his concerns about his relationship with the therapist. For example, a voice told Albert, 'Tell Richard … you're in too deep.' Another voice said, 'Richard doesn't understand what you are going through. When the time comes, he will understand.' The latter led to a long discussion about whether or not Albert was indeed being understood by his therapist. Despite these difficulties, Albert continued to perform the increasingly elaborate focusing exercises which the therapist devised. For example, the therapist asked Albert to spend time every day writing down what his voices said. This drew Albert's attention to the fact that the content of the voices was sometimes quite banal, an observation which seemed to considerably moderate his anxiety about them. On another occasion, the therapist asked Albert to repeat in a whisper what the voices had said and to consider in what way this experience differed from the voices themselves. Throughout these sessions, a reduction in the frequency, loudness and distressingness of the voices was noted, both in Albert's account during the sessions and in his PQRST ratings.

The duration of therapy was constrained by the treatment protocol. However, in the final sessions much time was spent discussing Albert's guilt about his offence and his relationships with other family members. Albert contacted his family and arranged for them to visit him in hospital (although he was careful to deny that this decision was in any way connected to his therapy). He began to use the hospital gym. He also applied for parole. Just before the last session, the visit from his family took place and was judged to be a success. During the final session, Albert reported that his voices continued to be less troublesome, but that his visions (which remained highly sexual in content) remained a source of distress to him. The last time the therapist attempted a focusing exercise with him, he reported that his voices whispered two things: 'You're doing alright' and 'You're not a cucumber salesman.' The interpretation of the former is fairly straightforward. We leave the interpretation of the latter statement to the reader.

Discussion

The changes in Albert's perception of his voices were confirmed by an assessment undertaken by an independent psychologist at the end of treatment. However, a further assessment 6 months later indicated that these changes had not been maintained. At that stage, Albert was again finding his voices highly troubling.

A number of issues are raised by the account we have given. The first concerns the advantages and disadvantages of conducting treatments according to pre-established protocols. This is a requirement of clinical trials but greatly limits the flexibility of the therapist. The trial protocol limited the number of sessions the therapist was able to spend with Albert. Under routine clinical conditions, he would have probably extended the treatment in the hope that this would have facilitated a return of the 'insight' Albert appeared to enjoy during the early sessions. More importantly, concern about adherence to the protocol was responsible for the therapist's initial reluctance to explore forensic issues with Albert, which turned out to be a mistake. Albert himself clearly thought that these issues were important, and therefore brought them up after a few sessions. This presented the therapist with the difficulty of encouraging an appropriate account of Albert's offence. Over-vigorously encouraging Albert to take responsibility for his voices would have probably provoked a catastrophic loss of self-esteem. In the end, an illness model was accepted by Albert.

A strength of protocol-driven psychological intervention is that considerable thought is usually given to the monitoring of the patient's response. In the case of Albert, thorough assessments were conducted both at the outset and at follow-up, and questionnaires were used to monitor progress during therapy. In retrospect, the Present State Examination does not seem an ideal measure of psychopathology for these purposes; although it allows a broad range of symptoms to be assessed, these are usually classified as present, possibly present or absent, allowing little sensitivity to change. Other interview schedules, for example the Positive and

Negative Syndromes Scale (PANSS) (Kay et al 1986), developed originally for drug trials, are more suitable for this purpose and are employed in our ongoing research. In contrast, the questionnaire measures we have described should be useful in routine clinical work. The brief diary measure, in particular, proved to be acceptable to patients and simple to complete.

Albert's fluctuating attitude towards his voices and to his therapist would not seem surprising to a psychodynamic therapist. Indeed, much of the content of his voices seemed to concern his relationship with the therapist and his struggle to find an acceptable account for his past behaviour. This came as a surprise to the therapist, who found it difficult to maintain a positive therapeutic relationship once Albert had insisted that his voices were alien. Under these circumstances, there is a danger of provoking psychological reactance in the patient (the more the therapist pushes a particular point of view, the more likely it is that the patient will stick to his guns) and it seems probable that the therapist failed to avoid this danger in this case. Maintaining an adequate relationship with the patient is one of the most difficult tasks faced by the cognitive–behaviour therapist working with psychotic patients (Fowler et al 1995). Interestingly, the quality of the therapeutic relationship was found to be a major predictor of long-term outcome in a trial of psychodynamic therapy for schizophrenia patients (Frank & Gunderson 1990). Yet, the role of the therapeutic relationship in CBT has been the subject of very little research.

The relatively poor outcome of Albert's treatment raises the question of whether CBT is generally effective with hallucinations. In recent years, enthusiasm for the use of CBT with psychotic patients has been fostered by the positive results of increasingly rigorous clinical trials, beginning with the pioneering studies by Kingdon & Turkington (1991), Tarrier et al (1993) and Garety et al (1994) and progressing to the more recent (and generally larger-scale) studies (e.g. Drury et al 1996). The poor outcomes observed at the end of the 2-year follow-up of our own patients at first sight appear to stand in marked contrast to these findings. However, many of the above-mentioned clinical trials have reported aggregate measures of positive symptoms. Close inspection of the data from some of the trials (e.g. Garety et al 1994, Tarrier et al 1993) provides a clear indication that hallucinations are more difficult to treat than delusions. Although it would be wrong to conclude from these findings that auditory hallucinations are completely resistant to psychological treatment, there certainly seems to be consistent evidence that hallucinations are relatively hard to treat compared to other symptoms.

It is possible that this difficulty reflects our lack of understanding of the psychological mechanisms responsible for hallucinations. Although we have drawn attention to the consensus view that auditory hallucinations consist of inner speech that is misattributed to an external source, very little is known about the *causes* of this kind of source monitoring error. This partly reflects our limited understanding of the developmental, cognitive and biological processes involved in effective source monitoring in ordinary individuals. Presumably, improved understanding in these areas will facilitate the development of novel therapies. Until this happens, therapy must proceed pragmatically.

Acknowledgement

The research described in this study was supported by a grant from the Medical Research Council.

REFERENCES

American Psychiatric Association (APA) 1987 Diagnostic and statistical manual of mental disorders, revised 3rd edn. APA, Washington DC

American Psychiatric Association (APA) 1994 Diagnostic and statistical manual for mental disorders, 4th edn. APA, Washington DC

Anderson D 1988 The delusion of inanimate doubles. British Journal of Psychiatry 153: 694–699

Asaad G, Shapiro B 1986 Hallucinations: theoretical and clinical overview. American Journal of Psychiatry 143: 1088–1097

Bentall R 1990 The illusion of reality: a review and integration of psychological research on hallucinations. Psychological Bulletin 107: 82–95

Bentall R, Haddock G, Slade P 1994. Cognitive behavior therapy for persistent auditory hallucinations: from theory to therapy. Behavior Therapy 25: 51–66

Cooklin R, Sturgeon D, Leff J 1983 The relationship between auditory hallucinations and spontaneous fluctuations of skin conductance in schizophrenia. British Journal of Psychiatry 142: 47–52

Drury V, Birchwood M, Cochrane R, MacMillan F (1996) Cognitive behaviour therapy for a cute psychosis. British Journal of Psychiatry 169: 593–607

Erickson G, Gustafson G 1968 Controlling auditory hallucinations. Hospital and Community Psychiatry 19: 327–329

Fowler D, Garety P, Kuipers E 1995 Cognitive behaviour therapy for psychosis: theory and practice. Wiley, Chichester

Frank A, Gunderson J 1990 The role of the therapeutic alliance in the treatment of schizophrenia: relationship to course and outcome. Archives of General Psychiatry 47: 228–236

Frith C 1992 The cognitive neuropsychology of schizophrenia. Lawrence Erlbaum, Hillsdale NJ

Gallagher A, Dinin T, Baker L 1994 The effects of varying auditory input on schizophrenic hallucinations: a replication. British Journal of Medical Psychology 67: 67–76

Gallagher A, Dinin T, Baker L 1995 The effects of varying information content and speaking aloud on auditory hallucinations. British Journal of Medical Psychology 68: 143–155

Garety P, Kuipers L, Fowler D, Chamberlain F, Dunn G 1994 Cognitive behavioural therapy for drug-resistant psychosis. British Journal of Medical Psychology 67: 259–271

Gould L 1948 Verbal hallucinations and activity of vocal musculature. American Journal of Psychiatry 105: 367–372

Gould L 1950 Verbal hallucinations and automatic speech. American Journal of Psychiatry 107: 110–119

Green M, Kinsbourne M 1990 Subvocal activity and auditory hallucinations: clues for behavioral treatments. Schizophrenia Bulletin 16: 617–625

Haddock G, Bentall R, Slade P 1993 Psychological treatment of chronic auditory hallucinations: two case studies. Behavioural and Cognitive Psychotherapy 21: 335–346

Haddock G, Slade P, Bentall R 1998 Cognitive–behavioural treatment of auditory hallucinations: a comparison of the long-term effectiveness of two interventions. British Journal of Medical Psychology 71: 339–349

Heilbrun A 1996 Hallucinations. In: Costello C (ed) Symptoms of schizophrenia. Wiley, New York

Hoffman R 1986 Verbal hallucinations and language production processes in schizophrenia. Behavioral and Brain Sciences 9: 503–548

Inouye T, Shimizu A 1970 The electromyographic study of verbal hallucination. Journal of Nervous and Mental Disease 151: 415–422

James D 1983 The experimental treatment of two cases of auditory hallucinations. British Journal of Psychiatry 143: 515–516

Kay S, Opler L, Fiszbein A 1986 Positive and Negative Syndrome Scale [PANSS] Rating Manual. Social and Behavioural Sciences Documents, California

Kingdon D, Turkington D 1991 Preliminary report: the use of cognitive behaviour therapy and a normalizing rationale in schizophrenia. Journal of Nervous and Mental Disease 179: 207–211

Margo A, Hemsley D, Slade P 1981 The effects of varying auditory input on schizophrenic hallucinations. British Journal of Psychiatry 139: 122–127

Miller L, O'Connor E, DePasquale T 1993 Patients' attitudes to hallucinations. American Journal of Psychiatry 150: 584–588

Mulhall D 1978 Manual for the Personal Questionnaire Rapid Scaling Technique. NFER Nelson, Windsor

Romme M, Escher S (eds) 1993 Accepting voices. MIND, London

Sartorius N, Shapiro R, Jablensky A 1974 The international pilot study of schizophrenia. Schizophrenia Bulletin 1: 21–25

Schneider K 1959 Clinical psychopathology. Grune & Stratton, New York

Sims A 1995 Symptoms in the mind, 2nd edn. WB Saunders, London

Slade P, Bentall R 1988 Sensory deception: a scientific analysis of hallucination. Croom Helm, London

Tarrier N, Beckett R, Harwood S, Baker A, Yusupoff L, Ugarteburu I 1993 A trial of two cognitive–behavioural methods of treating drug-resistant residual psychotic symptoms in schizophrenic patients I: outcome. British Journal of Psychiatry 162: 524–532

Tien A 1991 Distribution of hallucinations in the population. Social Psychiatry and Psychiatric Epidemiology 26: 287–292

Wing J, Cooper J, Sartorius N 1974 The measurement and classification of psychiatric symptoms. Cambridge University Press, Cambridge

CONTENTS

Cognitive–behaviour therapy for delusions

Paula Ewers, Karen Leadley and Peter Kinderman

Introduction

There is now a growing body of research that demonstrates the efficacy of cognitive–behaviour therapy (CBT) for people with psychosis. Some of this work has specifically focused on particular symptoms such as delusions. However, there is little work that has covered the application of such therapy to a forensic population, with conflicting evidence linking delusions to risk or criminality. These discrepancies may be mostly due to methodological differences. Although there are several factors contributing to crime which cannot be addressed directly in therapy (e.g. poor family history, poverty), a person's delusional beliefs can be treated with the aim of reducing the likelihood of them being acted upon. Such a case study is described here. Using a series of standardised assessments, there was a change in symptoms that was maintained at 3-month follow-up. There was a marked change in delusional beliefs, which we would hope would reduce the risk of further serious assault. The role of supervision in the therapy is reflected upon.

CBT and psychosis

CBT for psychosis has developed considerably in practice and in related research. Beck (1952) reports early case work, yet it is only in recent years that the approach has developed on a large scale. Possible reasons for this are complex and varied. Sellwood et al (1994) suggest that schizophrenia was previously considered to be outwith the scope of psychological practice, though such views have changed as a result of inadequacies in singularly biological models and weaknesses in medical treatment. Despite the prominence of medication, many patients still have residual positive symptoms (Curson et al 1985, Curson et al 1988, Harrow et al 1985). Garety et al (1994) state that 'the cost of positive symptoms to the individuals' life in terms of distress, disruption, potential, family burden and service use is very great.' With increasing moves towards community care and user empowerment, it is possible to see why psychological approaches, which may modify distressing symptoms and improve the individual's understanding and ability to cope, are so attractive.

Over the last 20 years, there have been numerous case studies which have reported success in using CBT with psychotic individuals (Slade & Bentall 1988, Johnson et al 1977, Watts et al 1973). Fowler et al (1995) suggest that one of the reasons that CBT, so far, has had little impact on clinical practice is that it has failed to demonstrate that modifying psychotic experience results in meaningful change in a person's life. However, it is important to remember that CBT for individuals with psychosis is in its infancy when compared with other approaches and consequently much less research is available to demonstrate its efficacy. Only three randomised controlled studies have been carried out (Drury et al 1996, Kuipers et al 1997, Tarrier et al 1993) and two of these (Drury et al 1996, Tarrier et al 1993) did not offer long-term treatment.

Although some researchers focused on interventions for specific symptoms because of the heterogeneity of schizophrenia, other researchers have moved towards a 'person' approach rather than symptom approach (Chadwick 1997). These approaches attempt to form cognitive therapy which addresses wide and varying problems that people with schizophrenia might face. Kingdon & Turkington (1991) treated 64 patients aiming to normalise the individual's psychotic experience. Subjects were recruited from both out-patients, who presented with persistent residual positive symptoms, and patients in hospital during acute episodes. The individual patients were offered

a stress vulnerability (Zubin & Spring 1977) explanation of their experiences. Information was given to show them that hallucinations and delusions are common experiences, dismissed rapidly in the 'normal' population. However, under times of stress these psychotic experiences are not easily dismissed, especially if the individual is socially isolated and unable to discuss the reality of the belief. This 'normalising approach' also includes teaching anxiety-management techniques, homework assignments (e.g. monitoring of symptoms), cognitive strategies and early intervention on recognition of prodromal signs.

Working with staff to provide a consistent approach was important. It is to their credit that Kingdon & Turkington not only acknowledge this but address these difficulties. Similarly, Sellwood et al (1994) remark that 'specific details on individual therapy may end up being less important than a shift in professional attitudes that this kind of work is possible and can show improvements.'

Tarrier's research team carried out a controlled trial comparing the efficacy of coping strategy enhancement (CSE) against problem-solving treatment (Tarrier et al 1993). All the patients were experiencing persistent, treatment-resistant hallucinations or delusions. The CSE group was encouraged to develop effective coping strategies and monitor symptoms. The problem-solving group involved teaching patients to effectively solve difficulties, but the techniques were not used directly to target symptoms. Both approaches were successful in reducing anxiety and positive symptoms compared to the control group. However, there was a large drop-out rate, and, disappointingly, the results showed no impact on social functioning. The CSE group showed greater improvement, especially in reduction of delusional beliefs. The fact that problem-solving produced similar results was not predicted, giving rise to the question whether non-specific factors such as the increase in therapist contact could account for the symptom reduction. A strength of the approach is its basis in people's natural coping abilities, encouraging collaboration and recognition of the individual's strengths.

Fowler (1992) and other colleagues (Garety et al 1994, Kuipers 1996) have developed a comprehensive approach for the treatment of long-term psychosis. This emphasises engagement, reducing distress from positive symptoms, increasing the individual's knowledge and motivation towards their disorder and medication, short- and long-term goal setting, overcoming hopelessness and modification of dysfunctional assumptions and beliefs around self. Fowler (1992), in a trial involving 19 patients, found clear improvements in positive symptoms and accompanying affective problems, but little change was observed in negative symptoms. Reducing depression and lifting self-esteem are central to this approach, which moves from the symptom model to a person model, based on individual case formulation. The results are encouraging as treatment effect generalises to other areas of the individual's life.

It has been argued that given the complexity of the schizophrenia diagnosis, it is more effective to concentrate research and therapy on specific symptoms, for example, auditory hallucinations (Bentall 1990). In a case study, Beck (1952) reports the successful treatment of a man with paranoid schizophrenia, where his belief in the number of people who were trying to harm him dropped significantly.

Watts et al (1973) termed their therapy 'belief modification'. This involves sensitively questioning the evidence underlying the belief, avoiding confrontation regarding the reality of belief itself. This small study used three patients, one as a control. The two who underwent belief modification showed significantly reduced conviction in their delusions. Milton et al (1978) compared the efficacy of belief modification and confrontation. Although, initially, both approaches were significant in reducing conviction, only belief modification had lasting results. Johnson et al (1977) observed in a single case study that delusional beliefs occur as a result of misinterpreting real life. Chadwick & Lowe (1990, 1994) used belief modification and reality testing to modify delusional beliefs. The treatment included identifying and assessing the nature of the delusions, sensitively helping individuals to question the evidence underlying their beliefs and developing behavioural experiences to test out the reality of the beliefs. Of 12 people, five rejected their delusion and a further five had reduced conviction.

As with all research, the quality of the evidence is open to scrutiny and some of these studies report on very small samples making generalisation difficult. There is a need for more randomised controlled studies to further demonstrate the efficacy of CBT with delusions. Bouchard et al (1996) after extensive literature review concluded that cognitive restructuring is more effective for delusions than hallucinations and noted from studies that many subjects became delusion-free. For delusions it may sometimes be appropriate in line with proper case formulation and supervision to make the primary goal a reduction of distress, rather than complete modification of the delusion.

Delusions and violence

Working with a person with delusional beliefs can be difficult and challenging. This becomes more difficult when trying to assess and work with the risk or danger that the client may act upon their beliefs. In forensic settings, this is a prominent theme. To some degree, risk has already been established because clients have committed an offence. However, the relationship between a person's delusional beliefs and associated risk can be complex.

Reed (1997) summarises the current evidence linking risk of violence and mental disorder as follows:

- The majority of mentally ill people do not present an increased risk.
- Factors that predict offending for the general population are the same for the mentally ill, for example, previous offending, criminality in the family, etc.
- People with schizophrenia when experiencing active symptoms are an increased risk to others.
- Those with serious mental illness who misuse drugs and have active symptoms may present an increased risk.

- Individuals with psychopathic disorder are an increased risk.

For our purposes, the third point is of particular relevance. Wessely et al (1993) concluded that violent behaviour in response to delusions was uncommon. However, they did identify several characteristics that increased the likelihood of acting upon delusions.

There appears to be a contradiction between criminologists and medical opinion on the association between crime and mental disorder, with the former believing that mental illness is not a significant cause of crime (Wessely 1997). However, in a review of the relationship between mental illness and violent behaviour, Link & Stueve (1994) concluded there was a robust pattern of findings, across studies using different designs, samples and measures, in favour of a causal connection between some types of mental illness and violence. They identified characteristics of delusion that might lead to an increase in risk, suggesting that violence is more likely when psychotic symptoms cause a person to feel personally threatened or involve the intrusion of thoughts that can override self controls. Other studies have found evidence for a relationship between delusional beliefs and violence. Hafner and Boker (1982) compared psychotic patients who had committed murder with those who had not and found a difference between the prevalence of the delusions. Among those with schizophrenia, 89% had been deluded at the time of the killing or attempted killing compared with 76% of the non-violent patients.

More recently Cheung et al (1997) found that there was no association between content of hallucinations and violence but that a violent group of subjects were more likely to have persecutory delusions compared to a non-violent group, who were more likely to have grandiose delusions. Moreover, those in the violent group were more likely to have been made angry by their delusions.

Referral and engagement

The following case study involves work with a person possessing delusional beliefs that led him to commit a violent offence. Through working on his delusional beliefs, it was hypothesised that his risk and dangerousness would be reduced.

CASE STUDY: JACK

Jack is currently an in-patient at a secure mental health unit. He has resided there for 3 years and has had a diagnosis of schizophrenia for 13 years. He was referred to the nurse specialist by his named nurse, who hoped that structured input could help with his distressing anxiety and give him a greater understanding of his illness. The clinical team was initially sceptical about the referral as Jack had previously refused to talk about his experiences. Bearing this in mind, and the general difficulties in engaging with this client group, a lengthy time was spent just to build engagement, getting him used to talking and building trust in a collaborative relationship. Initially, Jack was uneasy, but over time he appeared more relaxed and talkative. This initial time was essential in setting a foundation for future work. The fact that regular time had been given to Jack and that he was listened to and not told what was real and what was not seemed to be a powerful catalyst in therapy. The model of CBT employed was based on the work of Fowler et al (1995), driven by individual case formulation. This addressed not only psychotic symptoms but anxiety, depression, self-defeating behaviours, dysfunctional assumptions and core beliefs which maintain client difficulties.

Initial assessment

As the relationship developed, it became easier to explain to Jack that in order to be able to work on key problems it was important to first identify how he got to this stage in his life and what factors were crucial in developing and maintaining his life problems. A series of assessments needed to be accomplished, the results of which are summarised in Box 4.1. He was initially apprehensive that this would be monotonous, though this proved not to be the case. The assessment process provided the opportunity for guided discovery, active listening, reflection,

---

Box 4.1   Results of initial assessment

KGV (Krawiecka et al 1977)
Scored 4 for delusions
Had delusion of control with 100% conviction. He believed 'Sleepers' could totally control his emotions and actions. They put thoughts into his mind via computer. They were training him to be a killer to eliminate enemies of the State. If he did not obey, he could be dead in 1 to 2 minutes. He was unable to distinguish between his own thoughts and the 'Sleepers'.
Scored 2 for anxiety
Occurred frequently, described as terrible, often in response to delusional beliefs, could at times with limited effect turn his mind to other things, caused great deal of distress for him.

DELUSIONAL RATING SCALE (Haddock 1994)
Showed he thought about beliefs on an hourly basis, lasted

several minutes, causing maximum distress and severe disruption to his life.

LUNSERS (Day et al 1995)
Low score for side effects.

Hawton et al (1989)
Showed few coping strategies and he did not believe the illness explanation that he was given.

SECONDARY GAINS INTERVIEW (Yusupoff 1996)
Positive gains from 'Sleepers'
Sense of purpose, esteem and no responsibility for his actions.
Negative gains
Loss of control, happiness and hope for the future. The scoring demonstrated that the negative gains outweighed the positive ones by 2 to 1.

KGV: Krawiecka, Goldberg and Vaughn or Manchester Scale. LUNSERS: Liverpool University Neuroleptic Side Effect Rating Scale.

summarising and clarification to take place. Jack said he had not had the opportunity before to express himself to someone else who not only heard but was able to understand and make sense of his experiences. This seemed to really boost his confidence and was a very powerful normalising experience. He felt that he was not alone or so strange that he could not be understood.

Development history

A history was drawn up using Hawton et al's (1989) CBT assessment, supplemented with further information gathered from case notes, other professionals and, with Jack's permission, from his father.

Jack, now aged 30, was brought up by his mother and father until the age of 10. He describes this time as happy. When he was 10 years old, his parents divorced and he went to live with his father and sister. His brother remained with his mother, with whom he had regular contact. At school he performed badly and left at 16 to work first as a gardener and then in farming, but found that he could not cope with the work. He then found employment in a plant nursery and attended agricultural college. He says that he did well but decided to leave

the course for another job. However, others, including his father, suggest that the course was abandoned because he could not keep up with the academic work. Jack went on to obtain a grant to start his own gardening business but this venture went bankrupt.

It was around this time that Jack decided 'enough was enough', packed up and moved to London. During this stressful time, he began to feel very frightened and believed that a high-up agency who ran the country called the 'Sleepers' were out to attack him. He would relay these fears by telephone to his father, who became very concerned and travelled to see him. During the visit, Jack became convinced that his father was part of the conspiracy and attacked him. He was admitted to a local mental health hospital under section 2 of the Mental Health Act 1983. After persistent assaults on staff, he was transferred to a secure unit, where he was given electric convulsive treatment (ECT) and various antipsychotic medication. Although he refused to discuss his experience, the violent behaviour disappeared and he was eventually discharged into the community with follow-up.

For 8 years, Jack lived his life without incident. He had been receiving depot medication, but after coming into contact with a mental health user group, and thinking about various side effects, he refused to continue with medication. His father persuaded him to make an appointment to discuss this with his psychiatrist, though the earliest appointment was in 12 weeks time. In hindsight it appears that the psychosis was residual and now became active and stronger. Jack now reports that at the time he would not talk and that the 'Sleepers' controlled his thoughts and actions. They wanted him to be an 'assassin' who would 'eliminate enemies of the state'. Acting on this belief he assaulted a member of the hostel staff. He was arrested and sent once again to a secure unit. Whilst at the unit he was again very violent and was nursed in seclusion for long periods. He was eventually prescribed Clozaril, which appeared to help and his violent behaviour subsided. He was more willing to talk to people but refused to elaborate on his symptoms, except to indicate that the 'Sleepers' were still there, but that he no longer felt the need to attack anyone. For the last 3 years, Jack has stayed in the unit, moving from the intensive care ward to the rehabilitation ward, with a view to eventually being discharged to a long-term, less secure, unit.

Despite Jack's previous reluctance to talk, he did begin to discuss his experiences. Possible reasons for this were that engagement had taken place and that in the past people had made it clear to him that his experiences were not real and this seemed to lead to a sense of alienation. Now, his point of view was validated and taken seriously. This, coupled with the fact that he wanted to move on, enabled Jack to describe his problems more freely. He identified anxiety as a problem causing him a great deal of distress.

Formulation

A preliminary cognitive–behavioural formulation was developed, which is illustrated diagrammatically in Figure 4.2. On the basis of the information collected, it appears that Jack's delusional beliefs originally arose in the context of particular life stresses, related to real or perceived failure. Core beliefs included the view that he was a failure and that there was something inadequate and odd about himself. In this

light, Jack's difficulties at school, as well as insecurity and disruption in his childhood, may be seen as contributing significantly. The combination of these core beliefs, developed in response to Jack's difficult life experiences, can be seen as vulnerability factors, mediating his response to life stresses.

The initial development of Jack's delusional system is difficult to formulate with total confidence, as the first occurrence was over 13 years ago. However, a secondary needs assessment (Yusupoff 1996) suggested a number of potentially important elements. The belief in the persecutory existence of the 'Sleepers' appeared to make sense out of a chaotic situation. Although such a belief system made Jack anxious and insecure, it also gave him a sense of esteem and purpose. Jack was important, he was a 'secret assassin' for the 'controllers of the state'. These beliefs simultaneously removed or reduced Jack's perceived responsibility for negative actions, including the assaults on his father and medical and nursing staff.

Such a formulation is, of course, entirely consistent with an attributional model of paranoia (Kinderman & Bentall 1996). In this model, external, paranoid attributions accompanying persecutory delusions are believed to bolster a fragile or implicitly negative self-concept. Paranoid delusions are then considered to be a consequence of a pattern of causal attributions in which personal responsibility for negative events is avoided. It is important to stress that this formulation need not suggest that Jack did not necessarily report high self-esteem. Indeed, Jack reported that he frequently felt peculiar, insecure and inadequate. Nevertheless, his belief in the malevolent power of the 'Sleepers' appeared to be maintained, in part, by the consequences of this belief. These included the effect on his self-concept, rendering him less responsible (under the control of others) and simultaneously important.

In addition to such probable positive benefits, however, the belief in the malevolent power of the 'Sleepers' had negative consequences. Jack felt insecure and vulnerable, as well as inadequate and despairing. He also felt anxious in social situations, unable to communicate with

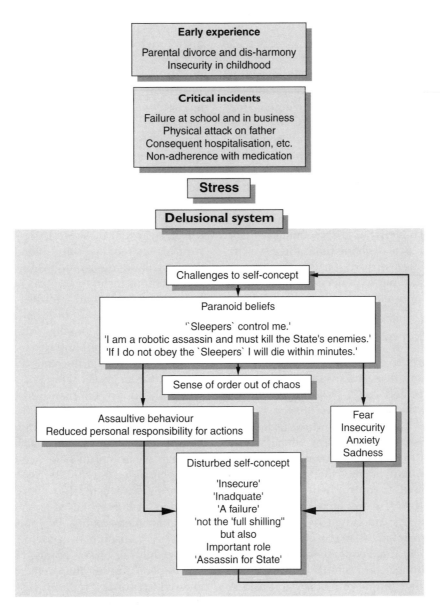

Fig. 4.2 Jack's life experiences and stress responses.

others and 'out of sync'. These negative consequences for Jack's self-concept may, paradoxically, also have reinforced his delusional beliefs, continuously recreating the situation from which the paranoid beliefs sprang. In addition, Jack's anxiety led to thoughts of being out of control, which served to increase his conviction in the reality of the 'Sleepers' control. His pacing and tendency to withdrawal also led to perceptible negative reactions from other people.

From a fragile and negative self-concept, and conflicting and chaotic experiences, a belief in the conspiracy evolved. The most striking negative consequence of Jack's delusional system was his offending. At the time of referral, Jack had been on a stable dose of neuroleptic medication for some time and he was no longer actively violent. However, although he was no longer commanded by the 'Sleepers' to kill, his belief in their presence and power and his role in the assassination conspiracy remained. Jack's belief system can therefore justifiably be seen as a major risk factor for future violence.

The assessments showed that the key problem areas were, first, to reduce anxiety caused by social situations. This could be an initial area, which would help socialise Jack to the model and generate hope and experience of success. The second key target at this stage was to enable Jack to have more control over the 'Sleepers'. Jack felt this would cause a weight to be lifted from him; he did not want to kill people but wanted to get his life back and have some normality again. These initial goals seemed realistic and although it was explained that there was no guarantee of success, just starting the task of making sense of his experiences appeared to generate hope and relief

Middle stages of therapy

To work on the problem area of reducing distress caused by anxiety, it was necessary to use guided discovery. It seemed that a typical cycle would start with Jack thinking 'I'm out of sync, people think I'm odd.' This would produce feelings of anxiety, restlessness and nausea, which would lead him either to pace up or down or withdraw. He would then have further thoughts like 'This is terrible, I'm out of control' which would further fuel and increase his anxiety. His behaviour of pacing up and down or withdrawing appeared to maintain this anxiety cycle as it drew attention to him. People would start to ask him 'What's wrong?', and act as if he was behaving oddly, giving him a wide berth and asking lots of questions. Sometimes his anxiety would be further fuelled when anxious by thinking that the 'Sleepers' had left him, believing that they provided security and that he was 'too dim' to survive without them, or to sustain conversation with people.

It was essential to demonstrate how thoughts affect feelings which affect behaviour. This was achieved through the guided discovery and then drawing a mini-formulation together. Jack was very relieved and impressed by the way his anxiety could be drawn out and made sense of. For

homework, he was first given information on anxiety which helped normalise his symptoms. He kept a simplified 3-column thought diary which he worked on in our sessions, helping to identify triggers which maintained anxiety. The anxiety was treated using behavioural techniques. From the formulation, Jack could see how pacing up and down exacerbated his anxiety, so, together, we devised new coping strategies, for example, the use of distraction and refocusing techniques like reading, thinking of calm scenes or slowing down breathing. Through considering his diary, and staff reports, it was clear that these strategies helped to interrupt his anxiety cycle and therefore reduce distress. This demonstrated that he had some control of his feelings, in turn creating a sense of hope that things could improve.

The next stage utilised a more cognitive approach. In one session, different thinking errors were explored and discussed. Jack recognised that he regularly catastrophised about his anxiety, for example: 'This is terrible. It's never going to end.', which increased the anxiety. Jack was helped to identify these thinking errors in the course of diary-keeping and in the sessions. He was then able to begin challenging thoughts, through weighing up evidence for and against. Role play aided a recognition of how anxiety can be normal and can affect everyone's ability to function. Jack then started to try to challenge his thoughts when anxious. He found the use of cue cards very useful in providing prompts to remind himself of key points. He also aimed to talk to people rather than avoid them when anxious which further reduced his thoughts about being 'out of sync'.

It was around this point in therapy that Jack seemed to make the connection that if initial thoughts and feelings were not always accurate, how could he be so sure about the 'Sleepers'? He asked the therapist 'Do you believe in the 'Sleepers'?' Using guidelines provided by Nelson (1997), the therapist first ascertained his motive, which seemed to be a genuine confusion. The answer given was that the therapist did not want to tell him what to think, but to find his own answers. Jack said that he found this response encouraging and wanted to find answers. At this stage, the secondary gains' assessment had shown that he had a sense of identity and security from the 'Sleepers'. It also showed there to be far more negative gains than positive ones, for example, loss of control and happiness. Jack was surprised at how much he stood to gain if, hypothetically, the 'Sleepers' were not around.

In supervision, it became clear to the therapist that if Jack was to move on from the 'Sleepers', his secondary gains' issues would need to be addressed by providing an attractive alternative. The next session involved Jack and the therapist looking purely hypothetically at what he might like to do with his life if the 'Sleepers' were not there. Jack was keen to participate as it was only hypothetical! A list of realistic and attractive goals was drawn up, for example, get fit, make more friends, move to the next rehabilitation unit, which seemed to increase Jack's motivation. At this point on the Personal Questionnaire Rapid Scaling Technique (PQRST) scale (Mulhall 1978) conviction had fallen from 100% to 80%.

The next stage involved using peripheral and guided discovery questioning to elicit evidence which supported the 'Sleepers' and to start gently to look at factors for and against this evidence. For example, 'If they communicate through noise from builders, why do they not approach him directly?' and 'How was it he had never been paid or met them, and had ended up in hospital?' Such questioning began to raise doubts. Since so much evidence came from his 'gut feeling', the Nelson (1997: 26) two-way processing model was relied on to explain and suggest that at times it is understandable, when feelings are very strong, that the brain needs to make sense of what is happening and jumps to conclusions. This notion was introduced in the context of the concept of stress vulnerability and normalised his experience. This model was linked to his own life and Jack felt it made sense of what had happened when he had had his first episode.

Further evidence for and against the 'Sleepers' was discussed. The evidence against them was overwhelming and Jack would read through the sheets used in therapy for homework. We also used a behavioural experiment to see if the 'Sleepers' could communicate with him via the television set. By setting up a no-lose situation, Jack watched TV and used cue cards to weigh up and challenge ideas of reference. He found that by challenging these thoughts and feelings, the sense of being controlled decreased. On the PQRST scale, his conviction rate dropped from 80% to 10%, with preoccupation rates also markedly reduced. He now believed the 'Sleepers' were a delusion and part of his illness. Through supervision, it was identified that this shift could possibly lead to depression or guilt because of his offence. The therapist closely monitored for this and informed the clinical team. However, there seemed no impact on mood and it appeared that Jack recognised that he could not have acted any differently as he had been ill. He now had the hope that he could be in control and learn ways to maintain staying well, which actually lifted his mood. This was the first time in years that he 'felt like himself, felt understood and in control.'

End stages of therapy: relapse prevention

At this stage, work began on Jack's core beliefs, which seemed pivotal in fuelling his anxieties. When he got anxious, his core beliefs about being of low intelligence would be fully activated with increases in his anxiety and catastrophising. These were also the only times now that his thoughts turned to the 'Sleepers'. The core beliefs had been identified early on in the case formulation and the initial hypothesis about them was confirmed in the course of therapy.

To address his low self-esteem and the belief that he was of low intelligence, he was asked to locate himself on a continuum of lowest IQ at one end and highest IQ (e.g. Einstein) on the other. We then went on to define certain idioms he used, like what it meant to be 'a full shilling'. Then we looked at which criteria Jack fitted and what were the advantages and disadvantages of viewing himself in certain ways. For instance, to see himself as having little or no intelligence meant he had little confidence and

---

Box 4.2   Jack's early warning signs and action plan

For short-lasting feelings and thoughts	For longer lasting, more intense thoughts and feelings
If you feel:	**If your anxiety and thoughts about the 'Sleepers' become:**
• anxious	• stronger
• worried	• more real
• start to think more about the 'Sleepers'	• last for a prolonged period
	• if you feel out of control
	• if you get the command to hurt someone
	• if you can't sleep at night/become withdrawn
Action	**Action**
• read over folder	• tell staff and doctor straight away
• keep up strategies	• read folder
• read cue cards	• follow strategies
• speak to staff	• read cue cards
• keep taking medication	• continue to take medication

Box 4.3   Results of assessments taken at the end of therapy

KGV (Krawiecka et al 1977)
Level of delusions dropped from 4 to 2
His conviction rate has dropped from 100% to 5%, the preoccupation and duration are also reduced. He now sees the 'Sleepers' as part of a mental illness.
Anxiety level dropped from 2 to 1
His anxiety levels are now less distressing, happen less often and he has a far greater degree of control.

DELUSIONAL RATING SCALE (Haddock 1994)
Pre-occupation dropped from 4 to 2
He now only gets thoughts about the 'Sleepers' once a day

rather than when first assessed he had thoughts about them every hour.
Conviction dropped from 4 to 1
See KGV results.
Distress dropped from 4 to 1
The 'Sleepers' now only distress on a minority of occasions. They used to cause constant distress when thinking about them. When distress does occur it has dropped from extreme distress to moderate.
Disruption dropped from 3 to 1
He now feels far more in control and able to get on with his life.

KGV: Krawiecka, Goldberg and Vaughn or Manchester scale.

got more anxious. After defining the terms used, the next stage was to look at evidence for and against his view of himself. This would often involve going back to the initial formulation and seeing where these views were formed and if they remained valid. Jack was able to see that many of these core beliefs were rigid, invalid and irrational, and contributed to maintaining his problems. This led to him moving himself up on the continuum scales. To maintain these gains in sessions, Jack undertook homework such as a positive log to consolidate the learning.

The final aim was to enable Jack to identify what he had learnt and how to use it in future. To achieve this, the therapist and Jack worked together to identify possible setbacks, early warning signs which would indicate impending relapse or increased risk and an action plan for the future (see Box 4.2). Setbacks were discussed as an opportunity to learn and to put skills into practice. The action plan identified what helped and what he had learnt from therapy, and what he could do if problems or early warning signs re-emerged. Jack found this very useful as it consolidated his learning and gave him an increased sense of control.

The therapist, with Jack's permission, spent time liaising with staff at the new mental health unit to inform them of his progress and optimum management strategies. They were given copies of the early warning sign work, reports on his progress and guidelines on how to work with him. There is also the facility for the therapist to maintain contact, providing monthly booster sessions in order to consolidate his skills, identify any setbacks and offer a way of overcoming difficulties. Box 4.3 summarises Jack's assessment scores at the close of therapy.

Reflections on practice

One of the strengths of this case was the effective engagement, establishing the foundation for therapy. This was achieved through time and by displaying core conditions of acceptance, warmth and genuineness (Beck et al 1979). Jack's shift away from rigid core beliefs led to an increase in confidence and a decrease in the distress caused by anxiety.

On reflection, there were particular aspects of this work that contributed to the successful outcome and maintenance of these gains at 3 months. However, with hindsight, certain aspects of the intervention could have proceeded differently. The pace of the sessions was initially too fast for the client. At times, the sessions were too long and demanding for him, and more flexibility in the therapist's expectations could improve this. It may have been useful to do some work with Jack's father, who was a possible part of a safety behaviour maintaining the client's problems. It became clear quite early in the therapy that the client had beliefs around wanting to please others and to be more acceptable. It might have been useful to tackle this issue earlier in therapy. Audio-taping the sessions helped the therapist make the most of clinical supervision. She saw that it would be helpful to summarise more often and check comprehension before moving on. The skills used in working with anxiety and depression were essential for working with this client group. The initial focus on anxiety brought a vital success and enabled Jack to relate the treatment model to his life.

The therapist has gained more confidence and skills from this clinical practice. Being able to move through the stages of therapy as guided by case formulation, Jack gained new skills. His distress from anxiety was decreased as his control increased. He was able to see that the 'Sleepers' were part of an illness and that under times of stress his thoughts may go back to them but that

he now has the skills to take a step back and test out what is real. The action plan has also supported Jack's sense of control. Perhaps just as important was the sense of being understood and the hope that it gave to Jack. Similarly, seeing that CBT for psychoses can work can positively affect the morale and therapeutic optimism of practitioners.

The role of supervision

Clinical supervision of the therapist was essential, as it provided a sounding board, learning resource and guide for practice. The supervision occurred once a week over the 3 months of therapy. All therapy sessions were taped and the majority systematically evaluated. The supervision was varied in format, including listening to part of a taped session together or using a whiteboard to draw out formulations or as an aid to teaching.

Padesky (1993) identifies several important factors in the teaching and supervision process. These include collaboration, guided discovery, conceptualisation and structure. The sessions also used the structure, style and techniques that underlie cognitive therapy. This involved negotiating agenda items, prioritising their importance and reviewing previous sessions including 'homework' that was given. The supervisor sought to use guided discovery by asking questions of the supervisee about various aspects of the therapy. This might involve examining the advantages and disadvantages of a particular intervention. A significant amount of supervision was devoted to case formulation. A discussion about any intervention or problems in the therapy would always be explored with reference to the initial conceptualisation. The formulation was seen not as static and fixed, more something that was evolving and changing.

The assessment of the therapy tapes was particularly helpful at highlighting specific skills development. The tapes also helped the therapist to be more flexible and tailor the session to the client. Learning new skills can be a difficult task, so it is important that a supervisor can offer guidance without making the therapist feel underskilled, devalued or patronised. The therapist felt able to be open with the supervisor about issues related to the therapy and felt encouraged and supported in the supervision.

The relationship between therapist and client is obviously important and any issues that could be hindering progress needed to be addressed. In the course of therapy the relationship between the client and therapist was often discussed, particularly with reference to his quite rapid progress. The issue of dependency and need to please the therapist was explored using a CBT framework. These issues were then explored with the client.

REFERENCES

Beck A 1952 Successful outpatient psychotherapy of a chronic schizophrenic with a delusion based on borrowed guilt. Psychiatry 15: 305–312

Beck A, Rush A, Shaw B, Emery G 1979 Cognitive therapy of depression. Guilford Press, New York

Bentall R 1990 Reconstructing schizophrenia. Routledge, London

Bouchard S, Vallieres A, Toy M, Maziade M 1996 Cognitive restructuring in the treatment of psychotic symptoms in schizophrenia: a critical analysis. Behaviour Therapy 27: 257–277

Chadwick P 1997 Schizophrenia: the positive perspective. Routledge, London

Chadwick P, Lowe C 1990 Measurement and modification of delusional beliefs. Journal of Consulting and Clinical Psychology 58: 225–232

Chadwick P, Lowe C 1994 A cognitive approach to measuring and modifying delusions. Behaviour Research and Therapy 32: 355–367

Cheung P, Schweitzer, I, Crowley K, Tuckwell V 1997 Violence and schizophrenia: role of hallucinations and delusions. Schizophrenia Research 26: 181–190

Curson D, Barnes T, Bamber R, Platt S, Hirsch S, Duffy J 1985 Long term depot maintenance of chronic schizophrenic out-patients. British Journal of Psychiatry 146: 464–480

Curson D, Patel M, Liddle P, Barnes T 1988 Psychiatric morbidity of a long stay hospital population with chronic schizophrenia and implications for future community care. British Medical Journal 297: 819–822

Day J, Wood G, Dewey M, Bentall R 1995 A self-rating scale for measuring neuroleptic side-effects: validation in a group of schizophrenic patients. British Journal of Psychiatry 166: 650–653

Drury V, Birchwood M, Cochrane R, MacMillan F 1996 Cognitive behaviour therapy for acute psychosis: a controlled trial and impact on psychotic symptoms. British Journal of Psychiatry 169: 593–607

Fowler D 1992 Cognitive behavioural therapy in the management of patients with schizophrenia: preliminary studies. In: Werbert A, Cullberg J (eds) The psychotherapy of schizophrenia: facilitating and obstructive factors. Scandinavian Press, Oslo

Fowler D, Garety P, Kuipers E 1995 Cognitive behaviour therapy for psychosis: theory and practice. Wiley, Chichester

Garety P, Kuipers L, Fowler D, Chamberlain F, Dunn G 1994 Cognitive behavioural therapy for drug resistant psychosis. British Journal of Medical Psychology 67: 259–271

Haddock G 1994 Delusions Rating Scale. Thorn Initiative, University of Manchester

Hafner H, Boker W 1982 Crimes of violence by mentally abnormal offenders. Cambridge University Press, Cambridge

Harrow M, Carone B, Westermeyer J 1985 The course of psychosis in early phases of schizophrenia. American Journal of Psychiatry 142: 702–707

Hawton K, Salkovskis P, Kirk J, Clark D (eds) 1989 Cognitive behavioural therapy for psychiatric problems. Oxford University Press, Oxford

Johnson C, Ross J, Mastria M 1977 Delusional behaviour: an attributional analysis of development and modification. Journal of Abnormal Psychology 86: 421–426

Kinderman P, Bentall R 1996 Self discrepancies and persecutory delusions: evidence for a model of paranoid ideation. Journal of Abnormal Psychology 105: 106–113

Kingdon D, Turkington D 1991 The use of cognitive behaviour therapy with a normalising rationale in schizophrenia. Journal of Nervous and Mental Disease 179: 207–211

Krawiecka M, Goldberg D, Vaughn M 1977 Standardised psychiatric assessment scale for chronic psychiatric patients. Acta Psychiatricia Scandinavica 36: 25–31

Kuipers E 1996 The management of difficult to treat patients with schizophrenia, using non-drug therapies. British Journal of Psychiatry 169 (Suppl 31): 41–45

Kuipers E, Garety P, Fowler D et al 1997 London–East Anglia randomised controlled trial of cognitive behavioural therapy for psychosis. Institute of Psychiatry, London.

Link B, Stueve A 1994 Psychotic symptoms and the violent/illegal behavior of mental patients compared to community controls. In: Monaghan J, Steadman H (eds) Violence and mental disorder: Developments in risk assessment. University of Chicago Press, Chicago, p. 137–159

Milton F, Patwa V, Hafner R 1978 Confrontation vs belief modification in persistently deluded patients. British Journal of Medical Psychology 51: 127–130

Mulhall D 1978 Manual for the Personal Questionnaire Rapid Scaling Technique. NFER, Windsor

Nelson H 1997 Cognitive behavioural therapy with schizophrenia. Stanley Thornes, London

Padesky C 1993 Staff and patient education. In: Wright J, Those M (eds) Cognitive therapy with inpatients developing a cognitive milieu. Guilford Press, New York

Reed J 1997 Risk assessment and clinical risk management: the lessons from recent inquiries. British Journal of Psychiatry 170 (Suppl 32): 4–7

Sellwood W, Haddock G, Tarrier N, Yusupoff L 1994 Advances in the psychological management of positive symptoms of schizophrenia. International Review of Psychiatry 6: 201–215

Slade P, Bentall R 1988 Sensory deception: a scientific analysis of hallucination. Croom Helm, London

Tarrier N, Becket R, Harwood S, Baker A, Yusupoff L, Ugarteburu I 1993 A trial of two cognitive behavioural methods of treating drug resistant residual psychotic symptoms in schizophrenic patients: I outcome. British Journal of Psychiatry 162: 524–532

Watts F, Powell E, Austin S 1973 The modification of abnormal beliefs. British Journal of Medical Psychology 46: 359–363

Wessely S 1997 The epidemiology of crime violence and schizophrenia. British Journal of Psychiatry 170 (Suppl 32): 8–11

Wessely S, Buchanan A, Reed A, Cutting J 1993 Acting on delusions: I prevalence. British Journal of Psychiatry 163: 69–76

Yusupoff L 1996 Motivation interview. Thorn Initiative, University of Manchester

Zubin J, Spring B 1977 Vulnerability – a new view on schizophrenia. Journal of Abnormal Psychology 86: 103–126

CONTENTS

Family work

Ged McCann and Mick McKeown

Introduction

This clinical case study describes a series of assessments and subsequent interventions with a psychotic offender and his family at a Special Hospital. It covers a period of about 1 year during which Greg, and his brother Bill, were engaged in working together as a family, as well as individually. The study briefly discusses the relevance of involving family members in clinical work, by referring to particular studies undertaken in the management of schizophrenia in the community. It draws on the key elements of these studies and attempts to apply their principles within an in-patient secure environment. An outline of the main interventions is given, as well as an evaluation of their effectiveness. The problems of involving families within a forensic setting are discussed and some solutions are suggested. Importantly, an account is provided of the benefits for both service users and family members of working in such a collaborative way.

Theoretical background

The rationale for involving family members directly in the clinical management of schizophrenia can be drawn from a number of recent studies (Falloon et al 1985, Hogarty et al 1986, Leff et al 1982, Tarrier et al 1988). This research has demonstrated that factors such as levels of criticism and emotional over-involvement amongst family members are highly predictive of relapse. In these studies family involvement was, therefore, aimed at reducing the effects of these factors through engaging relatives in clinical interventions. These interventions principally include a sound assessment of each family member's needs, education about schizophrenia and its management, and communication and problem-solving training to reduce stress. Such interventions have been rigorously evaluated and demonstrate effectiveness in reducing relapse rates.

Within a forensic in-patient setting, the home environment is replaced by lengthy periods of institutional life and contact with family members is severely reduced. Often, the roles performed by the significant members of a patient's normal family are assumed by professionals. It may seem unclear exactly what benefits might ensue by involving a person's family members in their care, or how this family involvement may be undertaken, as families can often live a great distance from the hospital, or may, for a variety of reasons, have reduced or lost contact.

It is clear that family members can experience a great deal of stress in their dealings with a Special Hospital (McCann 1993, McCann et al 1996). It is possible that their levels of stress may have a detrimental influence on their relative, particularly during visits to the hospital which, although infrequent, may be highly significant to everyone concerned. It is also expressly relevant in this case as Greg's offence involved his mother, so it seemed necessary to try to assess the effects of this on the rest of Greg's family, particularly in determining future needs and problems.

The aims of involving Greg's family members were thus:

1. For Greg to maintain contact with a significant family member.
2. To attempt to engage and involve Greg's family in his present and future care.
3. To assess the impact of Greg's offence on his family members and how this may affect the course, and future management, of his care.

CASE STUDY: GREG

Greg is one of a family of five brothers, all of whom had a turbulent childhood as their father had a history of alcohol misuse and violence toward his family. His father left home when Greg was 3, but later returned when all the boys had left home. Greg left school with no formal educational qualifications and started an apprenticeship as a butcher, staying for 2 years before joining the army. He remained in the army for 9 years where he trained further as a butcher, but he left to care for his mother when his father died.

His first psychiatric referral was whilst in the army when he was referred for psychological help and assessment for alcohol misuse. His time with the army was largely uneventful although Greg states that he was often involved in fights and he describes himself as having had an alcohol problem throughout his army career.

After leaving the army, Greg worked as a general labourer on building sites for about 3 years but then began to behave oddly, misusing alcohol, and eventually left home to live as a vagrant. It was during the next 2 years that Greg travelled the country, living and sleeping rough, occasionally returning home to see his mother and brothers. At this time, he described being followed by a group of men, and felt that other people were conspiring to do him harm. Eventually in 1980, he was referred to a reception centre for treatment of his alcohol problem and assessment of his mental health. He left because he felt others were talking about him, but was admitted to a psychiatric hospital several months later after becoming terrified that the devil was after him. Discharging himself from here 2 weeks later, against medical advice, he went home and, believing his mother was the devil, stabbed her to death.

Greg was then admitted to a Special Hospital with a diagnosis of paranoid schizophrenia. Throughout the court case, and subsequent admission to hospital, Greg did not speak to any of his brothers, some of whom attended the court hearings. In fact there has been little contact with any of Greg's family throughout his 14-year stay within the Special Hospital. Each of his brothers is now married with children and has no history of mental illness.

By the time the input described in this case study commenced (when GM was allocated as key-worker), Greg had already been detained in the Special Hospital for 12 years and had a reputation for being insular and frequently aggressive. He had a long history of assaulting fellow patients and being verbally abusive towards staff. His motivation was poor, he was reluctant to engage in any off-ward activities and he remained in his own room for much of the day. However, he was able to engage in conversation and he would discuss topics that interested him. Often he would appear preoccupied and would occasionally speak out loud to himself.

Initial engagement and assessment

Establishing some rapport with Greg was not too difficult as the key-worker relationship extended previous, more peripheral, involvement in Greg's care. He was also very familiar with the key-worker system having lived within a clinical setting for one-third of his life. It was proposed to Greg that the intended therapy would proceed quite intensely for a number of sessions, something he was not used to, and that efforts to involve other members of his family were felt to be important and potentially beneficial. At first, he was very sceptical about this family involvement and felt that his brothers would have nothing to do with him. He did agree, however, that he would prefer that his brothers did have some contact with him, although he suspected that his eldest brother felt so strongly he would probably try to kill him.

Initial assessments with Greg focused on both his past and present circumstances. These broad discussions aimed not only to engage and strengthen the therapeutic relationship, but were a chance for Greg to provide his story. Information was sought not just to record a chronological diary of events but to gain an insight into the thoughts, beliefs and values that Greg held towards his past and how they affected his present. More importantly, these early discussions set the tone for future sessions in that they were focused, clear about their purpose and collaborative.

A number of more structured assessment tools were also employed because of their reliability and validity and to provide accurate information upon which a number of outcomes could be evaluated. The Manchester Scale or KGV (Modified) (Krawiecka et al 1977) was used to furnish information about Greg's mental state. This is a semi-structured interview schedule which comprises a series of questions aimed to elicit enough information to rate the individual under a number of areas including anxiety, hallucinations and delusions. It also has a number of behaviour-rated items, including psychomotor retardation, incongruity and co-operation. Each section is rated on a range of 0 to 4, where 0 indicates an absence of the symptom and 4 indicates a high degree of severity. The Social Functioning Scale (Birchwood et al 1990) was used to assess Greg's social skills and competencies and to identify problem areas in relation to his interactions with others and his social activities. The Hospital Anxiety and Depression Scale (Zigmond & Snaith 1983) is a self-rating questionnaire which aims to indicate levels of anxiety or depression, showing changes in mood over a short timescale. The Liverpool University Neuroleptic Side Effect Rating Scale (LUNSERS) (Day et al 1995) assesses self-reporting of neuroleptic side effects and was useful as Greg was receiving large amounts of medication. The Maudsley Assessment of Delusions Schedule was also completed, together with questioning Greg in detail about how he makes sense of his experiences, particularly the evidence he draws on to support his beliefs.

All of these structured assessments were used to provide an accurate baseline of mental health need and engage Greg in monitoring his experiences more systematically. This was important as in future sessions Greg would be asked to discuss his symptoms in more depth and focus on working with him to exert more control over them himself.

These early discussions and assessments took about 4 months during which time we had established that Greg heard the voices of his brothers, and other patients and staff, talking to him and criticising his actions. These voices were abusive and derogatory, describing him, falsely in his view, as being homosexual. The voices were worse in the evening when he was on his own and occurred usually when there was no-one else about. Greg also believed that others talked about him behind his back, again making reference to his sexuality, and that these beliefs often resulted in him being abusive or aggressive in response. The assessment scores also indicated that Greg was clinically anxious and depressed most of the time and this resulted in him spending large amounts of his time on his own, avoiding the contact of others, which had the effect of exacerbating the voices.

A number of sessions were spent discussing these experiences and how Greg coped with them. He did not enjoy discussing the voices although he did welcome the opportunity to discuss them in an open and accepting way, helping him reframe these experiences. He progressed to thinking about the voices in terms of a range of experiences rather than singularly as a medical symptom.

It was at this time that Greg's brother, Bill, became involved in a ward-based, relative support group which had recently been initiated. He had been sent an invitation to the group as Greg had indicated that, out of his four brothers, he would be the one most likely to become involved. The group provided a forum for relatives to find out about a Special Hospital, but also to share their experiences and learn from others. It also provided an opportunity for Bill to meet with Greg following the group, and discuss how he might become more involved with Greg's care.

Following these early meetings, we agreed that we should try to work on some specific areas together. These initial areas reflected the worries that Bill held about Greg's alcohol misuse and how he felt this may cause problems later if he were released. These concerns were acknowledged and Bill engaged in some focused discussions in an effort to explore these views further. Two structured interview schedules were utilised, focusing on the special needs of relatives.

The Relative Assessment Interview for Schizophrenia in a Secure Environment (RAISSE)

(McKeown & McCann 1995) is a semi-structured interview which has been adapted from the Relative Assessment Interview (Barrowclough & Tarrier 1992) and the Schizophrenia Nursing Assessment Protocol (Brooker & Baguley 1990). It has been developed at Ashworth Hospital to assess the needs of relatives with regard to three areas:

• Information regarding the relatives' views about the illness
• Information relating to the patient's admission to a secure environment and associated stress
• Specific information regarding actual contact time during visits.

This interview was useful for Bill, as it focused more directly on the stress for him of having a family member detained within a high-security psychiatric hospital. The questioning allowed Bill the opportunity, the first in over 14 years, to discuss his feelings regarding the offence and Greg's subsequent court case and treatment. Several areas of concern were identified which had the potential to detrimentally affect the course of Greg's schizophrenia. It became clear that Bill understood the cause of Greg's illness in terms of him never wanting to accept any responsibility; that he became alcoholic, lived on the streets and had many disappointments in his life because he was basically irresponsible. He also stated that he never really knew about the extent of Greg's problems until the offence had been committed and the details emerged at trial. He also felt on reflection that the family did not give Greg any support at the time:

...if I had of known, I could have done something.

Some guilt about the offence was apparent, although Bill felt he had on occasion tried to help Greg out, but Greg would not have anything to do with him. The interview also picked up a lack of knowledge about the forensic hospital Greg was in and this in turn created worries and stress for Bill.

The Knowledge About Schizophrenia Interview (Barrowclough & Tarrier 1992) was also used. This is a semi-structured interview, which attempts to assess functional knowledge about schizophrenia. It is not designed to assess just what the relative knows, but rather how the views the relative holds may lead to effective or detrimental care of the individual with schizophrenia. For instance, Bill did not score highly in several areas, including symptomatology, aetiology, medication and course and prognosis of schizophrenia. These scores indicated that Bill had little knowledge about the environmental conditions that might make Greg's symptoms worse. He was not aware that it was an episodic illness or that symptoms might re-occur in the future. Bill was unaware that stopping medication might result in a relapse and held potentially problematic views of the cause of Greg's illness. He seemed to view schizophrenia as being caused by alcohol and irresponsibility. Views such as this may lead relatives to coerce individuals, or argue with them to alter certain behaviours, with little positive impact on the illness (Barrowclough & Tarrier 1992). Bill certainly felt that Greg's biggest aftercare problem would be alcohol and that he would have no hesitation in calling the authorities if he felt Greg was drinking too much.

Each of the assessments, taken together, identified a number of areas for intervention. It could only be speculated what effects the lack of previous intervention had had for Bill and Greg, especially how Greg might have benefited if his family members had been involved at an earlier stage in the care and management of his illness. The engagement and involvement of Bill directly in clinical work are taking place 13 years after the offence took place. It therefore follows many years of institutional life for Greg and years of non-involvement for Bill. The lack of information provided to relatives, their lack of involvement in care and the disregard of the value of relatives by professionals at Ashworth are a sad indictment of a closed institution, specifically criticised in this regard in the damning report of the 1992 Public Inquiry (Committee of Inquiry 1992).

Interventions

Because Greg was an in-patient within a large forensic hospital, he made use of a range of hospital-based activities, both recreational and occupational, and he received varying degrees of input from a full multi-disciplinary team. All of these formal and informal interventions comprised Greg's care plan but this study will discuss in detail only four aspects of his comprehensive care.

Psychoeducation

The key approach with Greg had been one of collaboration, focused on specific problems. It is the basis for a cognitive–behavioural approach which includes openness, agreement on the process and in the objectives of the work. This was difficult because Greg understood so little about various aspects of his experiences, about the aims of our work together and about how to consider improving the way he coped with his problems. For these reasons, we spent a number of sessions discussing the nature of schizophrenia and psychotic problems and what the range of Greg's experiences might be. These sessions were relatively unusual in that they were conducted on a group basis, involving other patients, who were also experiencing similar symptoms.

The advantages of doing this work within a group were that the participants could draw upon experiences of others and view their symptoms as experiences that other people also may share, rather than being unique to individuals. In total, 10 hour-long sessions were undertaken. Initial sessions were spent discussing in general the different views of schizophrenia, what the causes might be, the symptoms and treatment. Video- and audio-taped materials were used together with large and small group discussions. As the group progressed, and participants became more relaxed and trusting, the sessions focused more specifically on the experiences of individuals and their coping strategies. Attention was given to thoughts and feelings rather than symptoms and to a range of coping strategies rather than a singular reliance on medication.

These sessions provided a foundation upon which we could discuss symptoms in more depth in a more open and normalised way than before. It also built upon a trust that enabled Greg to explore and report on his experiences without fearing his medication would be increased or the chances of his liberty would be reduced.

Individual work

Following the group work, a series of focused sessions were undertaken with Greg aimed at fully understanding his positive symptoms and enabling him to cope with them more effectively. Initial descriptions of his 'voices' were of others being critical of him and calling him 'gay' or 'queer'. Greg found the voices so distressing that often he spent his time in his own room away from others. Further sessions were spent in discussing these experiences in more depth, in defining when they occurred and precisely what the experience was like. Greg managed to keep a diary, which recorded who the voices were, what they were saying and what Greg was doing at the time. This proved useful in determining that the voices were actually worse when he was on his own, so Greg's coping strategy was not at all effective.

Greg also held firm beliefs about who the voices were and why they were saying what they did. He was convinced that the voices were his brothers who were acting out their hatred of him by verbally abusing him. He felt they were justified in doing this because of the misery he had caused them. Further sessions discussed these beliefs and the evidence Greg drew upon to convince him that the voices were his brothers. This evidence included the facts that his brothers had not been in touch with him, that they were bound to feel hatred towards him because he had killed their mother and the little contact he had had with his brothers in the past had been negative.

A further belief Greg held, which was problematic and had resulted in him being aggressive, was his conviction that others talked about him and also whispered to each other that he was 'gay' or 'queer'. Greg would 'overhear' these comments as he walked past other patients or staff, or when staff were in the ward office with the door closed. Greg would react by going to his room or by assaulting patients or staff. Further sessions again focused on evidence which supported this belief, but also his own thoughts and feelings about why he believed others would discuss him in this way.

Greg openly discussed the disappointments in his life. His difficulty in establishing and maintaining intimate relationships, his feelings of being the odd one out from his brothers, who had all married, his feelings that he had lost out in his life and that he would never form a relationship again. He also felt that others might think he was gay because he had never married and he had joined the army.

Group family work

Bill became involved in two groups following the early assessment work. The relatives' support group was an open forum in which relatives and friends of patients could discuss any subject matter they wished. Although patient and staff representatives were present, relatives organised and facilitated the group themselves. Bill became an active member of this group, which not only supplied information about the hospital, but also created emotional support between the participants and provided an opportunity to learn from other relatives who had experienced similar problems. Some relatives, including Bill, stated that in all the years, this was the first time they had been provided with a forum to discuss their feelings and thoughts.

The second group was a closed psychoeducational group for relatives, which was organised by staff, and which focused on issues surrounding the care of someone with schizophrenia. Sessions drew on the educational material of Birchwood & Smith (1991), although this was adapted to relate more to the particular problems of a forensic setting. Bill found the sessions very informative and contributed a great deal to the discussions surrounding each of the topics raised. The seminars demonstrated that educational material needed to be interactive, with staff learning as much from relatives as relatives from the staff. There were four seminars in all and the programme again moved from being very general to being more specific about individual experiences and coping strategies.

Working with Greg's family

The individual family work aimed to pull together the individual sessions which Greg and Bill were involved with, to pursue in more depth some of the issues raised and to anticipate the future needs of both Greg and Bill. It was during these sessions that Greg was able to test out his beliefs about his brothers with Bill and to begin to understand what they were actually thinking and feeling about him and the offence. It was also an opportunity for Bill to discover more about the symptoms that Greg was experiencing and how they resulted in his behaviour, rather than to maintain the view that they were due to alcohol or being irresponsible.

Coping strategies began to change as Bill suggested writing to him and his other brothers and phoning him when Greg's voices or beliefs were bothering him. Greg also began to have more confidence as his relationship with his brother became stronger. His thoughts that others were calling him gay were still there but they were not as distressing as before. Further work, outside of these sessions, involved grief counselling for Greg and other confidence-raising strategies.

More importantly, as Greg approached a transfer to a regional secure unit, his family members were now actively engaged in his care and were able to anticipate and plan for changes which would arise. One of the most prominent issues was the possibility of Greg moving back to his local area, to where the rest of his family members were still living. Anticipation of this was causing some concern for other members of the family. Effective pre-discharge work allowed most of these concerns to be allayed and other members of Greg's family were engaged in the planning process.

These interventions were therefore of benefit not only whilst Greg was an in-patient, but were a necessary part of his transfer process and in reducing the risk of him ever needing to return to a secure environment.

Conclusion

This case study has demonstrated how psychosocial interventions developed for mainstream community settings can be adapted for use in secure conditions. The approach involves attempting to meet both the separate and joint needs of detained, mentally disordered offenders and their families. Group work allows services to maximise resources and facilitate engagement of different families, who may live considerable distances away from the host institution, limiting the frequency of their visits. Traditional family work has to be adapted to take account of the special needs which arise in a forensic context, not least of these being the issues around the offence, and the effects of this for relatives and their close relationships. This can be most extremely evidenced when the offence is committed within the family.

REFERENCES

Barrowclough C, Tarrier N 1992 Families of schizophrenic patients: cognitive behavioural intervention. Chapman and Hall, London.

Birchwood M, Smith J 1991 Understanding schizophrenia. Bromsgrove and Redditch Health Authority

Birchwood M, Smith J, Cochrane R 1990 The social functioning scale: the development and validation of a scale of social adjustment for use in family intervention programmes with schizophrenic patients. British Journal of Psychiatry 157: 853–859

Brooker C, Baguley I 1990 SNAP decisions. Nursing Times 86(41): 56–58

Committee of Inquiry into Complaints about Ashworth Hospital 1992 Report of the Committee of Inquiry into complaints about Ashworth Hospital, vol 1. (Blom Cooper Report) Cmnd 2028. HMSO, London

Day J, Wood G, Dewey M, Bentall R 1995 A self-rating scale for measuring neuroleptic side effects: validation in a group of schizophrenic patients. British Journal of Psychiatry 166: 650–653

Falloon I, Boyd J, McGill C et al 1985 Family management in the prevention of morbidity of schizophrenia. Archives of General Psychiatry 42: 887–896

Hogarty G, Anderson C, Reiss D et al 1986 Family psychoeducation, social skills training and maintenance chemotherapy in the aftercare treatment of schizophrenia. Archives of General Psychiatry 43: 633–642

Krawiecka M, Goldberg D, Vaughan M 1977 A standardised psychiatric assessment scale for rating chronic psychotic patients. Acta Psychiatrica Scandinavica 55: 299–308

Leff J, Kuipers L, Berkowitz R, Eberlein-Vries R, Sturgeon D 1982 A controlled trial of social intervention in the families of schizophrenic patients. British Journal of Psychiatry 141: 121–134

McCann G 1993 Relatives' support groups in a special hospital: an evaluation study. Journal of Advanced Nursing 18: 1883–1888

McCann G, McKeown M, Porter I 1996 Understanding the needs of relatives of patients within a special hospital for mentally disordered offenders: a basis for improved services. Journal of Advanced Nursing 23: 346–352

McKeown M, McCann G 1995 A schedule for assessing relatives: The Relative Assessment Interview for Schizophrenia in a Secure Environment. Psychiatric Care 2(3): 84–88

Tarrier N, Barrowclough C, Vaughn C et al 1988 The community management of schizophrenia: A controlled trial of a behavioural intervention with families to reduce relapse. British Journal of Psychiatry 153: 532–542

Zigmond A, Snaith R 1983 The hospital anxiety and depression scale. Acta Psychiatrica Scandinavica 67: 361–370

Self-harming behaviours

CONTENTS

Women who self-harm in a high-security hospital

Helen Liebling and Hazel Chipchase

Introduction

This case study is informed by an extensive research project into self-harm carried out at an English Special Hospital between 1992 and 1996. The work provided a foundation for a feminist therapy group which ran for 18 months and whose process was qualitatively evaluated. Individual and generic formulations for this group of women were devised concurrently. These used a woman-centred framework and gave an in-depth insight into individual and institutional factors in self-harm. The results of this and previous self-harm research, combined with the clinical experience of working with women in this context, enabled us to develop recommendations to promote positive strategies for women who self-harm in secure settings. It is hoped that the case study illustrates how theory and practice can be integrated as a strategy of resistance and change, supporting those whose lives have been constructed and controlled by dominant discourses.

Background to the project

The empirical work, which underpins this case study, included:

- Semi-structured interviews with 40 women patients about their self-harm (Liebling & Chipchase 1993, 1995b, 1996a, Liebling et al 1997a, 1997b)
- Semi-structured interviews with 96 staff in the service, regarding their support and training needs (Liebling & Chipchase 1995a)

- Case note study of 63 women at the same hospital and later comparison with case file information from women in two other Special Hospitals (Chipchase 1996, Chipchase & Lovelock 1995, Dolan & Bland 1996)
- The process of facilitation, and institutional context, of a feminist therapy group for women who self-harm in one Special Hospital (Liebling 1998, Liebling & Chipchase 1996b).

From the case note study, it emerged that a number of women currently detained in the Special Hospitals had not committed an index offence (in two of the hospitals this was over 20%). These women were often admitted through psychiatric or learning disability services. The commonest index offence was arson. At one of the hospitals, for all cases of arson, there was no record of the fires causing loss of life. Most of the fires had been small and caused little damage, with some deliberately set to access a place of safety. With respect to classifications, at one hospital nearly half of the women were legally classified under psychopathic disorder. Similarly, a Special Hospital Services Authority (SHSA) document (1995) noted: '… a greater proportion of women than men were categorised as suffering from personality disorder (34% of women to 23% of men) in the three Special Hospitals.'

This concurs with the review by Williams et al (1993) who discussed evidence that a history of sexual and physical abuse for women was associated with a high probability of misdiagnosis and greater levels of distress such as higher rates of depression, suicidal thoughts and attempts and self-harm. Likewise, our study (Liebling & Chipchase 1995b) found that 92.5% of a group of 40 women linked their self-harm to previous distressing life experiences. In order of importance, these were:

- Sexual abuse
- Family stress, rejection, or blame
- Physical and emotional abuse
- Illness of a family member or close friend
- Bullying at school.

Over 80% of women patients in the three Special Hospitals have deliberately harmed themselves at some point in their lives. The case note review showed most women had suffered disruptive childhoods; in one hospital 60% were placed into care during childhood (Chipchase 1996). Many women evidenced signs of distress at a very early age. Over 60% of women at the three Special Hospitals were sexually abused as children, with a significant proportion being physically or emotionally neglected and hurt. In addition, a number of women were also abused in adult life. Yet, in the confined world of the Secure Hospital, these women are placed in close proximity to male patients, some of whom have committed sexual and physical offences against women and children (Liebling et al 1997b).

Context of care

There have been long-standing concerns about the appropriateness, and quality, of services for women patients in the Special Hospitals. One example of this is the findings of the Public Inquiry at Ashworth Special Hospital (Committee of Inquiry 1992), which concluded: 'The culture is offensively "macho" in style and insensitive to their (women's) needs.' It further described the women's services as '… infantilising, demeaning and anti-therapeutic.' More recently, a national newspaper (Ackroyd 1998) reported that a previously suppressed report of an independent external advisory group carried out to review the provision of services for women at one of the Special Hospitals during 1993 concluded: 'We have felt it necessary to consider whether the women's services at Ashworth should continue. We have concluded that it should not.' Initial findings from our work support this sentiment, revealing that the therapeutic needs of women are not being adequately met (Liebling & Chipchase 1995a).

There is little evidence on the effectiveness of therapy groups for women who self-harm and this is particularly lacking for women in Special Hospitals. However, previous research has supported the provision of group therapy in this area. Lovaas & Simmons (1969) cited the need for interpersonal therapy for women who self-harm. The effectiveness of cognitive–behavioural approaches, and skills enhancement, has been shown with women who self-harm in the community (Linehan 1993). Babiker & Arnold (1997), though, are opposed to Linehan's assumption that a necessary starting point is for the person to be told that self-harm is unacceptable; seemingly a form of control at odds with the approach of not blaming the victim. They go on to state: 'We can see no advantage in being negatively judgmental and unsupportive. We consider the therapist always needs to be aware of the danger of undermining the patient's autonomy and responsibility' (Babiker & Arnold 1997).

Research has also shown that therapies which draw on feminist principles demonstrate success (Burstow 1992). It has been suggested that emotional empowerment in women is essential, as it helps to combat and reduce the shame women feel about the power they use. Although there is no clearly delineated feminist methodology as such, and feminist work is evaluated in relation to its purposes or goals (Burman 1994). Worell & Remer (1992) define five principles used in feminist therapy. These are:

1. Recognising the politics of gender as a central concern, reflected in women's lower social status and oppression in society
2. To value and seek knowledge about women's experiences
3. To seek equal status and employment in society
4. To acknowledge that values shape all human experience, and that neither science nor practice can be value-free
5. Being committed to action for social and political change.

Walsh & Rosen (1988) state that there are advantages to running therapy groups exclusively for women who self-harm. Within a group context, individual women may learn more effective skills, particularly interpersonal communication. They may also find greater self-understanding through sharing common experiences and common fears.

Whatever approach is used with women who self-harm, the relationship between the woman and the therapist is of paramount importance.

Noting the centrality of open and mutual discussion and goal-setting, Babiker & Arnold (1997) say of the therapist: 'She encourages the patient to cope, putting her in charge of her own recovery, and fostering security and continuity in the relationship. The therapist answers questions appropriately and honestly, offers feedback; and reorients towards reality when necessary.'

Identified needs of women who self-harm

From the 40 women who were interviewed as part of our project (Liebling & Chipchase 1993), the following needs were identified:

- 88% wanted involvement in planning their future
- 85% wanted positive goals in treatment
- 83% wanted help to express feelings and solve problems
- 80% wanted a regular listener.

When asked about specific therapy needs, the women wanted:

- Someone to listen to them (85%)
- To talk to other women who self-harmed (68%)
- Anger control (63%)
- Psychological therapy (63%).

Areas found to be significant antecedents to self-harm (Liebling & Chipchase 1995a) included:

- Severe depression
- Poor internal locus of control (i.e. a belief that events are not under one's personal control)
- Anxiety
- Anger
- Poor communication skills
- Difficulty solving problems.

Based upon the views of the women, and research findings reported in the literature, it was agreed that there were very good grounds for attempting to develop a therapy group for women who self-harmed within a Special Hospital. Planning sessions were established where women patients were fully involved in making decisions about the structure and composition of the group. It was deemed essential to involve the women owing to lack of control being identified as a major factor in women's continued self-harm (Burstow 1992, Liebling et al 1997b).

Interventions

The pilot group

A therapy group, using feminist principles, was established with five women patients in one of the Special Hospitals. Women chose to take part and selected the four women facilitators by interview with previously formulated questions. The women wanted staff with previous therapeutic experience who demonstrated an interest in the group. Collectively they felt that male staff generally did not understand self-harm and suggested one man should be involved. Despite reservations expressed by facilitators, it was agreed to try this initially, though for complex reasons it did not work out and he was replaced by a female assistant psychologist whom the group knew. The pilot group ran weekly from January to April 1995 in the Rehabilitation Department of the hospital. At first the structure was quite focused and used psychometric assessment of group change, but this proved unpopular with the women. The facilitators' perception was that this increased control over the women, contradicting the philosophy and theoretical base of the group. One woman described the assessments as a 'wind-up' and another said 'I thought you were trying to catch me out', referring to the repetitious nature of the instruments. These types of assessment were discontinued and more qualitative measures introduced.

Group sessions allowed an opportunity for women to discuss their concerns in the present, as well as issues related to self-harm. Each session included informal relaxing events which were selected by the women. The group also utilised discussions, role plays and educational material produced by Bristol Crisis Service for Women.

CASE STUDIES

Five women volunteered to take part in the group. All had histories of self-harming from an early age. They are briefly described below:

Mary had been at the hospital for 7 years. She still heard the voice of a man who had sexually abused her. She was in hospital following an index offence of criminal damage but had previously set a fire to escape an abusive situation.

Joanne had been at the hospital for 6 years. Part of her childhood had been spent in care and she had later suffered postnatal depression. Her index offence was attempted murder but she had previously set a fire to escape from an abusive situation.

Jennifer had been at the hospital for 11 years. Her index offence was arson and she had previously spent time in a Special Hospital.

Caroline had been at the hospital for 9 years. She had been placed into care and adopted as a baby. Her index offence was arson, after setting a small fire in prison.

Lindsey had been at the hospital for 8 years. It was her second admission. Her mother suffered with mental illness and her childhood was spent in a number of care homes. Her index offence was grievous bodily harm (GBH) following an incident in prison. She was still tormented by the voice of a male abuser.

The main group

Based upon the principles outlined above, the therapy group continued weekly from May 1995 with the same five women. It lasted for a total of 18 months but was unfortunately stopped abruptly, when the group leader was suspended and a facilitator withdrew from the service. During the life of the group it was not possible to audio-tape the sessions as originally anticipated because of understandable concerns by women patients. Instead, the facilitators' discussions about the proceedings of the group after each session were recorded.

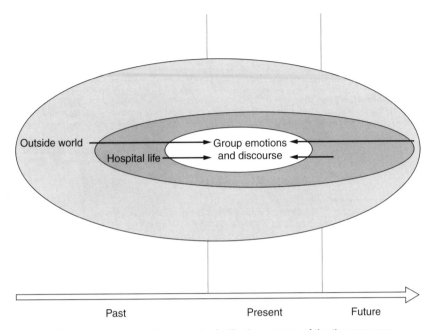

Outside world

Hospital life

Group emotions
and discourse

Past   Present   Future

Fig. 5.1   Representation of major clusters manifested in the facilitation process of the therapy group.

Table 5.1

Main categories	frequency recorded
Concerns of group members	147
Communication	138
Sources of distress	89
Coping strategies used in the group	70
Self-harm	69
Organisational constraints	28
Responses to distress	19

Outcomes and evaluations

The pilot group

Content analysis was used for the pilot group sessions and the main categories which emerged are shown in Table 5.1.

Concerns of group members included how they were treated on the wards, transport to and from the group and issues related to the women's futures. Despite finding it difficult to communicate feelings in the hospital environment, it was noticed as the group progressed that women were more able to express themselves clearly and disclosed more personal information about their lives. Exploration revealed that sources of distress included pressure, feelings of being punished (often for self-harming), being mistreated and the lack of positive goals. Women were reluctant to use hospital transport owing to the length of time it took to travel short distances and because of harassment from men. Security problems were varied and included women being sent to the wrong part of the hospital despite their request to attend the group, escort staff interrupting sessions and women being taken to sessions when they had been cancelled.

The main group

The narrative accounts of the women were analysed using the basic principles of grounded theory (Glaser & Strauss 1967). The main categories that emerged were:

• Hospital life (50%)
• Experiences within group (33%)
• Emotions (12%)
• Impact of the outside world (5%).

Discussions about aspects of hospital life dominated the group. These included ward issues, relationships with staff, gender issues, the

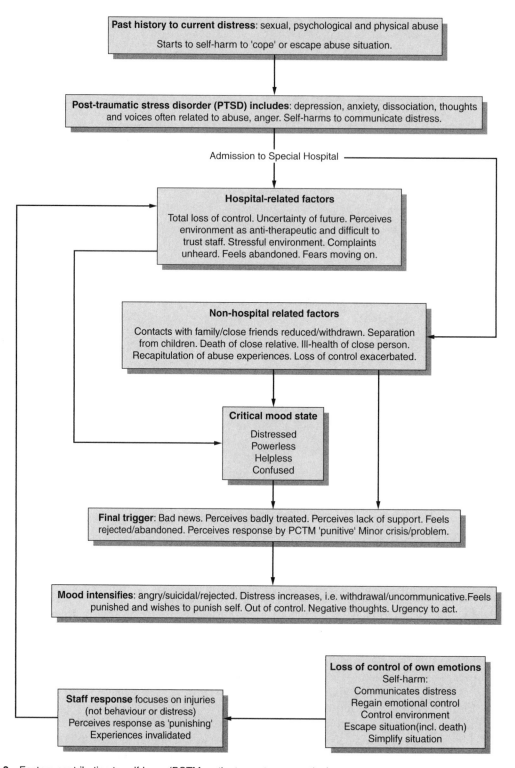

Fig. 5.2 Factors contributing to self-harm (PCTM: patient care team meeting).

physical environment, control/lack of control, threats to therapy and obstruction of the group process by emotional and systemic obstacles. This is represented in Figure 5.1.

The fact that women are physically contained within the hospital is self-evident. However, what emerged most powerfully from the group therapy was that they are contained in a way that not only obstructs therapeutic progress but also replicates their abuse experiences. Figure 5.1 attempts to reflect the relative significance of different aspects of the women's lives by both proximity to the group process and the size of the relevant area. Thus, the future is, for the women in the group, principally an anticipation of continued containment.

It is very difficult to undertake therapeutic work that requires a realistic perception of a future outside the hospital. The group served to contain the emotions arising from whatever source, past, present and future. What was disturbing was how much therapeutic effort had to be invested in dealing with issues relating to the 'here and now', challenges to therapeutic progress or even the survival of the group itself. Threats to therapy, and obstruction of the group process, accounted for over 25% of the total content. This was an indication of the anti-therapeutic environment in which the group attempted to function.

A generic formulation for the women involved in the group is shown in Figure 5.2. All suffered sexual, physical and psychological abuse prior to their admission to a Special Hospital. These were significant factors related to the commencement of self-harm. This included previous abuse histories and a wide range of trauma symptoms:

- Depression
- Suicidal feelings
- Anger
- Anxiety
- Dissociation
- Experiencing the 'voice' of an abuser
- Overwhelming sense of a lack·of control over internal and external events.

Once admitted to the Special Hospital, women experienced a loss of control and entered a 'critical mood state' exacerbated by hospital and non-hospital factors. Within these conditions, a minor trigger could result in self-harm as women attempted to regain control, communicate their distress or escape their situation. Responses to self-harm were perceived by the women as punishing, invalidating of their distress and experiences. Women were caught in a 'no-win' situation where self-harm served many functions (Liebling 1998).

Discussion

Women with extremely abusive pasts, few supports and histories of institutional care may end up being admitted to a Special Hospital, sometimes without having committed an index offence. Because of the dearth of adequate gender-sensitive facilities in the community for women who self-harm they may feel unsafe and out of control. This can result in behaviour designed to access 'a place of safety'. Having been admitted to such facilities, women are then seen as 'dangerous, disordered and doubly deviant' (Deu & Roberts 1997).

It is clear that psychiatric and medical labels have served to exacerbate women's distress (Arnold 1995, Ussher 1991) and current reports indicate women's care in Special Hospitals is completely inadequate (Ackroyd 1998, Committee of Inquiry 1992). The current judicial inquiry (Fallon 1998) is reviewing 'management arrangements for assuring effective clinical care' at the Special Hospital discussed in this case study.

Despite what benefits the therapy group held for individual women, the invalidating environment (see Linehan 1993) constantly impinged on its effectiveness and demanded a disproportionate amount of effort from all group members. It is questionable whether any successful therapeutic input can occur in such circumstances. Women's experiences outside the group conflicted with the progress they made within it and this resulted in overwhelming confusion. There was institutional resistance to the philosophy of the group and the environment did not assist women to label their experiences, tolerate distress or problem solve. Additionally, the punishment of women's behaviours, including self-harm, taught them to oscillate between emotional inhibition and extreme emotional states. Finally, the environment failed to enable women to validate their own experiences as they were doing in the group (Liebling 1998). It is interesting to note that Kelland (1995) came across similar difficulties in attempting to work therapeutically with women who self-harm at a women's prison:

There are practical, theoretical, ethical and personal issues to be addressed in trying to work therapeutically with women in a custodial setting. In spite of working from a feminist perspective, the notion of empowerment often becomes nonsensical, when women are locked in their cells at the end of a session or might be put 'on report' for trying out alternative coping methods.

It is acknowledged that a small number of women may need high security (11% identified by Maden et al 1995), but even for this group of women services could be developed in smaller, more therapeutic environments with better community links. There are well-documented gaps in current service provision in terms of the lack of medium- and low-secure settings for women which need to be addressed (Liebling & Lovelock 1995). At the same time, it is completely inappropriate to 'force-fit' women into medium-secure facilities which are predominantly 'designed for and dominated by male offenders' (Adshead & Morris 1995). Such gender-insensitive policies can have disastrous consequences, such as the death of a young woman patient at Reaside Regional Secure Unit (Channel 4 1995). She was the only woman on a ward of male patients at one point in her stay. Current literature stresses that women should be given a choice of residing on integrated or women-only wards (Liebling & Chipchase 1997b, Vishnick et al 1995).

In conclusion, the following changes need to take place:

- Women's histories need recognition and sensitive treatment.
- Changes need to be made in the way women's past and present lives are recorded and documented in medical records.
- They need to be offered the opportunity to add their own perspectives and stories.
- Small units should be created for women who self-harm, offering safety, containment and a real choice for women (*see* McCabe 1995).
- Development of a gender-sensitive service, for staff and patients, with a woman-centred vision and core values, is essential.
- Women's preference for segregated services should be respected (Liebling et al 1997b).
- Training, selection and staff mix are crucial.

REFERENCES

Ackroyd R 1998 Hospital inmates drugged. Daily Express 23 March

Adshead G, Morris F 1995 Another time, another place. Health Service Journal 9 February: 24–26

Arnold L 1995 Women and self-injury: a survey of 76 women. A report on women's experiences of self-injury and their views on service provision. Bristol Crisis Service for Women & Mental Health Foundation, London

Babiker G, Arnold L 1997 The language of injury: comprehending self-mutilation. The British Psychological Society, Leicester

Burman E 1994 Feminist research. In: Banister P, Burman E, Parker I, Taylor M, Tindall C (eds) Qualitative methods in psychology: a research guide. Open University Press, Milton Keynes

Burstow B 1992 Radical feminist therapy. Sage, Newbury Park

Channel 4 1995 Documentary about Reaside RSU, Birmingham

Chipchase H 1996 A study of self-harm amongst 63 women in a Special Hospital. Unpublished thesis, Liverpool University

Chipchase H, Lovelock C 1995 Describing the women in the three special hospitals. Paper presented at the Division of Criminological and Legal Psychology Annual Conference

Committee of Inquiry into Complaints about Ashworth Hospital 1992 Report of the committee of inquiry into complaints about Ashworth Hospital (Blom Cooper Report) Cmnd 2028 HMSO, London

Deu N, Roberts L 1997 Dangerous, disordered and doubly deviant, selected papers from the Special Hospital Psychology Advisory Group (SHPAG). Annual Conference 1994. Issues in Criminological and Legal Psychology

Dolan B, Bland J 1996 Who are the women in special hospitals? In: Hemingway C (ed) Special women?: the experience of women in the special hospital system. Ashgate, Aldershot

Fallon P 1998 Ongoing inquiry into the functioning of the Personality Disorder Unit at Ashworth Special Hospital

Glaser B, Strauss A 1967 The discovery of grounded theory: strategies for qualitative research. Aldine, Chicago

Kelland D 1995 Working with women who self-injure: therapeutic optimism vs therapeutic pessimism. Unpublished MSc in Applied Criminological Psychology, University of London

Liebling H 1998 The process of facilitation and the institutional context of a feminist therapy group for women who self-harm at Ashworth Hospital. Unpublished MSc in Forensic Behavioural Science, Liverpool University

Liebling H, Chipchase H 1993 A pilot study of the problem of self-injurious behaviour in women at Ashworth Hospital. Division of Criminological and Legal Psychology Newsletter 35: 19–23

Liebling H, Chipchase H 1995a Women who self-harm. Counselling News 20: 28–29

Liebling H, Chipchase H 1995b Research with women who self-harm, and the training needs of staff who work with them. Special Hospitals Research Bulletin 4: 4–17

Liebling H, Chipchase H 1996a Why do women at Ashworth Hospital harm themselves? In: Hemingway C (ed) Special women?: the experience of women in the special hospital system. Ashgate, Aldershot

Liebling H, Chipchase H 1996b Feminist group therapy for women who self-harm: an initial evaluation. In: Clark N, Stephenson G (eds) Psychological perspectives on police and custodial culture and organisation. Selected papers from the Division of Criminological and Legal Psychology Annual Conference, 1995

Liebling H, Lovelock C 1995 Paper written on behalf of Special Hospitals Psychology Advisory Group. Response to third draft of Special Hospital Service Authority discussion document: Strategy for women requiring secure psychiatric services

Liebling H, Chipchase H, Velangi R 1997a Why do women self-harm at Ashworth Maximum Security Hospital? In: Deu N, Roberts L (eds) Dangerous, disordered and doubly deviant, selected papers from the Special Hospital Psychology Advisory Group (SHPAG). Annual Conference 1994

Liebling H, Chipchase H, Velangi R 1997b Why do women harm themselves?: surviving special hospitals. Feminism and Psychology 7(3): 427–437

Linehan K 1993 Cognitive–behavioural treatment of borderline personality disorder. Guilford Press, New York

Lovaas O, Simmons J 1969 Manipulation of self-destruction in three retarded children. Journal of Applied Behaviour Analysis 2: 143–157

McCabe J 1995 In: Lloyd A (ed) Doubly deviant, doubly damned: society's treatment of violent women. Penguin, Harmondsworth

Maden A, Curie C, Meux C, Burrow S, Gunn J 1995 the treatment and security needs of special hospital patients. Whurr, London

Special Hospitals Service Authority 1995 Discussion document: strategy for women requiring secure psychiatric services. SHSA, London

Ussher J 1991 Women's madness: misogyny or mental illness? Harvester Wheatsheaf, London

Vishnick C, Cross P, McGuire J 1995 Gender integration in a secure hospital: a survey of patient attitudes. BPS Psychology of Women Section Newsletter 15: 20–29

Walsh B, Rosen P 1988 Self-multilation: theory, research and treatment. Guilford Press, New York

Williams J, Watson G, Smith H, Copperman J, Wood D 1993 Purchasing effective mental health services for women: a framework for action. University of Kent, Canterbury

Worell J, Remer P 1992 Feminist perspectives in therapy: an empowerment model for women. Wiley, London

CONTENTS

Young people in forensic care

Maureen Burke

SHATTERED JIGSAW: SARAH'S STORY

Introduction: the 'picture'

In forensic psychiatric practice, the helping relationship is often a difficult one to establish because, in part, the end-point of the endeavour is often unclear and frequently changing with life's events. However, what we do tend to know is that in building such a relationship we need to understand the many and varied fragments of the person's life that have contributed to his or her present state. Once we see and understand as many of the 'pieces' as possible, and where they fit in the overall 'picture', we can then help the person to build, or re-build, his or her shattered life. Yet, even then, the overall 'schema' often remains obscured or blurred. The following case presentation is an example of such a shattered life and an attempt to salvage it.

CASE STUDY: SARAH

Early history: the 'corner pieces'

Sarah was born 4 weeks prematurely, by caesarean section, being the fourth child in her eventual sibship of six children. Sarah's mother was alcohol-dependent and drank throughout all of her pregnancies. She was a single parent, and Sarah and the other children were from different relationships.

Sarah was admitted to the Special Care Baby Unit with breathing difficulties immediately after birth. Sarah's mother did not see her newborn baby for 4 days, as the postoperative period had been complicated by her withdrawal from alcohol. When they were reunited on the postnatal ward, the midwifery staff noted that Sarah's mother rarely picked up, or cuddled, her new daughter. Indeed, her only real contact with the baby was during bottle feeding or nappy changing.

Mother and Sarah were discharged from hospital after 10 days. From here, Sarah's very early life is a little unclear. It would appear that Sarah's older sister, then aged 8, assumed the care-giving role, as she was always looking after Sarah when the health visitor called. Historical accounts gathered since have also supported these suggestions. The mother continued to drink heavily and was therefore largely unavailable to provide Sarah with the appropriate nurturing, physical care or emotional validation.

When Sarah was 3 months old, the health visitor became concerned about a number of matters regarding the mother and baby relationship; first, the mother's drinking, second, the child's poor weight gain, and third, the general lack of care that the baby was receiving evidenced by severe nappy rash and cradle cap. The whole family was referred to Social Services who then became involved in assessing the family. It was felt that Sarah's mother was severely depressed with an alcohol dependency and she was referred to a psychiatrist. All the children were placed on the 'at risk register', including Sarah who was now 4 months old.

Setting the parameters: the 'edges'

When Sarah was 6 months old, her mother met, and married, a man whom she quickly became pregnant by. The resultant child, a boy, was treated quite differently to the other children, in that he seemed to be loved by his parents. Social Services continued to have contact with the family and became very concerned when Sarah, aged 1 year, was not walking and had bruising that could not be accounted for. On fuller examination, Sarah was found to have a healing fracture of her forearm, which again could not be

explained. Sarah was removed from the family and placed with foster parents whilst all the other children stayed with their mother and stepfather. At first, Sarah had regular supervised contact with her mother, but these meetings were described as lacking in emotional content. At such times Sarah's mother remained distant from, and seemed hostile towards, her young child. After a short period, Sarah's mother began cancelling, or not attending, the supervised visits. Finally, at the age of 3 years, Sarah was put up for adoption by her mother. As a result, Sarah was adopted by the family with whom she had been fostered.

There appeared to be no significant dilemmas until Sarah was 8 years old when she began having problems at school with aggression, poor concentration and general under-achieving. This ultimately led to Sarah being excluded from school and her referral to an educational psychologist; a report from this time stated that Sarah was 'a very unhappy little girl with a moderate learning difficulty'. Although her reading age was assessed at 5 years, with support from a classroom aid, Sarah improved in her school work and, with one-to-one attention, began to achieve her milestones.

Sarah did not come to the attention of any official services again until she was 13 years old, when her adoptive parents contacted Social Services to inform them that Sarah had been missing all weekend and was generally becoming difficult to manage. After the weekend, Sarah returned home without offering a full explanation about where she had been staying, simply stating that 'it was her business'.

Sarah's behaviour deteriorated over the next 6 months. This included coming home drunk, and on one occasion smelling of glue, with some form of adhesive evident in her hair and on her clothing. Sarah, now 14 years of age, was placed into the care of the local authority but was moved from one children's home to another as she became more and more violent and disruptive, usually whilst drunk. After 12 months in care, Sarah assaulted another young person in the children's home and was placed in local authority secure accommodation.

Filling in the 'middle'

Almost immediately that Sarah was admitted to secure accommodation, she began to harm herself, which usually took the form of lacerating her arms and breasts. She was also violent and assaulted several members of staff, with one serious attack resulting in a nurse sustaining a fractured jaw. Sarah was referred for a psychiatric assessment to a local mental health secure unit for young people and a team was dispatched to undertake this. Following the assessment, it was agreed that a period of admission would be needed to fully appraise both Sarah's mental state, and her care needs, under section 2 of the Mental Health Act 1983 and section 25 of the Children Act 1989.

The 10-bedded unit that Sarah was admitted to was managed by a multi-disciplinary team. This included a consultant forensic psychiatrist, consultant clinical psychologists, specialist nurses, mental health nurses, approved social workers, occupational therapists, art and music therapists, a psychotherapist, support and ancilliary staff and a small school with four teaching staff. Sarah was allocated a key-worker, who was one of the specialist female nurses on the unit, and the team met prior to Sarah's admission to discuss the case and devise a care programme. Each member of the team was allocated a specific task to complete throughout the 28-day assessment period.

The psychiatrist would undertake weekly formal mental state examinations and co-ordinate the overall team approach. The psychologist agreed to establish Sarah's IQ, level of depression and self-esteem. As part of the team approach, the approved social worker (ASW) would undertake a full social history and the occupational therapist (OT) agreed to explore both Sarah's aptitude for social interactions and her social skills abilities. The psychotherapist agreed to see Sarah for six sessions to establish if she could engage in therapy and, in particular, the most suitable therapeutic approach. It fell to the nursing staff to observe Sarah in the social setting on the ward and attempt to maintain her personal safety (Green & Burke 1998). A case

conference date was scheduled for 1 month ahead and all services that were involved in the case were invited to that meeting, including her probation officer and Guardian ad Litem.

On admission, Sarah avoided all eye contact, was quiet and withdrawn and reluctant to speak. Her key-worker spent considerable time with Sarah talking to her about the unit and what the timetable of events was likely to be. In particular, she went into some detail about the assessment procedure, placing great emphasis on the fact that the team wanted to establish an understanding of Sarah and her struggles. Sarah merely responded with nods of her head.

The key-worker handed the relevant information over to the evening shift, asking them to be particularly vigilant in observing Sarah as she seemed quite low and unhappy. During the evening, Sarah asked to go to the toilet and, although escorted by nursing staff, once in the toilet cut her arms with a razor blade that she had secreted in her underclothes. Sarah's wounds did not require suturing and clean dressings were quickly applied. This was also seen as a good opportunity to talk to Sarah and to let her know that the act of self-injury could be understood as a reflection of her feeling lost, tense and unable to share these feelings with anybody on the unit. Sarah looked surprised when the nurses attempted to soothe her in this way. They remained calm, quiet and reassuring towards Sarah (NWSIIG 1998) who then spoke for the first time since her admission. This can be taken as further evidence that the time of self-injurious behaviour is not one for reproach, but one in which there is an opportunity for a therapeutic encounter. She then asked if she could go to bed as she 'felt tired' and it was tactfully established that Sarah had not secreted any more sharp instruments and was feeling at least a little more settled.

This first evening seemed to be a watershed for Sarah as the next day she was up and pleasantly talking to the night staff before they went off duty. When her key-worker arrived on the unit, Sarah looked genuinely pleased to see her. Sarah was introduced to the school and the teachers and spent the morning there deciding on topics and times for study over her proposed 1-month admission. With her key-worker, Sarah established her timetable for the week, which included meeting all the other members of the team involved in her assessment.

The next few days passed without any untoward incident and Sarah became increasingly more involved in the unit's activities, participating well in the community meetings held by the nurses at the end of each day. This latter event gives the young people time to share how they are feeling, to discuss how their day has gone and to raise any problems or ideas that they want to discuss. These meetings encourage social skills and increase both a sense of community and a feeling of ownership. Sarah developed a close friendship with two of the other residents on the unit: one a girl and the other a boy, which was to create a dilemma for Sarah and the team.

Young people who require a secure mental health setting usually have a complicated history, with not insignificant relationship problems. Adolescence is marked by the importance of peer relationships, so any service providing for young people needs to be able to 'walk the tightrope' between enabling young people to have friendships and monitoring the impact of those relationships. Sarah and her two new friends began to rebel against the unit staff by not adhering to the individual timetables and disrupting the community meetings. Over the next few days, this culminated in the two girls cutting their wrists and the boy assaulting a member of staff, all on the same evening. The unit staff had a sense of the gender differential in expressing anger; women act in, and men act out (Carmen 1984, Miller 1994). Each of the young people involved was given extra individual time with their key-workers to explore their feelings. They were also seen as a group on four occasions, over a period of 4 days, by the occupational therapist and specialist nurse. During these meetings they were encouraged to express themselves appropriately, house rules were discussed, their agreement re-established and the nature of responsibility to self and the community explored. This range of interventions had a positive effect as Sarah and her friends

quickly settled down and relative peace was restored.

Sarah's sessions with the psychotherapist were well underway and the team received an interim report. The psychotherapist felt that Sarah's emotional functioning was severely impaired making it really difficult for her to articulate feelings in the sessions. It was felt by the team, at this point, that Sarah could possibly engage much more easily in one of the non-verbal therapies to facilitate a link between her thoughts, her feelings and her actions. The unit's art therapist agreed to see Sarah for four sessions.

The psychologist reported back to the team 2 weeks into Sarah's admission. This assessment established that Sarah experienced bouts of severe depression, which the team felt probably overlaid a chronic depressive state, possibly since childhood. Furthermore, Sarah's self-esteem was very low and she had periods when she felt 'worthless'. Sarah was, by now, engaged in all her therapies and had developed a strong bond with her key-worker. The occupational therapy assessment concluded that Sarah had poor social skills and functioned at a much younger age in her social constructs. School was going well and Sarah was enjoying the work, with art and information technology being her favourite subjects. All appeared to be going to plan until Sarah's key-worker let it be known that she was leaving the unit to take up a position elsewhere. Sarah quickly deteriorated, her self-harming became a daily occurrence and she began to destroy property in the unit. There was one incident of aggressive behaviour when she punched a member of staff.

The difficult 'pieces' to place: some problems

The team held a crisis meeting to explore how to proceed. It was decided that Sarah's present key-worker should increase her meetings with Sarah and include in these sessions the new key-worker who was to take over Sarah's care (Walker 1994). The team understood this deterioration in Sarah to be an expression of her sense of loss at the news of her key-worker leaving. This would be a re-enactment of Sarah's early, profound, loss of both her mother and family, and therefore would be very traumatic and emotionally disabling for Sarah (Bowlby 1980). It was important that the team remained consistent with Sarah, and that they managed their own anxieties (Lion 1973, Main 1989) with regular team meetings and clinical supervision (Faugier & Butterworth 1992).

A chink of light was thrown onto this bleak period when the ASW established contact with Sarah's adoptive family who expressed a desire to meet with her. The team felt this would be a positive, albeit anxious, move for Sarah. They saw it as potentially reducing Sarah's feelings of isolation and loneliness in the world and that it might possibly help to improve her sense of worth. A series of facilitated meetings with the family were planned.

It is perhaps not without significance that Sarah's distressing behaviours reduced around this time which was viewed by the team as Sarah feeling validated and emotionally contained on the unit. This produced the prospect of Sarah feeling that she 'belonged' or at least that she had found a 'secure base' from which to grow (Bowlby 1988, Delaney 1992, Holmes 1997)

The end of Sarah's assessment period was drawing near and the team met for a case review prior to the planned case conference. This forum enabled the team to draw together all the aspects of the assessment process and provide a formulation of future outcomes.

The 'picture' becomes clearer: assessment process, future outcomes and theoretical overview

Based on the history from the ASW, the team were able to establish a clearer picture of Sarah's early life. It was easy to see why Sarah had not been able to establish attachments to her carers because of the history of abuse and neglect from her parents. This early experience of victimisation robs a child of developing an identity and the ability to maintain authentic feelings which Shengold (1979) describes as 'soul murder'.

In a study by Carmen et al (1984: 378) it was concluded that 'abused patients had difficulty in coping with anger and aggression, impaired self esteem, and an inability to trust'. We can see how Sarah's behaviour mirrored this. The team's decision to explore Sarah's inner world using art therapy also seemed to bear fruit. Sarah's pictures depicted an isolated and lonely person with a poor sense of self which, again, linked into her history. Early neglect and abandonment had left her with a desolate inner landscape and an impoverished emotional repertoire (Burke 1997). Feelings of low self-worth, isolation and angry rejection had been turned inwards resulting in self-injury (De Zulueta 1996). Much of Sarah's presenting difficulties were understood as unconscious responses emanating from her 'felt experiences' as a child and infant (Connors 1996a 1996b). There were parallels to Sarah's behaviour and her early experiences, which the team felt were represented in the fact that she assaulted another young person in the children's home after 12 months in care. This equated with the same length of time that she had been in the 'care' of her biological family (Perry 1992).

It is always useful for any mental health team to be aware of, and make links to, the patient's unconscious calendar. Sarah's misuse of alcohol and other substances was discussed and it was concluded that this was Sarah looking for an escape from her intolerable, overwhelming psychic pain (Curtis Jenkins 1997). Van der Kolk (1989) would suggest alcohol and substance abuse produce natural endorphins that help the person 'feel soothed'. Self-soothing is mastered as part of the attachment phenomena during infancy (Bowlby 1980). Where there is rejection, abandonment and lack of attunement, particularly from the mother, the infant does not develop ways of modulating arousal and therefore cannot feel soothed. This is supported by a research study (Arnold 1995) which provided data about 76 women who injured themselves. These subjects spoke of a range of functions that self-injury served: 57% reported that it 'relieved feelings' and 13% claimed that they gained 'comfort'. So, this biological perspective is yet another lens through which the team could view Sarah's self-injurious behaviour.

Wise (1990) argues that victims of childhood abuse will develop survival responses to this trauma which may produce problems later in life. Families immersed in the 'shame' of alcoholism are more likely to produce children who develop escape/release patterns such as becoming alcoholics themselves, self-abusing or injuring others. She goes on to say 'self injury patterns continue to carry the coded truth of buried pain, fear, betrayal and loss' (Wise 1990: 193).

From this assessment, it was established that Sarah was currently depressed and an assumption was made that this depression was an acute phase that probably existed alongside a chronic, longer-term, depressive illness. Sarah was prescribed antidepressants and her acute depression, based on follow-up assessments, began to lift. We should always remain mindful to the possibility of an undiagnosed depression, particularly in an aggressive, assaultive, self-injuring young person (or adult). Sarah had been lurching from one interpersonal crisis to another for many years and this chronic state is likely to result in self-injury, particularly in times of an acute crisis (Curtis Jenkins 1997, Reder 1991).

Sarah's reaction to her key-worker leaving was considered at the review. Adshead (1998) considers psychiatric staff as bonding characters and points out: 'where mental health care professionals are seen as attachment figures, threats to relationships with them may produce anger and violence'. This would be experienced by the patient/client as a re-enactment of the initial trauma of abandonment and the person would re-experience 'felt' neglect. Sarah seemed overwhelmed in this way at the prospective loss of her key-worker. Although some of our patients/clients may struggle during significant workers' days off, annual leave, or even time off duty, we, then, as potential attachment figures, ought to use this position to provide our patients with a positive corrective, emotional experience.

Sarah's first evening in the unit could be seen as pivotal. When she self-injured at this time, it was managed in a way that maintained and encouraged empathy. Sarah was not rejected or 'punished' for her actions and a clear, early message was given that the unit staff could, and would, 'hold' Sarah and regard her with compassion and warmth. The team were pleased to report that Sarah and her adoptive family had met on three occasions and that these had gone well, and although there were clearly bridges to be built, this contact was viewed as a good sign for Sarah and her future.

The last 'piece': conclusions

The team concluded that their formulation of Sarah would enable the local authority to care for her and, with some outreach support from the unit, they would recommend Sarah was re-assessed regarding her accommodation requirements. There was a hope that she would be managed in a less secure environment. It was considered that there may even be a possibility of Sarah being re-united with her adoptive family at some time in the future. After the case conference, Sarah was discharged from the unit.

Our patients have much to teach us. Sarah's story is not unique and many of our patients have traumatic and impoverished early lives. We have a responsibility to know and understand our patients' early experiences in order to make sense of how they present in the 'here and now'. Nothing makes sense if we do not discover and pay attention to the context within which we are working. Putting together the pieces of our patients' internal puzzle, or 'shattered jigsaw', allows for clarity and direction to be made explicit.

Working with Sarah took courage, commitment and a cohesive team. The outcome will be that Sarah should not now spiral into a lifetime of episodic or even long-term psychiatric care. A tragedy exists in that many patients cannot access a relatively early range of interventions. Indeed, for Sarah, we can see how support in infancy might have helped to reduce the misery that she was later to endure.

REFERENCES

Adshead G 1998 Psychiatric staff as attachment figures. British Journal of Psychiatry 172: 64–69

Arnold L 1995 Women and self injury: a survey of 76 women. Bristol Crisis Service for Women, Bristol

Bowlby J 1980 Loss: attachment and loss, vol 3. Penguin, Harmondsworth.

Bowlby J 1988 A secure base: clinical applications of attachment theory. Routledge, London

Burke M 1997 Women's rage and self injury. Conference Presentation at International Nursing Conference, St Thomas Isle, Virgin Islands, August 1997

Carmen E 1984 Victims of violence and psychiatric illness. American Journal of Psychiatry 141: 378–383

Connors R 1996a Self injury in trauma survivors 1: functions and meanings. American Journal of Orthopsychiatry 66(2): 197–206

Connors R 1996b Self injury in trauma survivors 2: levels of clinical response. American Journal of Orthopsychiatry 66(2): 207–216

Curtis Jenkins G 1997 Depression in childhood and adolescence. In: Dwivedi K, Varma K (eds) Depression in childhood and adolescence in primary healthcare. Whurr, London

Delaney K 1992 Nursing in child psychiatric milieus. Journal of Child Psychiatric Nursing 5(1): 10–15

De Zulueta F 1996 From pain to violence: the traumatic roots of destructiveness. Whurr, London

Faugier J, Butterworth T 1992 Clinical supervision and mentorship in nursing. Chapman and Hall, London

Green J, Burke M 1998 The ward as a therapeutic agent. In: Green J, Jacobs B (eds) The inpatient psychiatric treatment of children. Routledge, London

Holmes J 1997 Attachment, autonomy, intimacy: some clinical implications of attachment theory. British Journal of Medical Psychology 70: 231–248

Lion J 1973 Countertransference reactions to violent patients. American Journal of Psychiatry 130(2): 207–210

Main T 1989 The ailment. In: Jones J (ed) Psychoanalytical essays. Free Association Books, London

Miller D 1994 Women who hurt themselves: a book of hope and understanding. Basic Books, New York

North West Self Injury Interest Group (NWSIIG) 1998 Self injury: a resource pack. Ashworth Hospital Authority, Liverpool, England

Perry C J 1992 Life events and recurrent depression in borderline and antisocial personality disorders. Journal of Personality Disorder 6(4): 394–407

Reder P 1991 The challenge of deliberate self harm by young adolescents. Journal of Adolescence 14: 135–148

Shengold L 1979 Child abuse and deprivation: soul murder. Journal of the American Psychoanalytical Association 27(3): 533–558

Van der Kolk B 1989 The compulsion to repeat trauma: re-enactment, revictimisation and masochism. Psychiatric Clinics of North America 12: 389–411

Walker M 1994 Principles of a therapeutic milieu: an overview. Perspectives in Psychiatric Care 30(3): 5–8

Wise M 1990 Adult self injury as a survival response in victim survivors of childhood abuse. In: Potter E (ed) Aggressive, family violence and chemical dependence. Hawthorn Press, USA

CONTENTS

A problem-solving approach to the treatment of suicidal behaviour and self-injury

Syd Fraser and Sheila Rose

Introduction

A case study is presented of a self-injuring, sometimes suicidal, 21-year-old resident of a secure hospital ward. Problem-solving therapy, as a structured, short-term, directive therapy undertaken in the cognitive–behavioural tradition, was used to target reduction in interpersonal conflicts with significant family members. This prescriptive skills training model promoted the development of 'means end' problem-solving thinking in a patient whose prior means for coping with interpersonal, sometimes intrapsychic, problems involved self-injury and a recent incident of serious suicide attempt. Results suggested significant but variable improvement in affective functioning, notably in hopelessness, depression and suicide intent, as well as in problem-solving. Setting and client compliance factors are discussed with regard to their implications for the process, and progress, of therapy within the secure setting.

Theoretical background

The treatment of the suicidal individual, and those who evidence self-injurious behaviours, often tests the capabilities of clinicians and institutions alike. This case study focuses on the assessment and treatment of an individual presenting with suicidal and self-injurious behaviours in a secure hospital situation. The combination of maladaptive behaviours represents aspects of the complexity of the presentation and is not untypical of a sizeable proportion of patients in this setting.

The literature on suicide risk in psychiatric hospitals, secure institutions and prisons suggests that individuals in these environments are at significantly increased risk compared to the general population (Goh et al 1991, Hawton & Fagg 1988). High incidences of self-injury are reported among the learning disabled, autistic, brain-damaged, schizophrenic and eating and personality disordered. Within psychiatric populations a reported 7 to 10% of patients engage in self-injury (Favazza & Conterio 1988), of which an excess are females. In Arnold's (1995) survey of a sample of Bristol women who self-injured, up to 50% reported multiple forms of sexual and emotional abuse experienced in childhood. Family backgrounds characterised by violence, alcoholism and chaos were not unusual (Walsh & Rosen 1988). Similarly, Van der Kolk et al (1991) found from follow-up studies that self-injurious behaviour was most tenacious amongst those women who had the most severe histories of separation, lack of secure attachments and neglect.

Studies of the prevalence of self-injurious behaviours within the Special Hospital system (Burrow 1992, Ferry 1992) revealed that in a 6-month period over 20% of the population engaged in forms of self-injury, including head-banging and lacerating as the most common forms, with over three-quarters of those who self-injured being female. The personality-disordered woman tended to inflict more severe injuries. Similar findings have been reported in other studies (Favazza & Conterio 1988).

A clear distinction can be made between suicidal behaviour and self-injurious behaviours in terms of admitted intent, putative causation and real or fantasised outcomes. However, it is important for clinicians to note that the behaviours are not mutually exclusive and suicide intent is often reported in association with self-injury (Favazza & Conterio 1988). A summary of the various coping functions of self-injury (Babiker & Arnold 1997, Herpertz 1995, Miller 1994) includes regulation of distress and anxiety, facilitating the expression of aggression, using pain as a distraction from dysphoria, to communicate distress and to punish or influence the behaviour of others (Simpson 1976). Likewise, the motives for undertaking suicidal behaviours include the coping functions: to escape an unbearable situation, to punish others, to show how much you loved someone, to make others understand desperation, to influence another, to make things easier, to frighten or get even with and to die (Bancroft et al 1976).

Miller (1994) proposes that the experience of various forms of abuse in childhood interferes with the development of a secure sense of self and inhibits the development of language to communicate experiences and feelings. Self-injury was said to develop as a powerful coping mechanism in these individuals and has its origins in deficient coping skills and problem-solving (Walsh & Rosen 1988). Coping is important to mental well-being and is instrumental in the regulation and avoidance of distress. It is basically a problem-solving or set of problem-solving strategies. Simpson (1976) suggested that self-injury was an intense interpersonal act in the context of a tense interpersonal situation. It was seen to represent a maladaptive attempt to counteract, by a physical act performed against the self, an overwhelming situation.

Within the Special Hospital context, treatment responses to suicidal behaviour and serious self-injury have included prescribed medication to sedate, seclusion and special levels of observation, clearing a side room to reduce access to objects which could be used to self-injure and the use of restraint garments. The apparent intention was to bring these behaviours under rapid control (Burrow 1992).

Because of the interpersonal focus and the psychosocial context in which suicidal behaviour is enacted, research interest has turned to examining the social problem-solving characteristics of those presenting with suicidal behaviour. A summary of the findings suggests that suicidal patients have a consistent deficit in social problem-solving; do not expect problems to be a natural part of everyday life; have a passive problem-solving orientation; experience difficulty in generating potential alternative solutions to problems once identified; show deficiencies in implementing viable solutions; demonstrate a tendency to focus on the potentially negative consequences of alternatives generated; and, a tendency to view suicide as an acceptable or viable solution to problems (Fraser 1986, 1987, Ivanoff et al 1992, Linehan et al 1987, Rotheram-Borus & Trautman 1990, Sadowski & Kelly 1993, Sakinofski et al 1990, Schotte & Clum 1987, Weisharr & Beck 1990).

More recently, alternative empirically-based treatment approaches have been developed for use with the suicidal and self-injuring patient. Dialectical behaviour therapy (Linehan 1987, Linehan et al 1987) and cognitive–behavioural problem-solving therapy (Fraser 1987, Lerner & Clum 1990, McLeavey et al 1994, Salkovskis et al 1990) being the two front runners. This contrasts with general psychiatric interventions (Diekestra & Kerkhof 1994).

The following case study focuses on the use of problem-solving therapy with a client presenting with a psychotic illness and associated behavioural problems, notably suicidal behaviours and self-injury.

CASE STUDY: CAROL

Patient history

Carol is a 21-year-old female resident on a secure hospital female ward, to which she had been admitted approximately 16 months previously. Her admission followed the very serious assault and wounding of a member of her extended family. This incident took place during what appeared to be an acute phase of a, then, unrecognised psychotic illness and in response to command auditory hallucinations.

Carol was diagnosed as suffering a schizophrenic illness. There was recorded evidence of repeated self-injurious behaviours and one recent suicide attempt on the ward using a contrived ligature. At the time of the author's (SR) intervention, psychotic phenomena were well controlled using a typical neuroleptic. Some disturbance of mood was noted by staff and there was clinical concern about the further

management of the behavioural problems, notably self-injury and suicidal acting out.

Carol was the elder of two children and her parents separated when she was aged 6 years. Contact with her father had been lost and she tended to construe this as an example of being rejected. Carol was described as having an anxious attachment to her mother and doted on her younger sister to whom she was over-protective. She had reported being sexually abused at age 12, over a 2-year period, by her then stepfather. This allegation was never fully investigated at the time and, although her mother did separate from this man, Carol felt that her mother never really believed her accounts. Their relationship was noted for its reciprocal tensions, threats of rejection and anxious attachment through to young adulthood.

Carol had long-term difficulties in both the home and school settings, the latter disrupted by refusal to attend, truancy and finally expulsion. Academic achievement was poor, but her intellectual level was assessed by an educational psychologist as being within the 'bright to average' range. Her adjustment to outside social demands, including work, was equally problematic as were her attempts to foster extra-familial social relationships.

Identified problems

On referral, the clinical staff were satisfied with the progress made in moderating psychotic symptomatology, but the presenting behavioural problems were posing difficulties for the ward atmosphere, particularly for planning Carol's future. The initial assessment highlighted the main areas of current difficulty.

First, on the behavioural side, the repeated self-injury was an increasing worry. Carol used available objects to superficially scar her legs and arms. The concern was about the escalating frequency and the possibility of the scarring becoming more serious. An associated behavioural problem was the recent episode of suicide attempt by ligation. This was regarded as a serious escalation of Carol's problems as it was associated with admitted suicide intent,

Table 5.2 Assessment and treatment change scores

Week	1	2	3	4	5	6	7	8	12
Hopelessness	14	10	10	9	8	9	6	5	6
Depression	25	26	22	17	13	13	10	10	12
Self-injury (no. of instances)	4		3		1		0	0	0
MEPS	0							3	

MEPS: Means End Problem Solving (no. of relevant means).

concordant suicide cognitions and a certain planfulness.

The second area of difficulty could be summarised as emotional rather than behavioural. The emotional difficulties were characterised by acute periods of hopelessness associated with a negative evaluation that the future was futile and that she had no control over it other than by interrupting her life. There were also recurrent, but associated, feelings of abandonment/rejection linked to failure in visits from her mother and anticipated or real loss of telephone contact with her sister. Failure of these highly valued visits was shown to follow arguments with her mother.

The third area of assessed difficulties was summarised as longer term issues to do with unresolved emotional conflicts associated with childhood sexual abuse, poor personal self-worth and coming to terms with the expressed feelings of guilt surrounding her index offence.

The assessment suggested that there was a contingent relationship between disruption (real or anticipated) of interpersonal ties with her mother and sister, self-injury and suicide ideation. This was a re-enactment of past anxious attachments and a recognised failure to appropriately manage or transact interpersonal relationships. The failure or disruption of interpersonal ties was hypothesised to create conditions of stress at which time Carol became vulnerable to suicide ideation, suicide intent and self-injury. This formulation is in keeping with the diathesis-stress model (Clum & Lerner 1990) which suggests that people with poor interpersonal problem-solving skills are vulnerable at times of high stress to hopelessness and suicidal behaviour. A summary of formal assessments of

mood state, hopelessness and interpersonal problem-solving is given in Table 5.2.

Treatment intervention

It was agreed with Carol and the ward staff that the first two areas of difficulty would be the focus of short-term intervention. On the basis of the behavioural and psychometric evaluations, Carol was regarded as suitable for short-term, problem-solving therapy, and it was recognised that the longer-term issues identified may reasonably be a consideration for future psychotherapy. Her florid psychotic symptoms were also under some degree of pharmacological control.

Problem-solving therapy is a structured, time-limited, sometimes directive, cognitive–behavioural intervention. It provides an opportunity to learn strategies for resolving interpersonal problems in general, which can then be applied to more specific interpersonal problems. The overall aims of problem-solving therapy included:

- To improve problem-solving options for the interpersonal difficulties identified and to increase the likelihood that Carol would put these options into practice
- To reduce the regularised and heightened experience of emotional distress which often preceded and/or triggered the dysfunctional behaviours and cognitions related to suicidal behaviour
- To reduce significantly the occurrence of self-injurious behaviours and acute episodes of hopelessness and dysphoria.

The intervention (*see* Fraser 1987, Platt et al 1988 for detailed treatment scripts) was conveniently divided into three stages and 16 sessions spread over an 8-week (two sessions per week) period, with a follow-up session at 12 weeks. Each session lasted 40 minutes on average.

Stage 1

The two sessions of stage 1 involved the crucial tasks of risk assessment, patient socialisation for therapy and ward staff education about the treatment plan and its implications for everyday management of ward relationships. Risk assessment was seen as a crucial first task and included the use of specific psychometric tools to assess hopelessness (Beck & Steer 1985a) and depression (Beck & Steer 1985b).

Problem-solving skills were assessed by using a modification of the Means Ends Problem Solving (MEPS) Procedure (Platt & Spivack 1975) for two hypothetical, but realistic, interpersonal problems. This method was used to gain insights into Carol's ability to generate relevant means for solving such problems.

Treatment orientation or socialisation was also seen as a vital Stage 1 task. The establishment of a working alliance with Carol, and clarifying her motivation for and expectations of treatment would be vital to the collaboration that needed to develop.

Stage 2

In Stage 2 there were 12 sessions involving formal training in the various stages of problem-solving. A prescriptive model of problem-solving (D'Zurilla 1988) was followed, which involved opportunities to learn the component, interpersonal, problem-solving skills. These skills included developing an orientation that problems were potentially solvable; recognising when the individual had a problem; defining clearly the specific problem(s) being experienced and the realistic goal state which the individual wished to reach or achieve; generating alternative solutions or strategies to achieve this goal state; deciding which of the various alternatives would be used; implementing the selected strategy; and,

getting feedback about the effectiveness of the intervention.

Stage 3

The two sessions of this stage involved learning to maintain the problem-solving orientation, generalising this learning to other real-life situations, relapse prevention (anticipation of future problems, obstacles to maintaining problem-solving) and preparing the patient for termination. Three goal states were identified collaboratively:

1. Reducing the number of arguments during visits between herself and her mother
2. Getting her sister to make the telephone calls she promised
3. Dealing differently with 'distress' caused by arguments or lost visits.

Training sessions involved the use of hypothetical, but real-life, problem examples and the application of the techniques learnt and rehearsed to achieve the agreed goal states. Training employed a variety of strategies including direct verbal instructions, guided discovery and guidance in formulating conclusions; facilitating independent productive thinking, coaching, modelling, and behavioural rehearsal; between-session assignments (homework), performance feedback, shaping and positive social reinforcement.

Treatment outcome

This section will comment on the quantitative and qualitative impact of the intervention and consider issues to do with the context of the intervention that bore some relevance to the observed outcomes.

Table 5.2 reports on the initial assessment findings and the change scores for the two affective indices, hopelessness and depression. Problem-solving changes were assessed at Week 1 and at Week 8. Carol's case notes were perused for indications of reported self-injury and suicide attempts over the period of intervention.

The initial hopelessness scores suggested persisting degrees of clinically significant hopelessness about her future. Although Carol had been making gains with her training, and these were paying some dividends for improving the interpersonal ties with her mother, it was recognised that her current situation (being in a secure hospital) continued to be a source of upset. These scores decreased significantly across the time of therapy and reflected not only improvements in relating, but the realisation that with continued treatment her future could be discussed in a positive way. It remains a clear difficulty to be hopeful about the future if one feels that one is shut away from society and deprived of easy access to the outside world. This is a problem confronting most clinical efforts in this setting and is only balanced by the 'here-and-now' improvements which can be used to motivate persistent effort and undermine giving up.

Beck depression scores also showed a steady decline from the moderate range of severity to the non-depressed range by the end of the period of intervention. It is recognised that these affective scores are subject to inflation during the initial period of distress and tend to show rapid decline thereafter.

'Means–ends thinking', the ability to articulate relevant step-by-step means of solving a stated interpersonal problem, was the main, assessed, problem-solving deficit identified using the MEPS procedure. Table 5.2 shows that this specific ability had significantly improved at the end of the intervention. It is not unusual for problem-solving skills to improve with training; the real test would be their persistent use by Carol over the longer term.

Significant improvement was demonstrated in the reduction of episodes of self-injury as gleaned from case records over the period of intervention. Problem-solving for dealing with the affective states of anger, tension and dejection involved the contingent adaptive use of relaxation, distraction and activity to good effect. The periods of distress were also reduced in frequency as the stated goals were achieved or as Carol learnt to deal differently with what was once construed as a catastrophe or crisis.

Reported changes in effect and self-injury were maintained as assessed at the short follow-up period, at which time Carol had undertaken long-term therapy with an agreed other therapist. On the qualitative side, Carol was able to use burgeoning signs of distress to prompt problem-solving behaviour in herself and to seek advice from ward staff and her therapist.

The spontaneous verbalisation of suicidal ideas had not entirely ceased, but the regular assessments detected the absence of suicide intent. Carol admitted that she was still keen to find 'objects' which she could hoard to use creatively in the future to self-injure 'if necessary'. It was clear that self-injury had not lost all its functional utility for Carol and that she was still being influenced by its continued occurrence in others around her in the ward setting.

Although Carol anticipated that failure of visits from her mother was still possible, and she was now able not to catastrophise about their occurrence, general feelings of abandonment and rejection were still apparent and were clearly related to the more enduring aspects of low self-worth. A worthwhile achievement was Carol's willingness to participate in longer term therapy with another therapist. She recognised that she was not helpless in relationships and, while they carried risks, she could have some influence on how they progressed.

Reflections on practice

The use of problem-solving training has demonstrated clinical utility for a range of clinical problems. This case study does suggest that the session arrangements suggested in training manuals can be used flexibly depending on the patient's speed of uptake. In Carol's case, twice-weekly sessions were valuable in maintaining her motivation and for readily reinforcing adaptive behaviour.

It was deemed crucial to the success of the intervention that ward staff be educated about the treatment plan, and importantly about how their behaviour needed to be adjusted to facilitate the desired changes in Carol's behaviour. It was important that the intervention was not seen as remote from the ward and that the therapist was readily accessible for consultation. Consistent handling of self-injury which did not give out messages to Carol of disgust, manipulation, anxiety and disapproval was equally as important for the therapist as it was for the ward team.

The assessment of suicidal behaviour may be seen as an intervention in itself. The twice-weekly sessions allowed ready evaluation of suicide ideation, intent and planning and provided for appropriate therapeutic responses to be made in good time.

The process of the therapy session did not always run smoothly. The initial socialisation to therapy, and the building of a therapeutic relationship, had first to deal with a distrustful reluctance on Carol's part. The therapist had to recognise that for Carol the forming of another relationship carried with it the risk of being rejected from it. Also, because of the setting, relationships with their attendant hazards take on much more significance for the parties involved. This working relationship, or alliance, was seen as important for the conduct of the problem-solving therapy.

The role of supervision needs to be mentioned. This relationship was used to discuss technical aspects of the therapeutic process and the way the relationship was faring with Carol and to discuss anxieties about aspects of her self-injuring and hopelessness at times. Clinicians need to receive regular supervision when working with this group of patients and this is not always possible for the ward staff who are in regular and close contact.

Conclusions

Carol has made modest, but significant, gains and her introduction to longer term therapy was a very important next step. Improving problem-solving skills could provide an alternative coping mechanism that suicidal and self-injuring individuals can use at times of interpersonal stress. Hopelessness is an endemic and ubiquitous symptom characteristic of the secure population and settings, given the personal and organisational issues which both confront.

Demonstrating clinical impact on maladaptive coping behaviours which suicide attempt and self-injury represent is the therapeutic challenge. This case study suggests that short-term therapies, such as problem-solving therapy, may have clinical relevance both for reducing the maladaptive behaviours themselves and for enhancing quality of life in these settings. The wider use of this therapeutic strategy is recommended. The training of more therapists, particularly ward-based staff, in these methods would be a rational development.

REFERENCES

Arnold L 1995 Women and self-injury: a survey of 76 women. Bristol Crisis Service for Women, Bristol
Babiker G, Arnold L 1997. The language of injury. BPS Books, Leicester
Bancroft J, Skrimshire A, Simpkin S 1976. The reasons people give for taking overdoses. British Journal of Psychiatry 128: 538–548
Beck A, Steer R 1985a Beck hopelessness scale manual. Harcourt Brace, San Antonio
Beck A, Steer R 1985b Beck depression inventory manual. Harcourt Brace, San Antonio
Burrow S 1992 The deliberate self-harming behaviour of patients within a British special hospital. Journal of Advanced Nursing 17: 138–148
Clum G, Lerner M 1990 A problem solving approach to treating individuals at risk for suicide. In: Lester D (ed) Current concepts of suicide. Charles Press, Philadelphia

Diekestra R, Kerkhof J 1994 The prevention of suicidal behaviour: a review of effectiveness. In: Leventhal H, Johnston M (eds) International review of health psychology, vol 3. J Wiley, Chichester
D'Zurilla J 1988 Problem solving therapies. In: Dobson K (ed) Handbook of cognitive behaviour therapies. Guilford Press, New York
Favazza A, Conterio K 1988 The plight of chronic self-mutilators. Community Mental Health Journal 1: 22–30
Ferry R 1992 Self-injurious behaviour. Senior Nurse 12: 21–25
Fraser S 1986 Interpersonal cognitive problem solving training and suicidal behaviour. British Journal of Cognitive Psychotherapy 4: 39–47
Fraser S 1987 Cognitive and behavioural strategies in the management of suicidal behaviour. Doctoral thesis, University of Leicester

Goh S, Salmons P, Whittington R 1991 Hospital suicides: are there preventable factors? Profile of the psychiatric hospital service. British Journal of Psychiatry 152: 243–249

Hawton K, Fagg J 1988 Suicide and other causes of death following attempted suicide. British Journal of Psychiatry 152: 359–366

Herpertz S 1995 Self-injurious behaviour. Psychopathological and nosological characteristics in sub-types of self-injurers. Acta Psychiatrica Scandinavica 91: 57–68

Ivanoff A, Smyth N, Grochowski S, Jang S, Klien K 1992 Problem solving and suicidality among prison inmates: another look at state versus trait. Journal of Consulting and Clinical Psychology 60: 970–973

Lerner M, Clum G 1990 Treatment of suicide ideators. A problem solving approach. Behaviour Therapy 21: 403–411

Linehan M 1987 Dialectical behaviour therapy: a cognitive behavioural approach to suicide. Journal of Personality Disorders 1: 328–333

Linehan M, Camper P, Chiles J, Stroshal K, Shearin F 1987 Interpersonal problem solving and parasuicide. Cognitive Therapy and Research 11: 1–12

McLeavey M, Tutek D, Ludgate W, Murray C 1994 Interpersonal problem solving skills training in the treatment of self-poisoning patients. Suicide and Life Threatening Behaviour 24: 382–394

Miller D 1994 Women who hurt themselves: a book of hope and understanding. Basic Books, New York

Platt J, Spivack G 1975 Manual for the MEPS procedure. A measure of interpersonal problem solving skills. Hahnemann Medical College, Philadelphia

Platt J, Taube D, Metzger D, Duome M 1988 Training in interpersonal problem solving. Journal of Cognitive Psychotherapy 2: 5–34

Rotheram-Borus M, Trautman P 1990 Cognitive style and pleasant activities among adolescent suicide attempters. Journal of Consulting and Clinical Psychology 58: 554–561

Sadowski C, Kelly M 1993 Social problem-solving in suicidal adolescents. Journal of Consulting and Clinical Psychology 61: 121–127

Sakinofski I, Roberts R, Brown Y, Cummings C, James P 1990 Problem resolution and repetition of suicide: a prospective study. British Journal of Psychiatry 156: 395–399

Salkovskis P, Atha C, Storer D 1990 Cognitive behavior problem solving in the treatment of patients who repeatedly attempt suicide: a controlled study. British Journal of Psychiatry 157: 871–876

Schotte D, Clum G 1987 Problem-solving skills in suicidal psychiatric patients. Journal of Consulting and Clinical Psychology 55: 49–54

Simpson M 1976 Self-mutilation. British Journal of Hospital Medicine 16: 430–438

van der Kolk B, Perry C, Herman J 1991 Childhood origins of self-destructive behaviour. American Journal of Psychiatry 148: 1665–1667

Walsh B, Rosen P 1988 Self mutilation: theory, research and treatment. Guilford Press, New York

Weishaar M, Beck A 1990 Cognitive approaches to the understanding and treatment of suicidal behaviour. In: Blumenthal S, Kupfer D (eds) Suicide over the life cycle. American Psychiatric Press, Washington

Violence and aggression

CONTENTS

Anger management

Penny Schafer and Cindy Peternelj-Taylor

Introduction

This case study highlights the treatment of Bill, a 30-year-old offender with a violent criminal history dating back to his early teens. Bill learned very early in life that violence and substance misuse were an effective means of coping with the stressors in his life and these very quickly became an integral component of his cycle of violent behaviour and incarceration. Bill entered an intensive treatment programme, the Aggressive Behaviour Control (ABC) programme, designed to address his identified criminogenic needs. Although the multi-disciplinary team tailored treatment to match his personality and learning style, clinical challenges related to the environment, his interpersonal style and the treatment team were encountered. Innovative approaches utilised to address these issues led to clinical excellence in practice.

Theoretical background

Although there may be a multitude of theories to explain Bill's criminal behaviour, these can generally be classified into one of three theoretical perspectives:

- sociological criminology
- clinical criminology
- social learning theory (Bonta 1997).

Sociological criminology targets societal factors, an enormous, if not impossible, task. Clinical criminology targets factors like anxiety and depression which are not associated with reduced criminal behaviour (Gendreau 1996a, Gendreau & Goggin 1996, Serin 1995, Serin & Brown 1996). Furthermore, the model of treatment associated with clinical criminology is supportive, client-centered therapy, an approach which has demonstrated limited effectiveness in the treatment of criminal behaviour (Bonta 1997). Thus, sociological and clinical criminological perspectives are of limited value in the identification of criminogenic needs or the treatment of criminal behaviour (Andrews & Bonta 1994, Antonowicz & Ross 1994).

Social learning theory emphasises the role of situational and personal variables that the individual brings with them to any given situation, each containing potential positive and negative consequences. Personal variables consist of cognitive factors such as attitudes, values and beliefs, social support and associates, and social skills and behavioural history. Social learning theory maintains that criminal behaviour is learned in accordance with the same principles of learning as any other behaviour (Bonta 1997). Factors derived from social learning theory (antisocial attitudes and associates) show a stronger relationship to criminal behaviour than those factors derived from sociological criminology (e.g. social class position) or clinical criminology (e.g. personal distress or psychopathology) (Andrews et al 1990, Antonowicz & Ross 1994). Social learning theory is of value in the management of criminal behaviour, identifying factors or criminogenic needs that, when treated, reduce recidivism. It is suggestive of a cognitive–behavioural model of treatment, which has demonstrated effectiveness in the treatment of criminal behaviour (Andrews et al 1990).

Generally, social learning theory suggests the consideration of three principles for the intervention and treatment of offenders:

1. Interventions be targeted at criminogenic needs
2. Treatment be tailored to meet the individual needs or learning history of the offender
3. The level of intervention be matched to the offender's perceived risk level (Bonta 1997).

These are often referred to as the need, responsivity and risk principles and are repeatedly identified as critical to effective treatment with offender clients (Andrews 1996, Andrews et al 1990, Antonowicz & Ross 1994, Gendreau 1996b, Losel 1996, Voorhis 1997).

Failing to consider these principles may be harmful. Treatment that is not targeted at criminogenic needs is not likely to reduce recidivism, and treatment outcome may be limited if treatment is not matched to the learning style of the client. While interventions appropriately matched with risk level are effective, interventions inappropriately matched with risk are ineffective and may have a negative effect (Andrews & Bonta 1994).

Further principles of effective treatment include both programme and therapeutic integrity (Antonowicz & Ross 1994, Gendreau 1996a). Programme integrity is high when the intended content is adhered to. High therapeutic integrity is present when the therapist's approach is congruent with the model of treatment upon which the programme is based. Additional characteristics of effective treatment identified in the literature include: role-playing/modelling, cognitive skills training (negotiation, interpersonal skills and assertiveness), multifaceted programming, offering a systematic system of rewards and based in a sound conceptual model (cognitive–behavioural) (Antonowicz & Ross 1994, Gendreau 1996b). These principles of effective treatment will be highlighted as they relate to the case of Bill.

CASE STUDY: BILL

Bill presented with a history of antisocial, acting-out behaviour, coupled with long-standing difficulties in getting along with other people. He experienced a chaotic childhood filled with neglect and abuse. Reports indicate that his father, an alcoholic, was frequently verbally and physically abusive to his mother, although Bill claims to have no memory of this. His father died violently, the victim of a family dispute, when Bill was only 6 years old. Unfortunately, violence and abuse continued to plague his young life. His mere presence served to remind his mother constantly of the abuse she suffered from his father and, as a result, Bill was often beaten by her or confined in restricted areas. He frequently witnessed intrafamilial sexual and physical assaults and recalls feelings of anger and helplessness at being too small to intervene. He vowed that one day he would stop the abuse.

He had many difficulties adjusting to school and was frequently in fights with classmates and/or older boys, particularly when these individuals were harassing or bullying either himself, someone he cared about or someone he perceived as vulnerable. He gained a sense of power and control through his use of violence and learned early in life that this was the only way to avoid being a victim. School reports indicated that he had a 'short fuse' and that he frequently responded to others in a physically aggressive manner. He had academic problems and had to repeat grade five. He left school in grade seven at the age of 14.

Alcohol misuse was common in Bill's family and he first began to drink when he was only 8 years old. Initially, he would consume any leftover alcohol found in his home after parties held by his mother or other family members. Bill enjoyed the way that alcohol numbed his feelings of vulnerability and pain. He later experimented with marijuana, cocaine and amphetamines but his preferred formula was the combined effects of alcohol and anxiolytics. Bill had difficulty maintaining long-term intimate relationships and associated only with those who supported his use of alcohol and aggression. Family members and friends would call on him to help them reclaim stolen property or to 'even a score'. By the time he reached 24, Bill had nine convictions for violent offences; these he felt to be justified, stating that he was either protecting, or seeking revenge for, those he viewed as unable to defend themselves. A direct correlation existed between the intensity of his violence and the amount of alcohol he consumed, with each subsequent offence becoming more violent. His frequent periods of incarceration further exposed him to a violent milieu, where those perceived to be in control are either feared or respected; where manipulation and intimidation are deemed acceptable means of asserting power and control (Schafer 1997).

His perennial difficulties in getting along with others, coupled with a severe alcohol problem, culminated in a serious crime, of which he has no recollection. While on parole from a previous sentence, in a drug- and alcohol-induced 'blackout', Bill stabbed and killed one man and severely injured two others. He was convicted of manslaughter, aggravated assault and assault causing bodily harm and was sentenced to an additional 8 years. Bill was initially classified as a 'medium security' inmate, but was quickly re-classified as 'maximum security' because of his involvement with assaults on other inmates, verbal abuse of staff members and several institutional charges including fighting and misappropriation of funds. With deeply ingrained antisocial attitudes, a network of antisocial associates, a substance misuse problem and a lack of insight into his problems, Bill entered treatment.

Treatment context

Bill was referred from a maximum security institution to an intensive treatment programme for violent offenders, the ABC programme, at the Regional Psychiatric Centre, Prairies, a multi-level mental health facility operated by the Correctional Service of Canada. The ABC programme was established in 1993 to provide intensive treatment to male offenders serving federal sentences with the Correctional Service of Canada, who have an extensive history of criminal violence, anger control problems and/or serious institutional conduct. The programme based on social learning principles is anchored in a cognitive–behavioural framework and emphasises group therapy complemented by individual therapy. The programme can accommodate 24 male offenders, taking participants 6 months to complete. A multidisciplinary team of mental health professionals and correctional staff are involved in programme delivery (Wong 1997). All participants are volunteers and may withdraw from treatment at any time. Conversely, clients may be discharged from the programme for violation of the treatment agreement.

Programme goals include assisting offenders in changing their attitudes and behaviours, while helping them put together an individualised comprehensive relapse prevention plan. To facilitate programme implementation, the ABC Workbook (Ruest, in press) was developed by treatment staff to enhance programme integrity and to serve as a formalised guide for clients and treatment staff alike. Key modules include an orientation to treatment, guides to journal writing, the development of an autobiography, assertiveness training and anger management. As with all treatment programmes, it begins with an in-depth assessment. The majority of clients assessed are accepted into treatment, but there are occasions when the match between the treatment programme and the client's needs or risk are not consistent with the underpinning principles.

Problems/needs

Gendreau (1996b) asserts that a thorough assessment is an essential component of effective treatment. Bill's assessment consisted of a complete file review, one-to-one interviews, direct observation in a variety of activities, psychological testing and the use of the Violence Risk Scale – Experimental Version 1 (VRS–E1) (Wong & Gordon 1996). The VRS–E1, an actuarial assessment guide, is used by therapists to score both static risk factors, such as age of first violent conviction, and dynamic risk factors, such as antisocial attitude or emotional disinhibition. The results of the VRS–E1 are used to identify the offender's criminogenic needs upon admission and to assess any changes in dynamic risk factors at termination of treatment. Ultimately, this tool will be used to discern the offender's risk of re-offending violently. Bill was considered a good candidate for treatment in the ABC programme. His score on the VRS–E1 was indicative of a high-risk, recidivist offender and many of his identified, dynamic risk factors matched treatment targets in the ABC programme. The

following criminogenic needs became the focus of treatment:

- Antisocial attitudes
- Antisocial associates
- Substance misuse
- Lack of insight into his violent behaviour.

Interventions

An individualised treatment plan was developed to address the identified treatment needs. Interventions were targeted at criminogenic factors, and his learning style and personality were considered when his treatment plan was designed, and his primary therapists assigned. Social learning theory identifies variables that individuals bring with them to any given situation: behaviour history, cognitive factors (attitudes, values and beliefs), social supports and associates and social skills (Bonta 1997). Although Bill's history is a source of valuable information regarding behavioural patterns, it cannot be changed. Similarly, Bill could not simply control or avoid every situation in which he tends to use aggression, intimidation or violence. Bill had mistakenly attempted to avoid violence by controlling others, only to learn that his controlling behaviour created situations where he was more likely to use violence, as, for example, when someone did not agree to follow his rules. Clearly, priority interventions had to be anchored in a cognitive–behavioural approach and targeted at the remaining dynamic variables: cognitive factors, social support and associates and social skills.

Highlights significant to the case will be presented, though it is beyond the scope of this case study to outline all the interventions used to address Bill's problems. Likewise, many of the interventions utilised had general application and targeted more than one problem area.

Journalling, anger log and autobiography

Journalling, anger logs and autobiography are key components of the ABC programme and are intended to facilitate self-awareness and insight in participants. Journal writing is used in helping clients to gain an understanding of the relationship between thoughts, feelings and behaviours. Anger logs assist clients to develop an awareness of the frequency, intensity and duration of acting-out behaviour and the identification of precipitating events. Bill completed an autobiography to reveal the relationship of his present behaviour to his learning history. Bill also kept a feelings journal and completed anger logs but the benefits of doing so were limited. He was not a reflective or analytical thinker and simply recorded his activities and what he thought others should, or should not, do. Although he did not benefit from these exercises in the manner in which they were intended, his journal entries provided his primary therapists with insights into how to best develop a trusting relationship with him; and, more importantly, the opportunity to further explore his very rigid framework of values and beliefs.

Role plays and feedback

Given his concrete learning style, Bill learned well from role modelling and preferred specific instruction and direct feedback. Staff and group members shared the impact that his use of aggression, intimidation and violent behaviour had on them and encouraged him to evaluate the positive and negative consequences of his behaviour. Bill was video-taped role playing a number of situations which he identified as likely to provoke a verbal or physical aggressive response, such as watching someone 'target' weaker individuals. He would later review the video tapes with his primary therapist to identify his aggressive response, receive specific feedback and discuss possible alternatives.

Creating cognitive dissonance

The interventions targeted at changing Bill's attitudes were designed to create cognitive dissonance, which arises when two opposing beliefs, based on different role expectations, exist at the same time, creating a dilemma or discomfort in the individual (Eagly 1993, Festinger 1957). It was hoped that by creating cognitive dissonance

Bill would begir
his antisocial a†

Strategies u
included pro
and encoura
ities. One of
was that ev
say or, in p
was incorporatє
Bill was asked to make ɯ
group that he thought would dεɯ
person from embarking on a life of crime. тɪɪ
assumption was that by making prosocial statements cognitive dissonance would be created in Bill if he did not 'walk his talk', that is, behave in a fashion congruent with what he was saying.

Role modelling and skill building

Group sessions focused on skill development in the area of anger management, stress management and assertiveness training. The emphasis in these groups was on the practical application of each skill taught, and situations that arose on the unit (ward) were often used as examples. Furthermore, Bill role played situations specific to his problem areas, for example, how to assertively say no to alcohol or how to appropriately handle a 'put down'. When Bill reacted aggressively on the unit, he was required to address his behaviour in group by identifying thoughts, feelings, or beliefs triggering the reaction, to explore methods to avoid the escalation of anger and to discuss alternative ways to deal with the situation. He was also asked to explore his pattern of aggression, intimidation and violence in the community and to develop alternative plans.

Staff role modelled the appropriate skills, both in group and during individual interviews. Bill would occasionally engage in a game of cards or a board game with staff. He was also encouraged to develop a prosocial support system prior to his discharge. Bill had very few experiences associating with prosocial individuals and needed to be systematically reinforced for his use of socially acceptable language, rather than relying heavily on prison

. Interacting in a more socially
anner resulted in people respond-
ositively to him, thus reinforcing his
rosocial language. Furthermore, Bill
ed a number of community support
rces that he could use after his discharge
with assistance from staff he established
ontact with them.

Reinforcement

The team consistently reinforced appropriate behaviour with social praise. Milestone celebrations are incorporated into the programme and serve two functions: to validate the efforts of the group members and to provide a social opportunity which does not revolve around alcohol or drugs. Social praise, although an unfamiliar concept to Bill, was very effective, even though he initially doubted people and questioned their motivations or sincerity.

Substance misuse interventions

Initially, Bill had difficulties appreciating the extent to which his substance misuse was directly related to the intensity of his violence and his crime cycle. While in treatment, he attended Alcoholics Anonymous (AA) meetings which involved volunteers from the community. In addition to providing Bill with information and support regarding these problems, the meetings also served as an opportunity to practise newly learned social and assertion skills; and, perhaps more importantly, to engage with people from a wider social network. Individual and group sessions focused on the identification of positive and negative consequences of substance use. Bill was able to compare the dulling effect that alcohol had on his emotions as a short-term positive consequence of using alcohol with loss of inhibition and resulting violence as an overriding negative consequence. Furthermore, treatment staff assisted Bill in identifying his substance misuse pattern, collaboratively developing an intervention plan that focused on alternative means of meeting his needs.

Outcomes

Bill's progress was reviewed daily by his primary therapists and his treatment plan was formally reviewed by the multi-disciplinary team at least monthly. The formal review consisted of an interim evaluation of his progress, including input from all disciplines, Bill and his peers. Bill demonstrated insight into his aggressive behaviour as treatment progressed. Once he became aware of the wider impact of his aggressive and intimidating behaviour on others, he took the responsibility of assisting them to respond differently towards him by demonstrating an openness to their feedback. Interim assessments, which included attitude scales, indicated that he was making a positive shift in his attitudes. Change was also reflected in the post-treatment VRS–E1. Perhaps most importantly, he was finally able to identify that his perception of others being victims and perpetrators was a trigger for much of his aggressive and violent behaviour and he was further able to identify the thoughts and beliefs that contributed to this. He was able to participate in conflict resolution and problem-solve in order to improve his relationships with others. Despite the changes Bill made in treatment, he remained a high risk to re-offend as the changes had not been sustained for a significant period of time. However, the treatment team's hope was that with appropriate community support he would be able to sustain these changes and subsequently reduce his risk.

Reflections on practice

Providing treatment in a forensic milieu is a challenge in itself. Provision of treatment to a violent offender, whose typical pattern of communication involves intimidation and aggression, creates additional dilemmas. The trials and tribulations of caring for Bill have three chief sources:

• The prison/forensic environment
• Bill's interpersonal style/behaviour
• The treatment team.

Environmental challenges

Within the prison environment, manipulation is seen as an acceptable way to pass the time (Peternelj-Taylor & Johnson 1995). Given that the programme involves group participation, whereby offenders are expected to self-disclose, it becomes easy for offenders to prey upon one another to gratify personal needs. Bill's tendency to protect and seek revenge on others' behalf was easily exploited within the penal subculture. He adhered to a code of conduct among the incarcerated, the 'con code', with anyone breaking ranks being written off by Bill. Even though he was in a mental health treatment facility, the prevailing culture dominated. The treatment team found that an effective way to guard against issues arising from the 'con code' was to discuss them openly in group.

Initially, Bill's peers were reluctant to give him any kind of feedback. Although he was not a large man, he would intimidate others in the group through intense eye contact and clenched fists (especially when he did not agree with what he was hearing). This, coupled with his repeated references to his past use of violence in similar situations, gave a very strong message that dialogue with Bill was not safe. These behaviours were pointed out to Bill, with the expectation of change. With time, and reinforcement, these interventions were effective.

Interpersonal challenges

Bill's initial behaviour was extremely aggressive, raising concerns among team members regarding his suitability to remain in the group. This apprehension was shared with Bill and the treatment team elected to give him an opportunity to continue in treatment as long as he adhered to the conditions of a treatment agreement. This specifically outlined that he would not attempt to control other clients' activities, intimidate fellow clients verbally, physically or through others, interfere with the treatment of others nor to accept a position of authority in the institution. When he failed to follow the treatment contract, he was expected to address the group and

identify the situation, his thoughts, feelings, behaviours and interventions.

In addition to Bill's interpersonal style, his rigid system of values and beliefs presented a further clinical challenge. For example, his therapist being a few minutes late for a scheduled appointment created a significant rupture to the therapeutic alliance. Successful resolution involved an exploration of Bill's expectations, negotiating realistic expectations, the team's rationale for the treatment approach, the therapist's or team's commitment and apologies, when appropriate. Resolving disruptions to the therapeutic alliance successfully resulted in additional new experiences for him. Consequently, Bill eventually began to alter his schema and accept that individuals make mistakes as a feature of ordinary life.

Treatment team challenges

Andrews (1996) asserts that health professionals often operate under the erroneous belief that treatment is only effective with low-risk offenders. Team members may question the rationale for investing in offenders who they predict will re-offend. A poor prognosis may influence commitment to the treatment plan, as if treatment outcome was a personal reward rather than there being implicit value in the professional effort. High-risk offenders benefit the most from treatment, as they have the most to gain. However, their criminal history and aggressive interpersonal style can provoke strong reactions from the team.

No-one appreciated witnessing, or experiencing, Bill's verbal attacks. Although he did not engage in any physical altercations during treatment, his verbal assaults, coupled with aggressive non-verbal gestures (slamming doors, clenching his fists, punching his hand) made it difficult for staff to consistently enforce limits and set boundaries. Team members found it very difficult not to personalise his aggression. Some questioned the value of allowing Bill to remain in the treatment programme and continued to challenge his primary therapists to justify their investment in his treatment. In turn, his primary therapists were rigorous about reinforcing realistic expectations and continually provided illustrations of his progress.

Although diverse opinions make for a resource-rich team, when emotional reactions conflict with sound clinical judgements, a polarisation between team members may develop. This can have a negative impact on the overall integrity of the treatment programme, particularly when team members stop valuing each other's opinions. Staff were provided with opportunities to talk about their personal reactions to Bill during team meetings and were reminded how well he fitted the ABC programme. They were encouraged to view him as a clinical challenge and to work together as professionals. However, in reality, there were those who never did engage in his treatment.

Conclusions

The innovative approaches used in working with Bill resulted in increased confidence among treatment team members to intervene with challenging clients. This necessitated that team members examined their clinical proficiency in order to ensure programme and therapeutic integrity. Although absolute consensus did not occur, the controversy surrounding the treatment plan promoted increased dialogue among team members, thereby creating an informal learning milieu. The lessons learned have continued to be of use in working with other aggressive and intimidating clients.

Shortly after completing the ABC programme, Bill was discharged to the community under supervision. At this time, he acknowledged using alcohol (abstinence being a condition of his release) on at least one occasion for which his community supervision was suspended. After a brief period of incarceration, he was again released under similar conditions. Recent drug and alcohol screening indicates that he is maintaining his sobriety, but unfortunately he has re-offended. However, treatment is still considered a success because of the lack of violence associated with this most recent crime.

REFERENCES

Andrews D 1996 Criminal recidivism is predictable and can be influenced: an update. Forum on Corrections Research 8(3): 42–44

Andrews D, Bonta J 1994 The psychology of criminal conduct. Anderson, Cincinnati, Ohio

Andrews D, Zinger I, Hoge R, Bonta J, Gendreau P, Cullen F 1990 Does correctional treatment work? A clinically relevant and psychologically informed meta-analysis. Criminology 28(3): 369–404

Antonowicz D, Ross R 1994 Essential components of successful rehabilitation programs for offenders. International Journal of Offender Therapy and Comparative Criminology 28(2): 97–104

Bonta J 1997 Risk assessment module 1: Theories of criminal behaviour. In: Wong S (ed) Risk assessment and management self study manual. Correctional Service of Canada, Saskatoon

Eagly A 1993 The psychology of attitudes. Harcourt Brace Javanovich, Toronto

Festinger L 1957 A theory of cognitive dissonance. Stanford University Press, Stanford

Gendreau P 1996a Offender rehabilitation: what we know and what needs to be done. Criminal Justice and Behavior 23(1): 144–161

Gendreau P 1996b The principles of effective intervention with offenders. In: Harland A (ed) Choosing correctional options that work: defining the demand and evaluating the supply. Sage, Thousand Oaks, ch 5, p117

Gendreau P, Goggin C 1996 Principles of effective correctional programming. Forum on Corrections Research 8(3): 38–41

Losel F 1996 Effective correctional programming: what empirical research tells us and what it doesn't. Forum on Corrections Research 8(3): 33–36

Peternelj-Taylor C A, Johnson R L 1995 Serving time: psychiatric mental health nursing in corrections. Journal of Psychosocial Nursing and Mental Health Services 33(8): 12–19

Ruest B (ed) (in press) Aggressive behaviour control workbook. Correctional Services of Canada, Saskatoon

Schafer P E 1997 When a client develops an attraction: successful resolution versus boundary violation. Journal of Psychiatric and Mental Health Nursing 4(3): 203–211

Serin R 1995 Psychological intervention in corrections. In: Leis T, Motiuk L, Ogloff J (eds) Forensic psychology: policy and practice in corrections. Correctional Services of Canada, Ottawa, ch 4, p 36

Serin R, Brown S 1996 Strategies for enhancing the treatment of violent offenders. Forum on Corrections Research 8(3): 45–48

Voorhis P 1997 Correctional classification and the 'responsivity principle'. Forum on Corrections Research 9(7): 46–50

Wong S 1997 Aggressive behaviour control program. Let's Talk 22(5): 18–19

Wong S, Gordon A 1996 Violence risk scale – experimental version 1 (VRS–E1). Department of Psychology and Research, Saskatoon

CONTENTS

Critical incident management: aggression and violence

Brodie Paterson, David Leadbetter and Cheryl Tringham

Introduction

Unfortunately in forensic practice a proportion of critical incidents may involve violence directed to others or self. This case study explores the management of one woman, with a complex psychiatric history, during a critical incident involving violence. It is fictitious in that while elements and details from real incidents have been drawn upon, details have been changed to produce a composite study. The study attempts to place the description of the intervention, which focuses on an episode of violent behaviour, in context both by brief reference to the wider situation and to the literature on de-escalation and the management of physical violence.

Background literature

Responding to a crisis involves the nurse, and other members of the care team, drawing upon their wider knowledge and value base as well as that relating specifically to the management of acutely disturbed behaviour (Paterson et al 1997a). That wider knowledge and value base includes awareness of communication skills, knowledge of key helping strategies for individuals experiencing mental illness and a positive value base which expresses itself via empathy, honesty and unconditional positive regard towards individuals who may present with challenging behaviours (Leadbetter & Paterson 1995, Lowe 1992).

In addition, practice must reflect an understanding of the relevant ethical principles. Aiken & Tarbuck (1995) stress that nurses and other health care professionals must strive to promote rather than deny autonomy in all settings. This is represented by the legal duty to obtain consent prior to the provision of treatment or care (Mason & McCall Smith 1991). However, the requirement to respect another's autonomy is not absolute and can be overridden by competing moral considerations. Thus the autonomy of individuals can be restricted against their wishes, if their autonomous actions would unnecessarily place themselves or others at risk or fail to take account of the autonomy of others. Further, certain individuals may be considered 'non-autonomous' as a consequence of their mental disorder.

The principle of autonomy does not have automatic precedence over that of beneficence, which requires, in essence, the nurse to act in the patient's best interests (Edwards 1996). Complications can thus arise in situations in which the patient's expressed perceptions of his or her best interests conflict with the nurse's perceptions of the patient's best interests. On the one hand, the nurse is charged with a duty to foster and develop patient autonomy, and on the other has a duty to act always in the patient's best interests (UKCC 1992). The patient may make treatment choices at odds with that of the nurse, or exhibit behaviour which the nurse considers not to be in the patient's best interests or places the patient or others at serious risk.

In determining whether restricting the autonomy of an individual can be justified ethically, it is necessary to reflect upon the legal position. If physical violence is a foreseeable event, then practitioners need to know the legal parameters that affect their practice in that setting with that patient. These will vary between practice areas and will reflect relevant statute law (such as the Mental Health Act 1983 and Mental Health Act Scotland 1984) and common law (such as the definition of assault). Practitioners must recognise that any restriction of the liberty or autonomy of a patient unless a 'lawful excuse' exists could be an offence (Lyon 1994). The potential

charges a practitioner might face include false imprisonment or assault and battery.

False imprisonment has been defined as 'an act of the defendant which directly and intentionally or negligently causes the confinement of the plaintiff within an area delimited by the defendant' (Brazier Law of Torts: 28 cited by Lyon 1994; 76). Confinement does not necessarily imply actual physical restriction; any measure by which an individual was prevented from leaving a hospital including its grounds, a room, a vehicle, specific area or even a chair could potentially constitute confinement. The restriction on liberty has to be 'total', in that patients would risk injury if they tried to escape or it would be unreasonable to have expected patients to attempt to escape in the circumstances.

In English Law, an assault is defined as 'any act of the defendant which directly and either intentionally or negligently causes the plaintiff immediately to apprehend a contact with his person.' Battery is defined 'as any act of the defendant which directly and intentionally or negligently causes some physical contact with the plaintiff without the plaintiff's consent' (Brazier 1989 cited by Lyon 1994: 79). In both instances the type of contact, whether actual or anticipated, must clearly go beyond that liable to be experienced in everyday life.

Lawful excuse

In demonstrating lawful excuse for their actions, which could otherwise constitute a criminal offence, the practitioner needs to show that a legitimate reason to use force and/or restrict the liberty of that patient existed and that the actions taken were reasonable in the circumstances (Gostin 1986).

Hoggett (1985, 1990) proposes that there are five main legitimate reasons for the use of force which may serve as a lawful excuse:

1. *To prevent a crime from being committed.* The English Criminal Law Act (1967) states explicitly that: 'A person may use such force as is reasonable in the circumstances in the prevention of a crime.

2. *To prevent a breach of the peace.* Lyon (1994: 89) defines a breach of the peace as a situation where 'harm is done or likely to be done to a person or in his presence, to his property: or harm is feared through an affray, riot, assault or other disturbance.'

3. *To defend the self.* The law imposes a duty on any potential victim to attempt to make an escape, but concedes that it may not always be possible. In such a situation, the use of reasonable force to protect the self is likely to be considered legitimate (Martin 1990).

4. *To restrain a dangerous lunatic.* Common law gives powers to detain the 'insane' in certain circumstances where their behaviour places their own, or others', safety at risk which predate current modern mental health legislation (Brookshaw vs Hopkins 1790). In determining what constitutes lunacy, a modern interpretation of these concepts would generally include those individuals covered under the term mental disorder used in both the Mental Health Act 1983 and the Mental Health Act (Scotland) 1984. This would embrace both those experiencing mental ill health and/or people with learning disabilities (Hogget 1990, Lyon 1994: 87)

5. *Exercise of force derived from statutory authority.* For example, removing a person to hospital without their consent, where this is urgently necessary, all other options having failed or being impractical. In such cases force could be used as a last resort to carry out the hospital order. Staff members must still demonstrate reasonableness in their actions in both the decision to use force and the degree and nature of force to be used. Interestingly, this 'lawful excuse' would already be provided by the restraint of dangerous lunatic provisions in point four.

The existence of a legitimate reason to use force does not of itself make it lawful. The practitioner will still be required to demonstrate that the force used was reasonable in both degree and duration. In determining 'reasonableness' two criteria are likely to be used. First, was the use of force the only feasible option? If there were other options not involving force, then the use of force is questionable. Second, if force was the only

option, was it used in proportion to the harm it was intended to prevent? Physical force should not be employed either in excess to the harm which it is intended to prevent or in punishment or revenge (Dimond 1990). Where violence is a foreseeable event, risk assessment should consider the issue of physical intervention. This should identify the potential for inappropriate behaviour, the risk of harm to the patient or others arising from that behaviour and the potential risks of physical and psychological harm if force is used to restrain (Paterson et al 1997b).

A clinical algorithm is given in Figure 6.1 to guide decision-making in this area. It emphasises the need to attempt to intervene early and to attempt to de-escalate or to block attacks and escape in preference to using restraint (Conlon et al 1995). It can be helpful to review the work of Smith described by Kaplan & Wheeler (1983) as the 'assault cycle' (Fig. 6.2). Smith developed the model based on his work with prisoners in California. From an analysis of a large number of incidents involving violence, it was proposed that many violent incidents could be described as consisting of a series of five phases:

1. Triggering phase
2. Escalation phase
3. Crisis phase
4. Recovery phase
5. Post-crisis depression phase.

Arousal and cognition

Crucial to an understanding of this model is recognition of the role of arousal. Arousal is an innate response to anxiety-provoking situations with physiological features sometimes referred to as the 'fight or flight' reaction. Arousal in itself is not intrinsically associated with anger and hostility. Yet, it appears to be strongly linked to aggression and violence (Averill 1982), although violence can occur in its absence (Berkowitz 1993). It affects behaviour both indirectly via its influence on cognitions and directly via the instinctual desire to act to reduce high levels of arousal in the 'fight or flight' response (Breakwell & Rowett 1989).

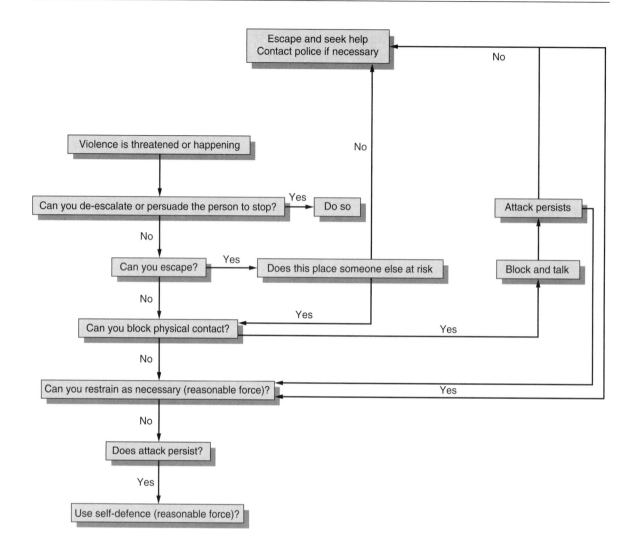

Fig. 6.1 Decision-making when responding to violence (adapted from Rowett & Breakwell 1992).

Novaco (1975) argues that events provoke anger only in the way that the individual interprets them. Individuals have their own unique way of interpreting the world around them which will determine their reaction to an event (Novaco 1977). Of note is the observation that the interaction between arousal and anger may be invidious. Whilst under stress, and thus aroused, individuals may be more likely to make negative attributions with regard to the actions or intent of others and thus likely to continually trigger thoughts maintaining and producing anger and high arousal (Mueller 1983)

Thus, either overt or covert events and their interpretation may function as triggers which act to move arousal levels upwards from some notional baseline towards a crisis. However, the factors which influence an individual's behaviour can change in nature and relevance, as the person's arousal level changes as a product of the interaction between arousal and cognition (Fig. 6.3). Behaviour in adults is usually under a degree of cognitive control. Thus, we can appraise a situation, make a judgement, consider our response and then act. Cognitive control, however, can rapidly decline as arousal increases

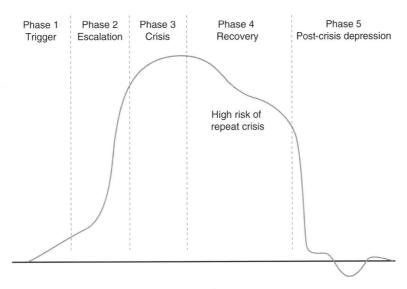

Fig. 6.2 The assault cycle (adapted from Kaplan & Wheeler 1983).

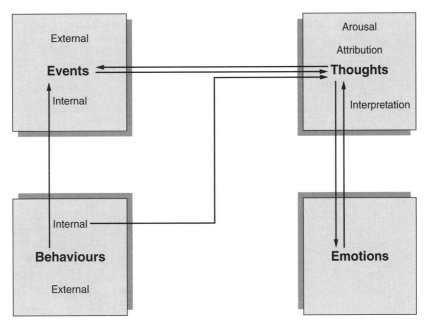

Fig. 6.3 Interaction between events' interpretation and arousal.

and emotion moves to become the predominant influence on behaviour. In the initial stages of a potential confrontation, therefore, rational argument may be a primary tool, but if the patient's arousal level is very high, other strategies such as distraction may be more viable (Leadbetter & Paterson 1995).

This insight is relevant not only in considering the behaviour of patients but in promoting awareness that critical incidents can create arousal in all the participants in a situation, particularly staff. The ability to recognise and manage one's own arousal is, therefore, a key skill in responding to potential crisis (Blair 1991).

Table 6.1 Summary care plan

Problem	Aim of intervention	Strategy
1 Auditory hallucinations. Main voice (only voice recognised is that of deceased daughter)	Reduce distress arising from experience of voices	Promote use of identified coping strategies and involve in coping strategies group: • listening to personal stereo • physical exercise • use of step machine
2 Motor agitation accompanied by poor concentration	Reduce motor agitation	Agitation believed linked to: • current medication regime *Medication to be reviewed via multi-diciplinary team* • alcohol withdrawal *Discuss with Community Detox Team*
3 Sleep disturbance	Promote normal sleep pattern	• facilitate use of relaxation tape and • milky drink at bedtime (ensure availability of caffeine-free coffee for Danielle's use) • promote access to exercise facilities; involve in exercise group • monitor sleep pattern
4 Paranoid misinterpretation of others' conversations	Acknowledge potential for misinterpretation. Discuss concerns with others	• modified anger management • contract covering behaviour
5 Risk of physical violence directed towards other patients. Known to use and construct weapons	Maintain safe environment	• assess via unit risk management protocol • communicate risk management guidance to all staff

Planning to manage potential confrontations should of course start before actual situations occur (Cox & Cox 1993) and one crucial element of de-escalation is to attempt to avoid triggering behaviours. If we know that particular situations are difficult or stressful for patients, then we can work with patients in the longer term to explore their perceptions and interpretations of those situations. If, however, patients are acutely unwell, then we may seek to prevent exposure to stimuli or situations which we anticipate may trigger violence.

CASE STUDY: DANIELLE

History and context

Danielle has been an in-patient in a local psychiatric intensive care unit for 2 days. She agreed to be admitted informally, for assessment, following concern over her deteriorating mental state and accompanying self-neglect and problems with self-medication compounded by alcohol abuse. She has a diagnosis of paranoid schizophrenia and substance dependency and was previously detained in a Special Hospital for 4 years following the death of her infant daughter aged 18 months when she was considered unfit to plead to a charge of manslaughter. Her partner, who is the father of her surviving son, was convicted at that time on a charge of manslaughter. She presently has no contact with her ex-partner or with her son, who was adopted during her period of detention.

When her mental health is poor, Danielle experiences auditory hallucinations in which she hears a number of voices. She cannot distinguish all the voices but believes the main one is that of her dead daughter. During acute episodes, she also becomes convinced that others, particularly women, are talking about her and calling her a murderer. She has previously carried out assaults on other women in-patients in which she has used, or attempted to use, weapons; she struck one person on the head with a radio and attempted to stab another in the eyes with a piece of stiff wire broken from a coathanger (see Table 6.1).

Critical incident

Phase 1 Trigger 2.00 am

Danielle is distressed and becoming increasingly agitated, saying she cannot sleep because her daughter is whispering to her. She has got up and is wandering up and down a small corridor outside other patients' rooms shouting. Her care plan (Table 6.1) has been followed regarding sleep promotion but she has been unable to settle. Danielle's key worker is currently on days, but one of her associate workers, Morna, has been working closely with her.

Morna, who is the senior registered nurse on duty, has been trying to calm the situation and her judgement at this point is that Danielle is experiencing, primarily, anxiety. Consequently, her interventions are targeted at trying to help Danielle relax. She has thus worked closely with Danielle but has been careful to respect her personal space (Turnbull et al 1990). She has tried to use a calm relaxed tone in conjunction with active listening skills (Paterson et al 1997a), being careful not to force eye contact (Burrow 1994). She has not sought to explore the reasons for Danielle's anxiety, her rationale being that at a time when Danielle is tired and distraught, this was not likely to be helpful. Instead, she has tried to actively problem-solve. In doing so, she has attempted to identify areas where she can help Danielle use positive coping strategies by suggesting activities to help her manage her voices. Unfortunately, all her suggestions have been rejected and an effort to explore the effect of stimulus change (La Vigna & Donnellan 1986) by involving a male care assistant, Lucas, has been similarly unproductive. Morna has, though, asked him to remain

immediately available should the situation deteriorate.

Phase 2 Escalation 2.20 am

Morna now becomes increasingly concerned by this situation. Danielle continues to pace up and down a small area of corridor and is now clearly angry, shouting loudly at her voices, staff and other patients. A number of other patients have been disturbed and are angry at being woken up. Morna has already sought the assistance of another care assistant to reassure those patients who have got up to investigate the commotion and to remove them to a quiet area in the interim. Danielle has rejected all offers of assistance, including suggestions to go elsewhere for a cup of tea and attempts to persuade her to return to her room. After about 15 minutes of this deteriorating situation, Morna decides there is a growing potential for a violent confrontation should other patients come out of their rooms. She now feels that she should offer Danielle her prescribed as required (PRN) medication. She has explained her concerns to Danielle, asking her firmly to comply, raising her voice momentarily, and 'mood matching' to gain Danielle's attention (Davies 1989), who was shouting over her.

Phase 3 Crisis 2.40 am

Morna offers Danielle her PRN medication but Danielle becomes extremely distressed by this. She starts to scream and shout at Morna who tries to withdraw but is grabbed by Danielle, rushing forward, trying to scratch and punch her. Morna blocks these blows and steps back triggering her personal alarm. Although Morna loudly tells Danielle to stop, Danielle persists with her attempt to assault her by punching and kicking at her. At this point, another member of staff arrives and Morna asks for help to initiate restraint, in which all staff had received training (Paterson et al 1992). After a struggle, Danielle is restrained on a sofa at the end of the corridor; Morna having decided that they could safely restrain her in a seated position, and that this would be less traumatic for Danielle than being restrained face down.

Phase 4 Recovery 2.45 am

Morna is aware that the effects of physical arousal following violence can mean there is a high risk of further violence, particularly for around an hour after incidents. Her aim therefore during this period is to cease the use of physical restraint as soon as is appropriate, without unduly compromising safety for staff and other patients. To this end, the restraint is gradually relaxed, as Danielle calms down and accepts the offer of medication. Morna and the other staff member involved consciously avoided premature discussion of the incident or the reasons for it. The intention here was to avoid re-igniting the situation or trying to engage in premature, and hence unproductive, post-incident analysis.

Phase 5 Post-crisis depression

Although post-crisis depression is reported after violent incidents and can be suggested to have a physiological basis (adrenaline levels dipping slightly below normal before returning to baseline), this was not evident in Danielle's case. The medication she accepted seemed to help her sleep and so any evident signs were masked. Morna carried out a post-incident review with staff involved and wrote up the incident detailing what had happened and passed on that information at shift handover. She discussed Danielle's observation status with the duty psychiatrist and they agreed that she should be closely supervised over the next 24 hours, pending a more systematic review.

The next day, the key-worker sensitively explored this incident with Danielle to identify perceptions of what had triggered the events. Danielle's account was incomplete and jumbled, but her foremost recollection was that Morna 'looked at me as if she thought I was a murderer' and this precipitated the attack. In trying to help Danielle learn from the incident, a collaborative plan was developed, exploring alternative

management strategies (Neizo & Lanza 1984) attending to the following issues:

a. *The setting conditions for the behaviour*
   Danielle was tired and her voice was whispering that she had killed her daughter. This was more significant than usual because she had recently heard of the birth of a niece.
b. *Alternative behaviours/cognitions which Danielle could employ to prevent recurrence*
   Danielle could talk about what she perceived to be happening with regard to the non-verbal expressions of others (rather than acting on the thought). She could explore and question her own interpretations and consider alternatives.
c. *How Danielle could be helped, and by whom*
   Her key-worker would work with Danielle to practice her self-management strategies. A behavioural contract would be negotiated, incorporating Danielle's agreement to talk rather than exhibit aggression.

Outcome

The review of the incident was positive. Danielle was able to discuss a manifestation of her illness not previously recognised, particularly her tendency to misinterpret other people's eye contact with her. This would be compounded when under stress, especially when hearing her persecutory voice. Therapeutic work focused on aspects of anger management, aiming to raise her awareness and to explore coping strategies. Complementary interventions targeted stabilisation of her medication and reduction of side effects. She was also supported in re-establishing links with Alcoholics Anonymous, where she had previously been helped in addressing her problem drinking.

Conclusions

The practice of de-escalation by teams and individuals forms, of course, only one part of the co-ordinated effort that should form a 'total organisational response' (Cox & Cox 1993). It encompasses issues such as building design, service culture and values (Fein et al 1981), operational policies, procedures and working practices (Rice et al 1989). This study has sought to give an example of practice in de-escaltion at the level of the individual practitioner. The actions of staff, even where exemplary, will not prevent all incidents. In any crisis, the actions of an individual member of staff, or even of a team, are only some of the variables (Steadman 1982) which will determine the ultimate outcome.

REFERENCES

Aiken F, Tarbuck P 1995 Practical ethical and legal aspects of caring for the assaultive client. In: Stark C, Kidd B (eds) Management of violence and aggression in health care. Gaskell/Royal College of Psychiatrists, London

Averill J R 1982 Anger and aggression: an essay on emotion. Springer Verlag, New York

Berkowitz L 1993 Aggression: its consequences, causes and control. McGraw Hill, New York

Blair D T 1991 Assaultive behaviour: does provocation begin in the front office? Journal of Psychosocial and Mental Health Services 29(5): 21–26

Breakwell G, Rowett C 1989 Violence in social work. In: Browne K (ed) Human aggression: naturalistic approaches. Routledge, London

Brookshaw vs Hopkins (1790 Lofft) at 234.

Burrow S 1994 Nurse-aid management of psychiatric emergencies: 3. British Journal of Nursing 3(3): 121–125

Conlon L, Gage A, Hillis T 1995 Managerial and nursing perspectives on the response to inpatient violence. In: Crichton J (ed) Psychiatric patient violence: risk and response. Duckworth, London

Cox T, Cox S 1993 Psychosocial and organisational hazards: control and monitoring. Occupational Health Series, no 5. World Health Organization (Europe), Copenhagen

Criminal Law Act. 1967 HMSO, London

Davies W 1989 The prevention of assault on professional helpers. In: Howell K, Hollis C (eds) Clinical approaches to violence. Wiley, Chichester

Dimond B 1990 Legal aspects of nursing. Prentice Hall, London

Edwards S 1996 Nursing ethics: a principle based approach. Macmillan, London

Fein A F, Garreri E, Hansen P 1981 Teaching staff to cope with patient violence. Journal of Continuing Education in Nursing 12(2): 21–26

Gostin L 1986 Institutions observed: towards a new concept of secure provision in mental health. King Edward's Hospital Fund for London, London

Hoggett B 1985 Legal aspects of secure provision. In: Gostin, L (ed) Secure provision. Tavistock, London

Hoggett B 1990 Mental health law, 3rd edn. Sweet and Maxwell, London

Kaplan S G, Wheeler E G 1983 Survival skills for working with potentially violent patients. Social Casework 64: 339–345

La Vigna G, Donnellan A M 1986 Alternatives to punishment. Irvington, Washington

Leadbetter D, Paterson B 1995 De-escalating aggressive behaviour in the management of aggression and violence in health care. In: Stark C, Kidd B (eds) Management of violence and aggression in health care. Gaskell, The Royal College of Psychiatrists, London

Lowe T 1992 Characteristics of effective nursing interventions in the management of challenging behaviour. Journal of Advanced Nursing 17(11): 226–232

Lyon C 1994 Legal issues arising from the care, control and safety of children with learning disabilities who also present severe challenging behaviour. Mental Health Foundation, London

Martin A 1990 The case for self-defence. Health and Social Service Journal 88: 697

Mason J, McCall Smith A 1991 Law and medical ethics, 3rd edn. Butterworth, Edinburgh

Mental Health Act (England and Wales) 1983. HMSO, London

Mental Health (Scotland) Act. 1984 HMSO, London

Mueller C 1983 Environmental stressors and aggressive behaviour. In: Green R, Donnerstein E (eds) Aggression: theoretical and empirical reviews. Academic Press, New York

Neizo B A, Lanza M 1984 Post violence dialogue: perception change through language restructuring. Issues in Mental Health Nursing 6: 245–254

Novaco R 1975 Anger control: the development and evaluation of an experimental treatment. Health Co, Lexington DC

Novaco R 1977 Stress inoculation: a cognitive therapy for anger and its application to a case of depression. Journal of Consulting and Clinical Psychology 45: 600–608

Paterson B, Turnbull J, Aitken I 1992 An evaluation of a training course in the short term management of aggression. Nurse Education Today 12: 368–375

Paterson B, Leadbetter D, McComish A 1997a De-escalation in the short term management of violence: a process based approach. Nursing Times 93(7): 58–61

Paterson B, Tringham C, McComish A, Waters S 1997b Managing aggression and violence: a legal perspective on the use of force. Psychiatric Care 4(3): 128–131

Rice M, Harris G, Varney G, Quinsay V 1989 Violence in institutions: understanding, prevention and control. Hoefgre and Huber, Toronto

Rowett C, Breakwell G 1992 Managing violence at work. National Foundation for Educational Research, Berkshire

Steadman H 1982 A situational approach to the understanding of violence. International Journal of Law and Psychiatry 5: 171–186

Turnbull J, Aitken I, Black L, Paterson B 1990 Turn it around: short term management of violence and aggression. Journal of Psychosocial Nursing and Mental Health Services 26(6): 6–12

United Kingdom Central Council (UKCC) 1992 Code of professional conduct. UKCC, London

CONTENTS

Changing the environment in the management of aggression

Richard Whittington

Introduction

What is the 'environment' in a mental health setting? How is this environment experienced by the people within it, both staff and patients, and what role does this experience have in generating anger and aggression? Evidence will be considered which implicates a number of environmental factors in increasing or reducing levels of aggression. This will be framed in a case study which illustrates some of the environmental processes which provoke, maintain and reduce aggression in mental health care. If environmental factors are as important as some of this evidence suggests, environmental changes should be urgently considered in any setting where violence is currently a problem.

Theoretical background

First, let us examine the concept of 'environment'. One common way of thinking about human aggressive behaviour is to divide the causes of such behaviour into factors which are largely biological and those which are largely environmental. By environmental factors, we mean events which impinge upon the person from outside of their bodies. Such events might include encounters with other people (the social or human environment) and encounters with certain types of physical environment (e.g. smells, decor). Environmental influences are made up of what people see and hear as well as what they smell, taste and physically feel. It should be acknowledged, however, that the

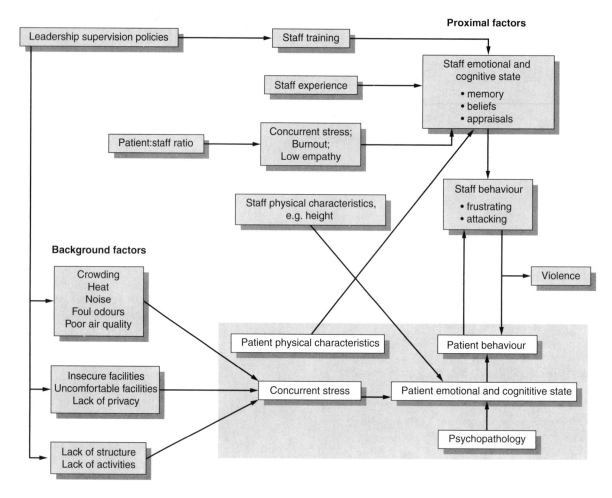

Fig. 6.4 Environmental factors influencing aggression in a mental health care setting.

relationship between environmental and biological factors in human behaviour is far more complex than this simple distinction will allow since the personal experience of all environmental events is mediated by cognitive processes such as appraisal (Lazarus & Folkman 1984). Therefore, any attempt to reduce aggression by environmental change must include consideration of such individual interpretations of the environment, especially when working with mentally disordered people whose perceptions of the environment may be very different from those of professionals. Notwithstanding this complexity, the focus of this case study is on the

'pure' external environment, separate from its mediated effect.

The importance of environmental factors in human aggression is emphasised by researchers working from a learning perspective (e.g. Bandura 1973). This model views aggression primarily as a learned behaviour largely developed through exposure to aggressive models (e.g. parents) and the reinforcement of imitation. Whilst such a developmental view is important as a framework for working with aggressive clients, it is probably more important in this context to think about how the current (rather than past) environment is important as an immediate trigger of aggressive behaviour in the mental health care setting. Figure 6.4 provides a summary of the main environmental processes which may be implicated in aggression in such settings.

The emphasis in Figure 6.4 is on aggression to staff, although most of the identified processes are operating in situations where patients attack other patients. All factors beyond the patient 'box' in this model are features of the individual's environment, although not all will be tangible and directly experienced. Some of the factors in this model have been demonstrated to be important in human aggression through basic psychological research using tightly controlled laboratory experiments where 'normal' (i.e. non-disordered) volunteers are exposed to aversive or other stimulation (Baron & Richardson 1994). Other factors are included because clinicians have argued that they are important in the generation of aggression specifically in mental health settings. Although empirical support for the importance of these latter factors is often weak, they are still useful as a basis for clinical and managerial decisions (Royal College of Psychiatrists 1998). Each of the factors identified in Figure 6.4 may be the focus of environmental change by professionals as part of an attempt to reduce levels of aggression.

In considering Figure 6.4, it is useful to distinguish background factors and immediate provoking factors in the patient's environment. The most important provoking factor is the behaviour of other people in close proximity to the mentally disordered person, both other patients and staff. Numerous studies have indicated that many violent incidents are immediately preceded by some sort of staff intervention which is perceived by the patient as either frustrating or as a form of attack and thus calling for legitimate retaliation (Cooper & Medonca 1991, Powell et al 1994, Sheridan et al 1990, Whittington & Wykes 1996). Such perceptions of staff behaviour as an attack may be 'normal' (i.e. most non-psychotic people would be angered by the experience) or may be exacerbated by psychosis. Examples of high-risk interventions include denial of requests, prevention of absconding, administering drugs and guiding, lifting or leading patients.

This is not a claim that staff are 'to blame' for violent incidents or are necessarily acting unprofessionally when their intervention leads to an assault. It is simply a recognition that receiving mental health care, especially in forensic settings, is often highly aversive and unpleasant, however well-intentioned the staff. It is important that professionals are aware of the effect of their behaviour on patients regardless of their benign intentions. This awareness will also increase levels of safety. One of the benefits of recognising the importance of staff behaviour in the generation of aggression is the opportunity it affords for behavioural change in staff. Management of violence training usually now includes refinement of verbal and non-verbal skills in defusion situations and there is some evidence that such training is associated with reductions in violence (Carmel & Hunter 1990, Infantino & Musingo 1985, Royal College of Psychiatrists 1998, Smoot & Gonzales 1995, Whittington & Wykes 1996). Moving beyond overt behaviour, it is clear also that staff beliefs about patients (e.g. stereotypes etc.) should be examined and opportunities to deal with strong emotions (e.g. fear, anger) should be provided, both as part of the violence training and as part of ongoing staff supervision.

The visual appearance of staff (as opposed to their behaviour) is also likely to be an important aspect of the environment as experienced by the patient. Again, some aspects of this dimension can be manipulated to achieve an environment which is less threatening to patients. Certain staff may acquire an 'aggressive cue value' (Berkowitz, 1974) in that they have a conditioned association for the patient with aversive stimulation and angry arousal. Repeated aggressive interactions with staff may lead to certain individual staff or certain general features of staff (e.g. gender, ethnicity, age, size, clothing, hairstyle in any combination) automatically eliciting aggression regardless of their behaviour in an interaction. Such associations may also have been developed through experience prior to admission, and staff may be entirely unaware of these effects of their appearance. Some aspects of staff appearance cannot be changed so an awareness of patient sensitivities should guide decisions on allocation of key-workers and staff involved in particular defusion situations. It is likely that such associations are usually not sufficient on their own to trigger aggression and some form of aversive behaviour by staff must be engaged in as well. Objects such as guns may also acquire this cue value and thus elicit aggressive behaviour when viewed by patients for instance on television. Waite et al (1992) report a significant reduction in violence following the banning of violent music videos (MTV) from an in-patient unit.

Other factors which may influence staff behaviour towards patients are morale and attitudes. Such factors could include concurrent stress loads, burnout as a result of heavy workloads and differing levels of experience. Way et al (1992) report no evidence of an association between staff–patient ratios and levels of aggression, but Whittington & Wykes (1994) found that assaulted staff were significantly less experienced than non-assaulted staff in a psychiatric hospital. A high turnover of personnel, with many temporary staff, has been associated with significant increases in violence (James et al 1990). These factors need to be taken into account when planning the staffing and skill mix on high-violence units.

The physical environment of the ward tends to play largely a background role in violence, rather than being a specific provoking factor. However, again, many aspects of this physical environment are relatively easy to adapt to reduce the likelihood of negative affect in patients (and staff) and thus levels of aggression. Experimental research has clearly demonstrated the aversive effects of excess heat, loud noise, foul odours (e.g. tobacco, excreta) and poor air quality, and the links between such unpleasant environments and aggressive behaviour. Crowding in mental health care settings has also been quite extensively investigated and there are strong suggestions that overcrowding generates irritability. Certain studies have involved reorganisation of procedures to reduce crowding at

certain times of day (e.g. mealtimes) and demonstrated reductions in assaults of up to 40% (Hunter & Love 1996, Lanza et al 1994, Negley & Hanley 1990, Palmstierna et al 1991).

The physical design of units may be adapted, without excessive cost, to contribute to a less threatening environment for patients and staff. The Royal College of Psychiatrists (1998) suggest that units should be designed to maximise a sense of safety, to provide opportunities for privacy as well as group interaction and to minimise physical discomfort. Most of these design principles for new and adapted units will be illustrated in the case study below.

Most of the processes outlined in Figure 6.4 can be influenced indirectly, for better or worse, by leadership quality and managerial decisions. Katz & Kirkland (1990) found that low-violence wards were characterised by good leadership, structured staff roles and predictable routines. The quality of leadership in a unit is often cited as the most important factor in adapting the patient's environment although empirical evidence is hard to obtain. Nevertheless, the Royal College of Psychiatrists (1998) emphasise a number of principles which again will be outlined below.

Overall, analysis of any violent incident involving a mentally disordered person should always include consideration of environmental factors alongside biological or 'illness' factors. We tend to explain our own anger and aggression by reference to environmental causes, and there is no reason to exclude such external irritants and provocations in understanding aggression by mentally disordered people regardless of psychopathology. Some of these issues will now be considered using a case study.

CASE STUDY: BARRY

Background

Barry is a 29-year-old man living on Paisley Ward, a 20-bedded unit built in the 1950s and located in a maximum security hospital in the UK. He is white, 6 ft 3 inches tall and somewhat overweight. He has a diagnosis of paranoid schizophrenia and a long history of violence. He was sexually abused as a child by his stepfather and became involved in petty crime from the age of 13. He stopped attending school and at 18 was sentenced to 5 years in jail for aiding a bank robbery. On release he became increasingly isolated and complained of hearing voices. At 23, he attacked a man in response to command hallucinations and was sent eventually to Paisley Ward. He is frequently physically aggressive to staff on this ward, complaining that they avoid him as much as possible and that they are hostile and abusive when they do talk to him.

Paisley ward

Paisley Ward has a number of environmental features which may exacerbate Barry's distress. Like the violent wards described by Katz & Kirkland (1990), there is a violent incident on Paisley Ward every day. Fewer than half of these violent incidents are recorded in daily notes and there is little effective communication about violence or other issues across the three nursing shifts. When incidents occur, there is little awareness of early signs of tension and little examination of incidents afterwards. The causation of violence is usually assumed to be the patient's 'illness' (Rosenhan 1973).

The ward atmosphere is characterised by fear, mistrust and tension combined with uncertainty and confusion amongst staff and patients: 'Staff and patients moved warily, staff members rarely left the nursing station and conversations among patients were few and usually hostile' (Katz & Kirkland 1990)

Routines on Paisley Ward are largely unpredictable for staff and patients. Meetings and activities take place occasionally and are usually ad hoc, hurried and cursory. They may be arbitrarily called by senior members of staff. The ward psychiatrist usually visits once a day for a few minutes, proceeding directly to the nurses' station and ignoring patients. The timing of her visits is entirely unpredictable for staff and patients. Staff responsibilities are unclear and patients are unaware of who they should approach with problems. Staff morale and perceived support are low and there are few training opportunities.

In one incident, Barry began the day feeling distressed. He felt that superior beings would remove part of his brain if he did not provide them with a 'sacrificial lamb'. These beliefs generated feelings of shame, humiliation and anxiety. He was angrily ordered out of bed by a member of staff who had verbally abused him in the past. This member of staff was tired after working on a late shift the previous night and angry at being allocated a task he did not enjoy. Barry got dressed and queued up for breakfast with the other patients. He felt a great thirst but was squeezed back in the queue by bigger men. After a drink, he returned to the dayroom, still experiencing unpleasant voices. He coped with his anxiety about these voices by pacing around the ward and occasionally resting his head on the wall. No staff were available in the dayroom. Those staff in the nurses' office who were aware of Barry's behaviour felt fearful that he was about to act aggressively and were reluctant to engage him in interaction. They felt little empathy and attributed his behaviour to his illness. Plans for 'preventive medication' were laid, staff from other wards called and a group of large male staff approached Barry. The team leader felt a mixture of annoyance and fear towards Barry which he communicated through a hectoring tone of voice, intrusive body movements and use of commands. Barry was informed he must take medication and go to his room. He willingly took the medication, but when a hand was put on his arm to guide him to his room, he panicked and struck the team leader.

If the environmental problems on Paisley Ward are identified, some changes could be made to the procedures and routines on the ward which should reduce the levels of aggression and improve staff and patient morale. Hunter & Love (1996) report how the introduction of a number of environmental changes based on 'quality management' principles led to a reduction in violence of 40%. A more radical solution involving 'going back to the drawing board' and building entirely new units is possible where resources allow. One such unit, hypothetically designed on the basis of guidelines provided by the Royal College of Psychiatrists (1998), is set out below. If Barry was transferred to such a unit, his levels of aggression would probably not be entirely extinguished but they may be extensively reduced.

Blair house

Blair House is a purpose-built, medium secure unit located in a large British city. Planning for the design of the unit began 5 years ago and involved user-representation on the planning team. Good physical design enables adequate amounts of natural daylight and fresh air, giving the impression of space. Ambient temperature is well-controlled. Sight-lines are clear, and movable objects are designed to be safe. The building is rectangular in shape with a central enclosed garden area. The following dedicated rooms are available: separate, open reception area with private interview room; smoking room available day and night; non-smoking room available day and night; time-out room with strong fabrics, secure fittings, reinforced glazing, sound insulation and nearby toilet/washing facilities; activity room with gym equipment; visiting rooms; interview rooms; 20 single-occupancy bedrooms with one-way locks; single-sex areas; adequate bathroom and toilet facilities; separate television area; staff office and other offices. Effective housekeeping ensures cleanliness of the environment.

Clear management policies were drawn up when the unit was established and are regularly updated, again in collaboration with service users. A philosophy of care emphasising optimal self-determination, dignity and protection from intimidation and violence is explicitly stated. A multi-disciplinary consensus on approaches to care has been developed and open communication of issues is encouraged amongst staff and between staff and patients. Full information on legal status, diagnosis, treatment, progress and discharge and post-discharge arrangements is available to patients. A clear policy on substance misuse, including police involvement and charging, has been developed. Staff responsibilities are clearly specified. Staff were recruited to match the gender and ethnic mix of the patient population and training includes sensitivity to ethnic and cultural values. A core group of staff has extensive experience of working with violent patients and mentors less experienced members of the team. There is regular supervision and appraisal of all staff and training needs are monitored. Authoritarian behaviour by staff is explicitly challenged. Staff job stability is facilitated as much as possible.

The procedures for dealing with violent incidents are well-known to all staff and form part of their induction programme. Alarms and doors are easily accessible and unobstructed. Collective response by all available staff to alarm calls is agreed and consistently applied. Critical review of every incident takes place. Recording of incidents, seclusion, restraint, supplementary medication, staff injuries, staff sickness and staff time-out is maintained and regularly audited.

Each day on the unit follows a well-structured and predictable timetable, including adequate handover time. Key-workers are regularly available for private discussions and ensure that appointments are kept. A member of staff is always available for distressed patients. All complaints are taken seriously and non-violent expression of angry feelings is encouraged. Visits from friends and relatives are also encouraged. Personal possessions are kept securely but are easily accessible by patients.

It is likely, if Barry was resident on this unit, that some general improvement in his mood would take place through exposure to the pleasant physical surroundings. More directly, the overall sense of clarity, order, open communication and predictability should promote a sense of trust and calmness. In addition, the confidence and empathy of staff should enable those incidents where both staff and patients feel under threat from each other to be dealt with sensitively and safely.

REFERENCES

Bandura A 1973 Aggression: a social learning analysis. Prentice-Hall, Englewood Cliffs, New Jersey

Baron R, Richardson D 1994 Human aggression, 2nd edn. Plenum Press, London

Berkowitz L 1974 Some determinants of impulsive aggression: the role of mediated associations with reinforcements for aggression. Psychological Review 81: 165–176

Carmel H, Hunter M 1990 Compliance with training in managing assaultive behaviour and injuries from inpatient violence. Hospital and Community Psychiatry 41: 558–560

Cooper A, Medonca J 1991 A prospective study of patient assaults on nurses in a provincial psychiatric hospital in Canada. Acta Psychiatrica Scandinavica 84: 163–166

Hunter M, Love C 1996 Total quality management and the reduction of inpatient violence and costs in a forensic psychiatric hospital. Psychiatric Services 47: 751–754

Infantino J, Musingo S 1985 Assaults and injuries among staff with and without training in aggression control techniques. Hospital and Community Psychiatry 36: 1312–1314

James D, Fineberg N, Shah A et al 1990 An increase in violence on an acute psychiatric ward. A study of associated factors. British Journal of Psychiatry 156: 846–852

Katz P, Kirkland F 1990 Violence and social structure on mental hospital wards. Psychiatry 53: 846–852

Lanza M, Kayne H, Hicks C, Milner J 1994 Environmental characteristics related to patient assault. Issues in Mental Health Nursing 15: 319–335

Lazarus R, Folkman S 1984 Stress, appraisal and coping. Springer, New York

Negley E, Hanley J 1990 Environmental interventions in assaultive behaviour. Journal of Gerontological Nursing 16(3): 29–33

Palmstierna T, Huitfeld B, Wistedt B 1991 The relationship of crowding and aggressive behaviour on a psychiatric intensive care unit. Hospital and Community Psychiatry 42: 1237–1240

Powell G, Caan W, Crowe M 1994 What events precede violent incidents in psychiatric hospitals? British Journal of Psychiatry 165: 107–112

Rosenhan D 1973 On being sane in insane places. Science 179: 250–258

Royal College of Psychiatrists 1998 Management of imminent violence. Clinical practice guidelines to support mental health services. Occasional paper 41. Royal College of Psychiatrists, London

Sheridan M, Henrion R, Robinson L, Baxter V 1990 Precipitants of violence in a psychiatric inpatient setting. Hospital and Community Psychiatry 41: 776–780

Smoot S, Gonzales J 1995 Cost-effective communication skills training for state hospital employees. Psychiatric Services 46: 819–822

Waite B, Hillbrand M, Foster H 1992 Reduction of aggressive behaviour after removal of music television. Hospital and Community Psychiatry 43: 173–175

Way B, Braff J, Hafermeister T, Banks S 1992 The relationship between patient–staff ratio and reported patient incidents. Hospital and Community Psychiatry 43: 361–365

Whittington R, Wykes T 1994 Violence in psychiatric hospitals: are certain staff prone to being assaulted? Journal of Advanced Nursing 19: 219–225

Whittington R, Wykes T 1996 Aversive stimulation by staff and violence by psychiatric in-patients. British Journal of Clinical Psychology 35: 11–20

CONTENTS

Chronically dangerous patients: balancing staff issues with treatment approaches

Greg Van Rybroek

Introduction

A case example involving a chronically dangerous psychiatric in-patient is used to illustrate the critical staff–patient inter-relationship in managing hospital aggression. The power of staff counter-transference is described and practical methods for managing it are outlined. Similarly, the potential for an interactive descent to protracted intractability on the part of patient and staff is described. Practical management and treatment interventions such as the use of ambulatory restraints, seclusion and restraints, behavioural programming and psychopharmacology are discussed. Finally, the important role of hospital administration is outlined and recommendations for realistic administrative support to frontline and clinical staff are offered.

Background

Most forensic hospitals are faced with at least a handful of psychiatric patients who are considered chronically dangerous (Lion & Reid 1983). Over time these patients are viewed as treatment failures. In the eyes of the staff they can become recalcitrant, repeat perpetrators who destroy the treatment milieu for everyone. These patients usually have name recognition to most staff and their negative reputations precede them and are very difficult to overcome (Fontana 1971). Once a chronically dangerous patient takes on a reputation of putting the safety of others in peril, staff dynamics can lock into counter-therapeutic responses.

Dangerous hospital patients are individuals who have a known, repetitive history of inflicting severe physical harm to other patients, to staff or to themselves (Harris & Rice 1986). When such patients become chronically dangerous to themselves or others, the real issues descend towards protecting the vital interests of safety and security rather than the psychiatric treatment of the patient (Dubin & Lion 1992). When unit staff are criticized by outsiders for their restrictive approaches towards such dangerous patients, their typical reaction is a defensive one inviting the sideline critic to 'spend a day' on the unit with the patient in question. Accordingly, outsiders are met with staff emanating a 'you don't understand' posture about the potential degree of harm the patient can deliver. And, in truth, a majority of outsiders do not have practical ideas to assist the staff in improving the psychiatric treatment for the patient. In summary, the dynamics of recurrent in-patient dangerousness have all the makings of long-term problems unless adequate interventions effectively break the cycle of aggression (Maier et al 1987).

How, realistically, can staff manage and treat repetitively aggressive patients who are sometimes known as the 'worst of the worst'? While there are no magical solutions, this case study offers some considerations for dealing with repetitively aggressive patients who are chronic in their manifestation of dangerous behavior. The intent is to briefly describe a comprehensive approach that captures the essence of key interventions available to psychiatric care staff.

CASE STUDY: BRAD

The hospital registrar calls the most secure unit in the facility and informs them that Brad Stevens is returning to their unit. Brad, known to all, has been admitted multiple times in the last several years. In the community, his interactions are never very serious but he is placed regularly into the hospital because his actions are the result of his mental illness. Over the years there has been disagreement about his diagnosis, but the general consensus is that he has a major mental illness, probably paranoid schizophrenia.

Brad does not like to take medication since he does not believe he has a mental illness and, to make matters worse, medication has not been very effective at remitting his psychiatric symptoms. In his multiple hospital stays, Brad has seriously injured both patients and staff. Usually the aggression is based on a paranoid belief that he is going to be harmed. But sometimes Brad becomes belligerent about a unit boundary and refuses to comply, prompting staff to have to enforce compliance. When staff hear that Brad is returning, they at once become angry and afraid. The usual complaints about the legal system come to the surface, with the prominent theme being that Brad belongs in jail or prison. Before Brad arrives, frontline staff create an impromptu plan that automatically restricts his freedom. They brace themselves for another round of injuries and commiserate about their lot in life. The discussion involves wondering 'How long will we have to keep him this time?' The staff feel abandoned and rationalise that all they can do is 'keep everyone safe'.

Staff issues

Staff counter-transference reactions

Any solutions for dealing with chronic patient dangerousness need to arise from the ability of the staff to understand their own counter-transference reactions to the patient. In cases involving dangerous patients, counter-transference can be described as negative staff emotional reactions. Most typically, the reactions are manifested by fear, frustration and anger (Winnicott 1949). When these counter-transferential feelings are left unaddressed or unchecked, they can become the driving force behind nearly every decision concerning the patient (Hansen & Berman 1991). Such negative reactions should be expected since there is a good deal of legitimacy to being fearful and angry when patients cause physical harm. If staff counter-transference reactions can be legitimised as natural and real, the issue shifts to how their feelings can be managed in the name of reasonable safety and proper patient care.

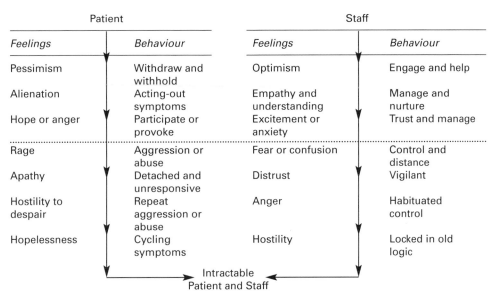

Patient		Staff	
Feelings	*Behaviour*	*Feelings*	*Behaviour*
Pessimism	Withdraw and withhold	Optimism	Engage and help
Alienation	Acting-out symptoms	Empathy and understanding	Manage and nurture
Hope or anger	Participate or provoke	Excitement or anxiety	Trust and manage
Rage	Aggression or abuse	Fear or confusion	Control and distance
Apathy	Detached and unresponsive	Distrust	Vigilant
Hostility to despair	Repeat aggression or abuse	Anger	Habituated control
Hopelessness	Cycling symptoms	Hostility	Locked in old logic

Intractable
Patient and Staff

Fig 6.5 Descending stages to intractability. Chronic patients and staff can simultaneously sink to various stages of intractability. Most psychiatric patients, however, improve in a hospital setting and do not descend into stages below the dotted line. With intractable cases, patient–staff regression presents a parallel process; the patient manifests cycling aggressive/abusive symptoms; the staff become lost in counter-transference reactions and habituated controlling responses. Intractability sets in when severe patient symptoms persist and staff utilisation of old and ineffective logic systems continues.

Since counter-transference reactions can inappropriately guide many decisions on a psychiatric unit, there must be concrete staff interventions which attempt to balance feelings of fear and anger against patient treatment needs. That is, administrative sanction needs to be given to the development of a *regular meeting* where all levels of staff can come together for open, honest communication about their feelings concerning difficult patients. The notion of an administratively supported meeting is to allow the staff an opportunity for catharsis regarding their fears about safety, while ultimately cultivating development of humane and effective management or treatment interventions to ameliorate the patient's aggressive symptoms. If such a meeting is permitted to occur on a regular basis, a process evolves in which staff come to trust each other enough to share their true feelings. With time, cathartic eruptions can be shifted to problem-solving directions which involve taking reasonable risks with the patient. Regular meetings of this kind need skilful facilitation, where the leader constantly balances staff

feelings about dangerous patients against appropriate intervention techniques. In the case of Brad's impending admission, it is imperative that staff have an opportunity to ventilate before any management and treatment planning occurs (Dubin 1989, Maier & Van Rybroek 1995).

Staff–patient intractability

When Brad makes his way onto the unit, staff are likely to be unaware that their actions can contribute to the extremely problematic situation. When a patient has the reputation of being too dangerous to treat, invariably there is the potential for a regressive interactive pattern between the staff and patient to take place. When the staff have not dealt with their own counter-transferences to the patient situation, they fail to recognise that their own interactive behaviours can inadvertently contribute to a regressive descent towards more dangerous behaviour (see Fig. 6.5). In exploring treatment alternatives for intractable patients, staff need to specifically analyse their own hand in contributing to the cycle of aggression. In the case of Brad, it is likely staff will react with habituated controlling responses that have not proven to be effective psychiatric measures, but have had some success at keeping everyone safe. While unilateral, overdetermined controlling responses may solve the 'here and now' issue, they also create the conditions for protracted problems.

To increase the probability of clinical change, it is necessary for staff to create an 'interactive shift' regarding dangerous patients (Caldwell 1994). Whereas the logic of the old controlling approaches may keep everyone safe for a time, a logic shift attempts to break away from ultimately ineffective methods. For example, rather than automatically applying the last 'successful' controlling intervention with Brad, the staff could organise a programme that allows him some choice about the degree of restrictiveness involving several new and different interventions. Once the staff allow themselves to reframe their own logic structure and embrace approaches that may be counter-intuitive to their usual habits, they open themselves up to interactive shifts which can free the patient from a predictable aggression cycle. The notion of shifting staff–patient interactions offers the possibility of breaking out of habituated responses to patient aggression (Van Rybroek et al 1995). If the staff can admit that the old methods of dealing with Brad have had no long-term efficaciousness, the groundwork has been readied for them to replace intractable practices with new, even paradoxical, management and treatment methods.

Physical intervention training

Psychiatric hospitals have not developed uniform methods of safely intervening in dangerous situations with patients (Maier 1996). Most hospitals are confused about what kind of training to give staff and have not learned from the much more systematic and established intervention programme coming from correctional systems. Correctional facilities have developed a more comprehensive and systematic continuum of 'how to' concretely deal with inmate verbal and physical aggression (Klugiewicz 1989). It appears that psychiatric hospitals, for ideological reasons, are resistant to fully embracing correctional concepts concerning the control of dangerous situations. That is, there seems to be an underlying stereotype that correctional facilities 'don't really care' about inmates, whereas conversely, psychiatric facilities 'really do care' about patients. However, state-of-the-art correctional interventions appear to be much more advanced and developed than interventions used in many psychiatric hospitals. Much greater examination of correctional emergency response techniques, such as the use of brief and focused compliance holds (to replace less than effective techniques used in many psychiatric hospitals) needs to take place.

The much more organised thrust of correctional physical intervention training is towards keeping everyone safe (Klugiewicz 1993). In contrast, many psychiatric facilities have half-hearted training and confused curriculums that delicately attempt to incorporate 'caring' concepts when patients are completely out of control. Current correctional interventions are designed to neutralise staff emotions while focusing on quick, safe and efficient methods (Klugiewicz 1990). If psychiatric hospital training does not place an emphasis on clear verbal and physical intervention techniques, unnecessary staff and patient injury will occur because of improper handling of such high-risk situations. Better training coming out of correctional facilities should not be viewed as criminalising interventions with the mentally ill. Instead, psychiatric facilities need to learn about safer intervention strategies arising out of correctional training programmes and make adaptations for the hospital environment.

Management and treatment approaches

Ambulatory restraints

One of the most common reactions to patient physical aggression is the use of seclusion (Fisher 1994, Tardiff 1984). While seclusion is very necessary and appropriate at times, its repetitive use can increase the social distance between patients and staff. With known dangerous patients such as Brad, staff can easily fall into a cycle of repetitive seclusion. The sequence of aggression–seclusion–social distance creates a dynamic which minimises contact and interaction between staff and aggressive individuals. Ultimately, repeated use of seclusion can become ineffective in creating long-term change with a patient. In fact, cyclic repetition of seclusion becomes a habituated response between patient and staff (Monroe et al 1988).

As an alternative to placing Brad in successive seclusions, ambulatory restraints have been developed as a safe intermediate step between seclusion and the unit milieu (Maier et al 1994, Van Rybroek et al 1987). Such restraints as leather wrist or ankle cuffs attached to belts by adjustable straps (Humane Restraint Co. 1998) permit the patient some range of motion in the unit milieu while still protecting others from significant physical aggression. Programmatic use of ambulatory restraints can assist in quickly re-integrating dangerous patients into the unit's milieu and unit treatment programmes. In addition, the use of ambulatory restraints greatly reduces staff and patient anxiety and leads to an increased willingness to interact with the formerly aggressive patient. If ambulatory restraints are used as part of a comprehensive intervention plan to support a patient's ongoing psychiatric treatment, they can become a powerful concrete tool that reduces staff counter-transference and increases patient participation in treatment.

Seclusion and restraint

Seclusion and restraint is a controversial and sensitive area where both clinicians and consumers need to stay aware of uses and practices. Unfortunately, the use of emergency seclusion and/or restraints continues to be a necessary measure in psychiatric hospitals (Gutheil & Shader 1994). Patients like Brad are the primary candidates for seclusion use. Even though the notion of using seclusion or restraint is disturbing to consider and unpleasant for staff to implement, there are clinical situations where no other safe alternatives are available. Whenever a clinician must balance the patient's need for safety against the desire for freedom, complex challenges are raised (Liberman & Wong 1984). In terms of using seclusion or restraint, problems arise when proper standards for application and monitoring of these techniques are not well established in the psychiatric facility. When staff are not well trained and are poorly monitored concerning seclusion and restraint practices, the conditions for abuse are ripe. If few expectations are set and enforced in terms of proper seclusion and restraint usage, a psychiatric facility can devolve into a culture that simply accepts improper utilisation of such techniques.

It is proposed that the *use* of seclusion and restraint, in and of itself, is not the fundamental issue. It is the misuse and overuse of seclusion or restraint that lead to serious problems (Robbins & Van Rybroek 1995). The hospital culture can accept that no other, less restrictive alternatives can be employed and not make vigorous attempts to find alternative measures to seclusion or restraint. When such passivity is coupled with inadequate monitoring and oversight, powerful conditions for future problems are created. Also, if staff are not aware of counter-transference reactions to aggressive and frightening patients, the use of seclusion and restraint can increase unnecessarily. The case of Brad's repeated admissions is an example of where staff could form a 'safety plan' that exclusively uses seclusion or restraint. Without proper balancing of staff emotional reactions and continuous training, and an express focus on such highly restrictive measures, seclusion and restraint bring with them very serious risks.

Behavioural programming

Generally, psychiatric units dealing with violent in-patients tend to be fairly closed systems without much access to less restrictive units or the community during the time the patient is considered dangerous. Research has shown that behavioural methods and approaches have been effective when dealing with violent psychiatric in-patients (Wong et al 1987). A specific recommended approach for Brad is the development of a behavioural programme with a short schedule of reinforcement. One approach, termed 'today–tomorrow' behavioural programming, is to design a milieu-based programme that provides for quick redemption on a daily basis. The today–tomorrow terminology is used because the programme calls for the patient to succeed or fail in targeted areas over a short period of time. That is, today's behaviour provides tomorrow's privilege level (Van Rybroek et al 1988). These kinds of programme can be developed on a standardised unit-wide basis and also can be individualised according to the needs of a selected patient. For the aggressive patient, a narrow, specific and time-limited approach using immediate reinforcers can be effective.

For example, a specific programme for Brad would expect that he meet behavioural criteria in (1) the ability to get along with peers, (2) the ability to get along with staff and (3) the ability to comply with staff re-direction. In exchange for accumulating a certain number of points based on pre-arranged definitions and thresholds, Brad would gain specific reinforcers that presumably are of some value to him. If, for instance, Brad is interested in receiving an evening snack or staying up later or making additional, long-distance phone calls, such reinforcers are built into his programme. It is the daily repetition of reaching high privilege levels that starts to change the habit of aggression. The critical feature with behavioural programmes is to train staff about objective ratings based on written behavioural definitions. To illustrate, the today–tommorrow programme is rated after the morning and afternoon shift. Brad would know by the end of the afternoon shift what his privilege level is for the following day. His progress can be mapped on a graph on a daily basis and followed over time. The notion of providing internal structured support on a programme that is success-orientated is important for both the patient and the staff. Using behavioural structure, staff counter-transferences can be reduced

because patient expectations are clearly spelled out in a fair and objective manner.

Psychopharmacology

While there have been few controlled studies on pharmacological treatments for antisocial or violent behaviour inside psychiatric facilities, there is reason to believe that pharmacological interventions have helped ameliorate aggressive symptoms in some cases (Eichelman 1988). In the case of Brad, research suggests that a combination of psychoeducational, behavioural and psychopharmacological treatments has a greater positive effect than any one intervention (Harris & Rice 1997). Numerous studies have demonstrated that the antipsychotic medication clozapine has been effective in reducing hostility and aggression in patients with a schizophrenic disorder (Cohen & Underwood 1994, Menditto et al 1996, Volavka et al 1993). As part of a comprehensive approach to treating Brad, certainly one would argue that a trial on one of the newer forms of antipsychotic medication is merited (Ratey et al 1992).

However, there is a tendency on the part of many frontline and clinical staff to bank on the hope that neurophysiological changes induced by medication will create a magical cure for the violent behaviour. But chronic cases such as Brad's are not usually successfully navigated within a unilateral approach. In addition to cognitively based social learning programmes (Beck et al 1991, Rhoades 1981), research supports attempts at psychopharmacological trials with the hope of finding an antipsychotic medication that contributes to the reduction of psychotic symptoms (Ratey & Gordan 1993). In Brad's case, if there is a behavioural programme running in parallel with a psychopharmacological approach, the daily ratings can easily be monitored to determine if and when any changes resulted from either approach (Harris & Rice 1992, Peniston & Kulkosky 1988). Ideally, the behavioural graphing would be marked so as to indicate when medication was initiated and terminated. Finally, there is some evidence suggesting that behavioural and social learning approaches have a greater effectiveness to the treatment of aggression once a patient has been stabilised through pharmacological interventions (Corrigan et al 1993).

Overarching issues

Specialised units

Many hospitals tend to divide extremely problematic patients among different units. The apparent strategy is to make certain no one unit has all the dangerous patients. One difficulty with this approach is that the unit staff do not have an ability to develop a focused identity and a common reaction is for unit staff to do everything possible to remove the problematic patient from their environment. If the patient cannot be moved, then staff may react by instituting more and more restrictive measures with the aim of keeping everybody safe. Of course, these responses ultimately make the ingredients for an intractable case.

One can imagine the multiple number of units Brad must have resided in during his psychiatric referrals. Instead of adopting a practice where problematic patients are spread throughout various parts of a hospital, it is recommended that one specialised management and treatment unit be developed. This unit would adopt an identity of dealing with difficult and aggressive patients. Under this strategy, the clinical and nursing staff will develop a mission and philosophy specifically geared towards dealing with very complex clinical cases. Patients who are extremely violent and aggressive are viewed as appropriate admissions to a unit when staff understand that their role is about dealing with this type of clientele. In turn, the staff become more familiar with effective, safe management and treatment interventions for very dangerous individuals. With the development of a specialised unit, Brad stands a much better chance of receiving proper psychiatric care. Under this scenario, specially trained staff would become sophisticated in managing their emotional reactions (i.e. counter-transferences) towards a patient like Brad and develop a treatment plan where clinical and safety issues

are balanced. The environment and culture of the unit will become one where the staff keep their collective eye on creating a comprehensive and effective treatment programme for Brad. The programme may use restrictive measures in the name of safety, while also employing other effective clinical approaches in order to assist Brad in the long term (Monroe et al 1988).

The creation of a secure, specialised unit needs the support of upper administration. While the development of such a unit may be difficult to institute at first, the hospital will profit greatly by removing problematic patients from multiple units and placing them on a specialised unit. It allows for the proper care and treatment of these problematic patients and simultaneously facilitates better internal operations on other psychiatric in-patient units.

Administrative sanction and support

All too often when extremely problematic patients revolve in and out of psychiatric facilities, the unit staff feel as though they are on their own in dealing with the situation. When the hospital administration is unaware or unconcerned about the extreme difficulties certain patients create on a unit, repetitive institution problems occur (Hunter & Love 1996). Upper level administrators can establish a certain degree of denial about problem patients (Maier & Van Rybroek 1990). Either these administrators have very little personal experience dealing with this kind of population and are not able to understand what the staff experience, or they settle into a laissez-faire posture that tacitly permits neglect or abuse. In either case, the passive acceptance of clinical work that is beneath the professional standard of care contributes to institutional tolerance of unacceptable practices and conditions (Miller 1996).

The case of Brad is a good example of how the administration can either embrace problem-solving approaches or settle for a continuation of extremely problematic conditions. Administrative leadership can assist clinical and frontline staff working with the most problematic cases:

- Develop systems in the hospital that allow for safe, effective and creative clinical approaches to the most problematic cases.
- Work within the larger administrative structure, as well as with law-making and regulating bodies, to facilitate policy and statutory modifications which ultimately provide staff with the ability to carry out

proper care and treatment in a safe environment.

- Recognise that nursing and clinical staff have a complex role in dealing with difficult and dangerous patients and provide them with the necessary resources and support to safely and successfully carry out their clinical work.

REFERENCES

Beck N, Menditto A, Baldwin L, Angelone E, Maddox M 1991 Reduced frequency of aggressive behavior in forensic patients in a social learning program. Hospital and Community Psychiatry 42: 750–752

Caldwell M 1994 Applying social constructionism in the treatment of patients who are intractably aggressive. Hospital and Community Psychiatry 45: 597–600

Cohen S, Underwood M 1994 The use of clozapine in a mentally retarded and aggressive population. Journal of Clinical Psychiatry 55: 440–444

Corrigan P, Yudofsky S, Silver J 1993 Pharmacological and behavioral treatments for aggressive psychiatric inpatients. Hospital and Community Psychiatry 44: 125–133

Dubin W 1989 The role of fantasies, countertransference, and psychological defenses in patient violence. Hospital and Community Psychiatry 40: 1280–1283

Dubin W, Lion J (eds) 1992 Clinician safety: Report of the American Psychiatric Association task force on clinician safety. American Psychiatric Press, Washington DC

Eichelman B 1988 Toward a rational pharmacotherapy for aggressive and violent behavior. Hospital and Community Psychiatry 39: 31–39

Fisher W 1994 Restraint and seclusion: a review of the literature. American Journal of Psychiatry 151: 1584–1591

Fontana A 1971 Patient reputations. Archives of General Psychiatry 25: 88–93

Gutheil T, Shader R 1994 Seclusion as a treatment modality. In: Shader R (ed) Manual of psychiatric therapeutics, 2nd edn. Little, Brown, Boston

Hansen J, Berman S 1991 The relationship of family and staff expressed emotion to residents' functioning of community residences. Psychosocial Rehabilitation Journal 4: 85–90

Harris G, Rice M 1986 Staff injuries sustained during altercations with psychiatric patients. Journal of Interpersonal Violence 1: 193–211

Harris G, Rice M 1992 Reducing violence in institutions: maintaining behavior change. In: Peters R, McMahon R, Quinsey V (eds) Aggression and violence throughout the life span. Sage, Newbury Park, California

Harris G, Rice M 1997 Risk appraisal and management of violent behavior. Psychiatric Services 48: 1168–1176

Humane Restraint Company 1998, 912 Bethel Circle, Waunakee, Wisconsin 53597, USA

Hunter M, Love C 1996 Total quality management and the reduction of inpatient violence and costs in a forensic psychiatric hospital. Psychiatric Services 47: 751–754

Klugiewicz G 1989 Principles of subject control training manual (Correctional personnel). ACMI Systems, 4011 South 90th Street, Greenfield, WI 53228

Klugiewicz G 1990 Principles of subject control training manual (Public Service Employees). ACMI Systems, 4011 South 90th Street, Greenfield, WI 53228

Klugiewicz G 1993 Correctional emergency response team (C.E.R.T.) training manual. ACMI Systems, 4011 South 90th Street, Greenfield, WI 53228

Liberman R, Wong S 1984 Behavior analysis and therapy procedures related to seclusion and restraint. In: Tardiff K (ed) The psychiatric uses of seclusion and restraint. American Psychiatric Press, Washington DC

Lion J, Reid W (eds) 1983 Assaults within psychiatric facilities. Grune and Stratton, New York

Maier G 1996 Training security staff in aggression management. In: Lion J, Dubin W, Futrell D (eds) Creating a secure workplace. American Hospital Publishing, Chicago, Illinois

Maier G, Van Rybroek G 1990 Offensive images: managing aggression isn't pretty. Hospital and Community Psychiatry 4: 357

Maier G, Van Rybroek G 1995 Managing counter-transference reactions to aggressive patients: a means to enhance clinician safety. In: Hartwig A, Eichelman B (eds) Clinician safety. American Psychiatric Press, Washington DC

Maier G, Stava L, Morrow B, Van Rybroek G, Bauman K 1987 A model for understanding and managing cycles of aggressive psychiatric inpatients. Hospital and Community Psychiatry 38: 520–524

Maier G, Van Rybroek G, Mays D 1994 Staff injuries and ambulatory restraints. Journal of Psychosocial Nursing 32: 23–29

Menditto A, Beck N, Stuve P et al 1996 Effectiveness of clozapine and a social learning program for severely disabled psychiatric inpatients. Psychiatric Services 47: 46–51

Miller R 1996 Legal issues for hospital administrators. In: Lion J, Dubin W, Futrell D (eds) Creating a secure workplace. American Hospital Publishing, Chicago, Illinois

Monroe C, Van Rybroek G, Maier G 1988 Decompressing aggressive inpatients: breaking the aggression cycle to enhance positive outcome. Behavioral Sciences and the Law 6: 543–557

Peniston E, Kulkosky P 1988 Group assertion and contingent time-out procedures in the control of assaultive behaviors in schizophrenics. Medical Psychotherapy 1: 131–141

Ratey J, Gordan A 1993 The psychopharmacology of aggression: toward a new day. Psychopharmacology Bulletin 29: 65–73

Ratey J, Sorgi P, O'Driscoll G et al 1992 Nadolol to treat aggression and psychiatric symptomatology in chronic psychiatric in patients: a double-blind, placebo controlled study. Journal of Clinical Psychiatry 53: 41–46

Rhoades L 1981 Treating and assessing the chronically mentally ill: the pioneering research of Gordon L Paul. US Department of Health and Human Services, Rockville, Maryland

Robbins K, Van Rybroek G 1995 The state psychiatric hospital in a mature system. In: Stein L, Hollingsworth E (eds) New directions for mental health services. Jossey-Bass, San Francisco

Tardiff K (ed) 1984 The psychiatric uses of seclusion and restraint. American Psychiatric Press, Washington DC

Van Rybroek G, Kuhlman T, Maier G, Kaye M 1987 Preventive aggression devices (PADS): ambulatory restraints as an alternative to seclusion. Journal of Clinical Psychiatry 48: 401–405

Van Rybroek G, Maier G, McCormick D, Pollock D 1988 Today–tomorrow behavioral programming: realistic reinforcement for repetitively aggressive inpatients. American Journal of Continuing Education in Nursing 2: 1–11

Van Rybroek G, Caldwell M, Robbins K 1995 Intractable inpatient aggression: new approaches to protracted emergencies. Emergency Psychiatry 1: 27–31

Volavka J, Zito J, Vitrai J, Czobor P 1993 Clozapine effects on hostility and aggression in schizophrenia. Journal of Clinical Psychopharmacology 13: 287–289

Winnicott D 1949 Hate in the counter-transference. International Journal of Psychoanalysis 30: 674–699

Wong S, Slama R, Liberman R 1987 Behavioral analysis and therapy for aggressive psychiatric and developmentally disabled patients. In: Roth L (ed) Clinical treatment of the violent person. Guilford, New York

Firesetting

CHAPTER CONTENTS

CONTENTS

Arson

Jack White and J. Thomas Dalby

Introduction

There has been a great deal of psychological interest over the years in examining the reasons why people illegally and maliciously light fires. Explanations relating to offences of arson have been put forward that relate to characteristics of the offenders. Such explanations include genetic factors (e.g. gender, chromosomal makeup), developmental factors (e.g. childhood firelighting play and parental separation) or clinical features related to personality and mental health. A number of motivation factors associated with arson have been identified. These include sexual gratification, fire fascination, revenge, anger, profit, politics and crime cover-up. This case study focuses upon a 28-year-old Australian male who committed a number of serious arson offences and discusses his case in light of contemporary research findings.

Background

Arson is commonly defined by US statute as the malicious and voluntary burning of property without consent. It is a very serious crime as it can indiscriminately kill many hundreds of people, destroy large amounts of property and cause millions of dollars of damage.

The Federal Bureau of Investigation (1997) reported that in 1996 there were 88 887 cases of arson in the USA that led to approximately 19 000 arrests. They stated that the average monetary value of property damage was $10 280 per incident. It was further indicated that each year in the USA there were over 700 deaths caused through arson (National Victim Center 1997). A statement made in US Senate hearings claimed that 'Arson is one of the easiest crimes to commit but one of the hardest to prevent or prove' (Geller 1992a).

The dangers of arson are especially known to people living in climates that experience weather that is hot and dry and in such places arsonists are feared more than almost any other offender. Adelaide, the capital city of South Australia, is one such place where arson has the potential to cause huge destruction. Adelaide is the setting of the case study to be examined.

CASE STUDY: ANDY

Andy was a 28-year-old Australian, divorced male who was pleading guilty to multiple charges of arson. His offending occurred over several months and involved the burning of inner city warehouses that caused damage in the order of many millions of dollars. No loss of life was reported from the fires.

Andy came from a family of three children that included a younger sister and an older brother. His parents were both alive, but had separated when he was 19 years of age. Andy attended a local High School to year 10 level, describing himself as an 'average' student. He left school at 17 to work for his father, who was a self-employed carpenter. After several months helping out in the family business, Andy was offered a job as a 'jackeroo' in the outback of Australia. He took the job but had great difficulty adapting to the work and, after only 3 weeks, returned to the city and rejoined the family firm until his father's retirement 2 years later. He subsequently had intermittent periods of employment working in a car wrecker's yard and as a kitchen hand. At the time of his arrest he was studying full-time to become a cook.

Andy reported an unstable and frustrating interpersonal history. He had his first 'serious' girlfriend at the age of 15 and several others followed, but none of these relationships were described as 'satisfactory'. At the age of 25 Andy got married, but this ended in separation just 16 months later. While married, Andy and his wife had tried, unsuccessfully, to produce a family. Various tests, which he underwent at this time, determined he was sterile and suggested a diagnosis of Klinefelter's syndrome. He had received hormonal treatment over a 16-month period, but this had been terminated at the time of his offence.

Andy first presented for psychological help when he was 19, after his third conviction for 'indecent exposure'. His first two offences were heard in the children's court, his third in an adult court. Andy re-offended a further seven times and was also charged with indecent assault against his 4-year-old stepdaughter. He strongly denied committing this latter offence and claimed it was subsequently dropped. In relation to the 'indecent exposure' offences, he attributed his behaviour to 'feeling depressed' because of his personal relationship problems and the distress caused by his parents' separation.

5 months after Andy's 10th sexual offence conviction, he was charged with the arson offences. On arrest, he admitted committing the offences, explaining that they occurred in the following way. At night, he walked the city streets checking the bins for bottles and cans which he collected in a hessian bag. When he came across premises that he felt were relatively easy to break into, he would make a mental note of the location. He would then return, on a later occasion, with a set of bolt-cutters and gear to assist him with the robbery. He claimed that he sold the stolen goods to 'friends', but said the most he ever received was about $75. After he committed the larceny, he would set fire to the warehouse/ building, usually by setting light to papers or burnable materials inside the property. He could not recall much detail from the time of his arrival at the crime scene to walking away from the burning buildings. He did not think about the cost of the damage caused, nor the risk to human life, since he maintained that the locations were not occupied. After the offence, he would quickly exit the scene either by foot or by car and travel home or to another place of safety.

When asked about his motivation for setting the fires, Andy offered a threefold explanation. First, he said that because he was not wearing gloves while committing the offences, the act of 'torching' the place would destroy any sign of his finger prints. Second, he said that he wanted to 'get back at the police' for what they had done, stating that he had been falsely accused of interfering with his stepdaughter and he still felt angry and humiliated by the charge. He said his parents were still unconvinced of his innocence regarding the child sexual assault charge and blamed the police for causing the whole problem. By lighting the fires, he believed that he was getting back at those in authority, such as the police and the Department of Family and Community Services. Third, he said he enjoyed watching the flames and the fire burn. Andy recalled that from around the age of 7, he and friends played with matches 'down by the creek' and that they would make 'Molotov cocktails' (putting a fuse into a bottle that contained a mixture of petrol and kerosene) which they would light and watch explode. Andy remembered that he enjoyed playing with explosives and fire. He also recalled fondly his childhood memories of watching the incinerator burn and reported experiencing a thrill when lighting it.

A psychometric profile was constructed from the results of several psychological tests that measured Andy's intelligence and clinical and personality features. The Kaufman Brief Intelligence Test (Kaufman & Kaufman 1990) indicated his overall level of intelligence to be in the 'low average' range. The Personality Assessment Inventory (Morey 1991) measured Andy's general clinical profile and indicated that he was highly elevated on the 'schizophrenia' and 'borderline features' scales. The high 'schizophrenia' scale score (elevated 'psychotic experiences' and 'thought disorder' sub-scales) indicated he reported experiencing acute psychotic symptoms that involved unusual perceptual or sensory events, as well as unusual ideas that included magical thinking and delusional beliefs. Andy reported thought processes marked by confusion, distractibility and difficulties in concentration. His elevated 'borderline

feature' scale was high on the sub-scales' 'negative relationships' and 'self-harm'. This indicated his history of involvement in intense and short-lived relationships, which often ended because he engaged in self-destructive behaviours. Andy was pessimistic about relationships and preoccupied with fears of being rejected. Morey (1996:99) suggested that individuals with this profile were typically presenting 'in a state of crisis and marked distress, often related to interpersonal disruption ... Because of their unhappiness, resentment, impulsivity, poor judgement, such individuals have increased risk of self harm or acting out behaviour.' On the 'treatment' scales, Andy had an elevated 'suicide ideation' scale score and saw people as being unsupportive towards him.

The Minnesota Multiphasic Personality Inventory-2 (Hathaway & McKinley 1989) indicated Andy was elevated on 'psychopathic deviate' and 'paranoia' scales. Carson (1969) described such people as 'angry, sullen people who utilise excessively a transfer of blame mechanism. Typically they are rigidly argumentative and difficult in social relations and are frequently seen as obnoxious.' Webb (1970) reported that individuals with this profile type made up approximately 1.7% of a population of 12 000 psychiatric patients.

Discussion

Andy's case illustrates a number of factors which have been identified in the literature that relate to arson offending. The relevance of gender upon offending risk has changed considerably since the very early arson writings (e.g. Platner 1797) that suggested arson was almost always perpetrated by females. The recent literature, consistently, has shown males to be the more prevalent offenders, an incidence of around 90% of arson offenders (Rasanen et al 1995b).

The chromosomal links with arson go beyond simply the male–female distinction. Andy had an abnormal chromosomal disorder, Klinefelter's syndrome, which is a condition where there is an additional one or two X chromosomes. Rather than the 'normal' male XY, the

Klinefelter male is XXY or XXXY. Danish researcher Johannes Nielsen (1970) first reported that a high proportion of patients with Klinefelter's syndrome exhibited criminal behaviour and that around 7% of his sample had a record of arson. US data collected by Miller & Sulkes (1988) indicated that approximately 20% of Klinefelter's patients had a history of arson. Kaler et al (1989) concluded that 'chromosome analysis should be an important consideration in the evaluation of young male arsonists'. Geller (1992b) found that in many of the studies that reported a relationship between arson and Klinefelter's syndrome, hormonal treatment produced favourable outcomes.

Andy indicated that he had great difficulty coming to terms with his parents' separation. Parental separation appears a common characteristic among arsonists. Virkkunen et al (1996) studied familial variables among recidivist arsonists and found they were more likely to have experienced parental separation. Saunders & Awad (1991) examined the parental characteristics of a sample of female firesetters. They found there was a high incidence of separation, domestic violence, drug/alcohol abuse and poor parenting skills among the parents. They also noted that the children, as a group of firesetters, showed little remorse or concern for their behaviours. Sakheim et al (1991) studied children with 'minor' and 'severe' firesetting histories. They found that of crucial importance was the relationship of the child to the parents. The findings indicated that the 'severe' firesetters had strong feelings of anger and resentment over maternal rejection, neglect, abuse or emotional deprivation.

Andy reported that in his childhood he enjoyed playing with fire and watching things burn. The literature would indicate that this is not an unusual childhood characteristic. Nurcombe (1964) showed children's interest in fire usually started between the ages of 2 and 3 years. Kafry (1980) suggested that fire interest was a universal childhood characteristic and that fire-play was common in approximately half the children he studied. Of those children who played with matches Kafry reported they tended to be more mischievous, adventurous, exhibitionist, aggressive and impulsive than their peers. Soothill (1990) noted that in children under the age of 12 years, firelighting usually took place in the home and 'excitement' was most commonly the motivating factor. He found that with older teenage children, arson was more commonly committed in pairs or small groups.

The similarities associated with Andy's aberrant sexual behaviour and his firesetting behaviour were probably more to do with the offending pattern than sexual motivation. Stewart (1995) found in his sample of arsonists there was 'no evidence of sexual arousal being associated with firesetting'. Similarly, Rice & Harris (1991) in a Canadian study of arsonists found that sexual motivation was very uncommon. Andy's modus operandi with his sex-offending behaviour was to wander the local streets and find suitable locations for offending that offered several exit points. He would then return to the location and wait until a victim appeared. When the victim appeared, he would expose himself and make a hasty exit from the area.

Andy's arson offending involved checking out potential premises to break into while walking the streets collecting bottles and cans. He reported that when he found an appropriate location he would return at a later time with his break-in equipment and carry out the larceny. He would then start a fire and exit the premises.

Both scenarios involve the stages: walking the streets, choosing the target location, returning to the target location, committing the offence and rapidly exiting the location.

Andy's intellectual level was in the 'low average' range. The literature indicated that most commonly arson offenders were at the lower end of the intellectual scale. For example, a Finnish study (Rasanen et al 1994) found the mean intelligence of a sample of arsonists to be in this range. They also noted two significant interaction effects: female arsonists were less intelligent than the male arsonists, and juvenile arsonists were more intelligent than the adult arsonists. Hill et al (1982) found that among the arsonists undergoing psychological assessment, one in five was mentally retarded.

Andy's clinical picture indicated he had significant psychological and personality-based problems. His clinical symptoms included psychotic experiences, personality disorder characteristics and strong suicidal ideations. Such general symptomatology appeared relatively common in the arson literature. Leong (1992) indicated that from a sample of court-referred adults charged with arson, around one-half had a psychotic disorder. Geller (1992b) found that firesetting was secondary to hallucinations among schizophrenics and was often part of a delusional system. Rasanen et al (1995a) compared arsonists with murderers and found arsonists were four times more likely to have a psychotic disorder; further, more than one-third of the arsonist sample claimed to have used firesetting as a suicide attempt. Of those studies that associated arson offenders and personality disorder, Laubichler et al (1996) concluded that 'most arsonists had a personality disorder, with insecurity and narcissism predominating'. Repo et al (1997), reviewing the characteristics of 282 convicted arsonists, found that alcohol dependence and antisocial personality disorder were the most common underlying features associated with lifetime recidivist offenders. Barnett et al (1997) compared the rate of arson recidivism among mentally disordered offenders and those without a recognised mental disorder. They found that after a 10-year follow-up, the relapse rate for the mentally disordered group was significantly greater.

Finally, Andy identified three distinct motivating factors behind his arson offending:

1. To cover up the larceny and destroy the evidence of the break-in
2. To get revenge and retaliate against the police for his perception that they had falsely accused him of interfering with his stepdaughter
3. To gain enjoyment from watching the fire.

These motivating factors have been commonly identified in the literature. Inciardi (1970) further quantified the relative percentage of occurrence of different motivational factors from a sample of convicted arsonists as: crime cover up (7%), revenge firesetting (58%), excitement firesetting (18%), institutionalised firesetting (6%), 'insurance claim' firesetting (7%) and vandalism (4%). Swaffer (1993) argued the importance of determining the motives behind the offending since 'diverse motives imply varying treatment needs and intervention tactics'.

Conclusions

In conclusion, the literature has identified a multitude of psychological factors associated with crimes of arson. Andy's case serves to illustrate many of these factors. The person's gender, chromosomal make-up, parental stability, childhood fire-play, intelligence, mental health and motivation to offend were all predisposing factors for arson offending. Given Andy's level of association with each of the factors, it was understandable (statistically at least) that he was strongly predisposed to offending.

Postscript

Andy received a 7-year prison sentence for his arson offences, with a 4-year non-parole period. In correspondence, soon after his imprisonment, he wrote to the writer to say he was quite happy in the prison environment. In relation to his rehabilitation, he wrote: 'I hope to do quite a few courses while I'm inside. It will be great! I will finally have completed a course and will have something to show for it! It's great!' After reading this letter, the writer queried whether mania was perhaps another clinical feature hitherto not noted!

REFERENCES

Barnett W, Richter P, Sigmund D, Spitzer M 1997 Recidivism and concomitant criminality in pathological firesetters. Journal of Forensic Sciences 42(5): 879–883

Carson R C 1969 Interpretative manual to the MMPI. In: Butcher J (ed) MMPI: research developments and clinical applications. McGraw-Hill, New York

Federal Bureau of Investigation 1997 Crime in the United States, 1996. Government Printing Office, Washington DC

Geller J L 1992a Pathological firesetting in adults. International Journal of Law and Psychiatry 15(3): 283–302

Geller J L 1992b Arson in review: from profit to pathology. Psychiatric Clinics of North America 15(3): 623–645

Hathaway S, McKinley J 1989 Minnesota Multiphasic Personality Inventory-2. Manual for administration and scoring. University of Minnesota Press, Minneapolis, Minnesota

Hill R, Langevin R, Paitich D, Russon A, Wilkinson L 1982 Is arson an aggressive act or a property offence?: a controlled study of psychiatric referrals. Canadian Journal of Psychiatry 27(8): 648–654

Inciardi J A 1970 The adult firesetter: a typology. Criminology 8: 145–155

Kafry D 1980 Playing with matches: children and fires. In: Canter D (ed) Fires and human behaviour. Wiley, Chichester, p 47–61

Kaler G, White B, Kruesi M 1989 Fire-setting and Klinefelter syndrome. Paediatrics 84(4): 749–750

Kaufman A, Kaufman N 1990 Kaufman Brief Intelligence Test manual. American Guidance Service, USA

Laubichler W, Kuhberger A, Sedlmeier 1996 'Pyromania' and arson: a psychiatric and criminologic data analysis. Nervenarzt 67(9): 774–780

Leong G 1992 A psychiatric study of people charged with arson. Journal of Forensic Sciences 37 (5): 1319–1326

Miller M E, Sulkes S 1988 Fire-setting behaviour in individuals with Klinefelter's syndrome. Paediatrics 82(1): 115–117

Morey L 1991 Personality Assessment Inventory professional manual. Psychological Assessment Resources, USA

Morey L 1996 An interpretive to the Personality Assessment Inventory. Psychological Assessment Resources, USA

National Victim Center 1997 Arson. Infolink Bulletin. Arlington, VA

Nielsen J 1970 Criminality among patients with Klinefelter's syndrome and the XYY syndrome. British Journal of Psychiatry 117: 365–369

Nurcombe B 1964 Children who set fires. Medical Journal of Australia 1: 579–584

Platner E 1797 De amentia occulta alia observatio quaedan. Leipzig

Rasanen P, Hirvenoja R, Hakko H, Vaisanen E 1994 Cognitive functioning ability of arsonists. Journal of Forensic Psychiatry 5(3): 620–625

Rasanen P, Hakko H, Vaisanen E 1995a The mental state of arsonists as determined by psychiatric examinations. Bulletin of the American Academy of Psychiatry and the Law 23(4): 547–553

Rasanen P, Hakko H, Vaisanen E 1995b Arson trend increasing: a real challenge to psychiatry. Journal of Forensic Sciences 40(6): 976–979

Repo E, Virkkunen M, Rawlings R, Linnoila M 1997 Criminal and psychiatric histories of Finnish arsonists. Acta Psychiatrica Scandinavica 95(4): 318–325

Rice M, Harris G 1991 Firesetters admitted to a maximum security psychiatric institution: offenders and offences. Journal of Interpersonal Violence 6(4): 461–475

Sakheim G, Osborn E, Abrams D 1991 Towards a clearer differentiation of high risk from low risk fire-setters. Child Welfare 70(4): 489–503

Saunders E, Awad G 1991 Adolescent female firelighters. Canadian Journal of Psychiatry 36(6): 401–404

Soothill K 1990 Arson. In: Bluglas R, Bowden P (eds) Principles and practice of forensic psychiatry. Churchill Livingstone, Edinburgh

Stewart L A 1995 Profile of female firesetters: implications for treatment. British Journal of Psychiatry 163: 248–256

Swaffer T 1993 A motivational analysis of adolescent firesetters. Issues in Criminological and Legal Psychology 20: 41–45

Virkkunen M, Eggert M, Rawlings R, Linnoila M 1996 A prospective followup study of alcoholic violent offenders and firesetters. Archives of General Psychiatry 53(6): 523–529

Webb J T 1970 The relation of MMPI two-point codes to age, sex and educational level in a representative nationwide sample of psychiatric outpatients. Presented at the Southeastern Psychological Association, Louisville

CONTENTS

Cognitive analytic therapy: learning disability and firesetting

Philip Clayton

Introduction

This case study describes how a brief, time-limited intervention, cognitive analytic therapy (CAT), benefited a 22-year-old man with a learning disability and history of firesetting. The approach was instrumental in exploring a way of dealing with the repetitive thinking which underpinned his offending. The individual discussed is currently detained under section 37 of the Mental Health Act 1983 in medium-secure provision. The legal charges that precipitated his admission into secure care were arson with intent to endanger life and assault.

Theoretical background

Cognitive analytic therapy is an integrative mode of short-term psychotherapy, the conceptual basis deriving from both cognitive psychology and psychoanalysis (Leiman 1994, Ryle 1993). This method aims to identify, in a language the patient can share, those mental constructions which underlie the patient's symptoms and difficulties. Therapy involves a challenge to rigid patterns of thinking which become self-defeating and offers alternative strategies of coping and change (Ryle & Bennett 1997).

The conceptual tools which provide the vehicle for therapy in CAT provide the client and therapist with a structure where collaboration is implicit, focused on the target problem(s) and those patterns of thinking and behaving

175

(target problem procedures (TPP)) which re-inforce it.

The first of these is the 'psychotherapy file' which the patient is asked to complete in order to help identify areas of difficulty in terms of 'traps, dilemmas and snags' (Ryle 1993):

- *Traps* can be summarised as: negative assumptions generating acts which produce consequences that reinforce the original assumptions.
- *Dilemmas* can be defined as: the person acting as if possible roles were restricted to polarised alternatives (false dichotomies) usually being unaware that he/she is thinking in this way.
- *Snags* can be described as: the abandonment of appropriate goals or roles on the (true or false) assumption that others would oppose them; or, regardless of the views of others, as if they were forbidden or dangerous. The individual might be aware that he/she acts in this way, but be unable to relate this to feelings such as guilt.

(Ryle 1993)

A second therapeutic strategy is the 'reformulation letter' (Ryle 1993, 1995) (or tape), which is a tentative account of the patient's problem(s) and the context in which it occurred. This is normally written after the first four sessions and reflects a collaborative exploration of the problem. It is, arguably, the most powerful aspect of CAT and lays emphasis upon the formulation of dense descriptions of those 'procedures' that cause or maintain problems over time. In developing and sharing these descriptions with the patient, it is possible to extend awareness and develop skills and capacities for self-understanding and control.

Two further features of CAT are the 'sequential diagrammatic reformulation' (SDR), a visual representation of the procedures and the use of 'rating sheets' in order to measure recognition and revision of procedures. Finally, there is the 'goodbye letter' in which the therapist summarises the therapy and the patient reflects on his/her experiences of the relationship and any outcomes. These letters are exchanged at the last session.

CASE STUDY: ABDUL

Abdul's birth was normal. He began school at the age of 5 years, when it was first recorded that he had behavioural problems. It was suggested that he had learning difficulties and an assessment of his educational needs was made. At 9, Abdul was involved in a road traffic accident, subsequent to which he developed epilepsy. School reports documented increasingly antisocial behaviours towards other pupils and at 11 he was referred to a specialist educational service for children, where he also received treatment for his epilepsy.

From the age of 12, Abdul began to engage in self-injurious behaviour. He was referred to, and subsequently placed in, a residential school some distance from his home. Here he continued to display disruptive behaviour and sometimes extremely serious life-threatening episodes of self-harm. Over time, Abdul's behaviour began to improve. The reasons why are not noted but will be postulated later.

Abdul's recollection of experiences in infancy is limited, but he remembers that the relationship between his mother and father was quite distant. It appears that his father tended to control other members of the family, who in turn acted passively. Abdul is the only surviving male of five children. His two sisters accepted traditional domestic roles and Abdul feels that his father still seeks to actively dominate him.

When Abdul left the residential school, his time in the family home was extremely short and he was relocated in a nearby council flat. There seems to have been an ongoing conflict between Abdul and his father, which culminated in his setting fire to his flat in anger. Abdul later disclosed in therapy that he had set a fire in the home when he was 8 years of age because his father disapproved of local services having to be involved in his son's life and the stigma which this imposed on the family. His mother is emotionally very close to Abdul and extremely protective towards him. This created a tension for Abdul, in that although she had great respect for him, it appears she was powerless in her relationship with the father.

Abdul was also involved in assaulting a member of the public whom he states was harassing him over issues that concerned his cousins, which became the focus for the anger despite his non-involvement. The only way to resolve this issue for Abdul at that time was, he says, to attack the person physically.

Different life events that Abdul has experienced, having grown up in a predominantly Asian community and then transferring to an English residential school, appear to have influenced how he relates to family members and others. It also appears that his perceptions are in conflict with those of his father. Abdul believes himself to be a 'British Muslim' and sees himself living in a 'Westernised' Asian community. He wants to remain in Britain, but his father constantly urges Abdul to return to Pakistan to marry his cousin.

Intervention

CAT was indicated as a first therapy because Abdul presented as someone whose problems might originate in a personal construction of reality, perpetuated by beliefs which were sequential and personality based, rather than purely problem-orientated.

The first four of 16 sessions dealt with Abdul's perception of the problems and his understanding of the offences. Identification and descriptions of the procedures that potentiated Abdul's distress were the main aim of the therapy.

The initial session with Abdul indicated that he had some awareness of why he had set the fire. During the process of therapy, an exploration of Abdul's experiences and major life events facilitated an understanding of events prior to the firesetting and then focused on alternative behaviours. This is termed 'recognition and revision'. With this in mind, alternative cognitive strategies were explored as possible coping mechanisms should the same setting conditions and personal situations re-occur.

The reformulation letter (see Box 7.1) was read to Abdul over one complete session, slowly and carefully to facilitate understanding. One or two words needed explanation or placing in context. Although it was a lengthy letter, at two pages, the time and substance of the session supplied an understanding of the content. It should also be noted that the focus was on the summary throughout the sessions, in relation to past and contemporary relationships. Obviously variations will occur, but in this case there happened to be a trap, a dilemma and a snag.

Abdul's response to the reformulation was an acknowledgement that someone could be empathic with his situation, commenting, 'You know me don't you, but what can I do about it?' Throughout therapy, the client–practitioner relationship was interpreted in transferential terms and Abdul was able to reflect on past relationships and what they meant to him. These were also explored in relation to Abdul's 'eliciting', or reciprocal, role procedures (Ryle 1993) and the notion that 'she/he is there for me' (see Fig. 7.1).

At this point, rating sheets were introduced and weekly ratings were made as to how Abdul was recognising and revising his procedures. The SDR (Fig. 7.1) was also introduced as a visual representation of procedures.

Both the Reformulation and the SDR are used in sessions to exemplify the patient's target problem, and target problem procedures, to enable the focus to remain in the room. Any deviation from this focus may be interpreted in relation to the procedures.

In the weeks that followed, Abdul showed an increased capacity to relate to others rather than self-injure. However, the firmly embedded snag still echoed in Abdul's responses at times of despair, 'What can I do, if only ...' Constant reminders of Abdul's self-denigration to staff and therapist confirmed his being caught in a low self-esteem trap. Alternative ways of thinking were explored and towards the end of therapy it emerged that Abdul might benefit from group work. An assertion group was felt to be most appropriate and this was organised as our sessions came to a close. Abdul subsequently participated in the group and evaluation measures indicated a significant shift in thinking. Self-report, and reports from staff in all areas of the hospital, confirmed this change.

Box 7.1   Reformulation letter

Dear Abdul,

It would seem that you have been in many situations in your life which have probably been beyond your control, and that have perhaps been unsettling for you. Your family may have been absent at times when you needed them most, their place being taken by other people, some of whom you respected and saw as being like parents to you. Some of your experiences have been nice, such as the stability of school, but some have not. There were times when you felt your family have been against each other, and other times when you felt that your family was against you. It is the circumstances around your family that you may feel are the reasons for your being admitted into hospital. Could it be you feel as though your father and mother have been in conflict with other members of your family, and that part of the reason is to do with the way in which some members of the family have been dishonest with each other, including being dishonest with you?

It would seem that you have taken responsibility for your family's problems. You seem to feel that your voice is not heard within the family because of the way it is organised; your father being very powerful and your mother being quiet and accepting of how your father deals with family matters. Sometimes it is as if the pressure is too hard to bear, and that you feel as though there is nothing you can do about the family problems. You then feel powerless and unable to confront those people you feel hurt you. This then becomes like a problem that cannot be solved, and you begin to think 'What can I do?', questioning how effective you can be with others. You then become angry and resentful and sometimes either hurt yourself, blame other people, or set fire. It would seem that it is when you are most unhappy that you will set a fire, and perhaps this is because it is a powerful way of expressing your anger without hitting a person. It appears that the only times you have actually set a fire is after an argument with your father, who you see as powerful and in control of the family, but not respecting you as a person. Perhaps it is useful for you to look back in time to earlier conflicts in the family, however I wonder how helpful that is for you, given that you have no control over the past and those relationships.

Could it be that sometimes you think of your mother, as your father makes all the decisions, and feel there is nothing you can do about it. That part of you that acts like your mother then gives in and withdraws, feels powerless and controlled. You then turn the anger in on yourself, as if in an attempt to say 'See now what you have made me do', and you may self-injure (hurt yourself) because you feel that you have been let down. The powerful and angry part of you that is like your father will set the fire to show that you can control something and be powerful.

I feel that you are perhaps searching, trying to find a real sense of belonging to a family, much like school was for you, and like the hospital often is now, safe, secure and respectful. It is this feeling of security that you crave, and often you might think of the past and wish you could turn the clock back. However, I feel that by beginning to look at the problems you brought into hospital you are taking a step in the right direction. By looking at alternative ways of dealing with relationship problems, you are actively working towards helping yourself be 'stronger' with other people.

I feel that the main 'target problem' is the snag of 'I want things to be better, but ... what can I do?' As well as this is the low self-esteem trap of believing that good things are not going to happen because 'It won't happen anyway, why would anything good happen to me?', It seems that you have felt like this for as long as you can remember. Since the age of 8 you have felt as though your life is out of your control, and that the only way to cope with a problem is to be in control, blaming others, being angry, in the extreme setting fire, or, to withdraw and self-injure. In other words you 'either take it out on others or take it out on yourself.'

The target problem procedures, or the patterns that lead you to think 'but what can I do?' are perhaps the feelings of hopelessness. They are a way of addressing the problems that you sometimes come across and a means of coping, which do not solve the problem, but make it worse: 'either I kick off and win' (but nobody likes me) or 'I sulk and try to get sympathy'. You will become aware, by talking to others in a direct but polite way, that we can get what we want (if it is reasonable!).

There may be times during our work together when you feel anxious and worried about going back into the past, and you may feel as though I am not being fair with you. You may also feel like getting angry at me for letting you down as the therapy comes to an end and you may feel like blaming me for leaving you. Perhaps we will be able to talk about this during the sessions.

I hope you find this letter useful as a starting point in our work together and I look forward to seeing you at our next session.

Yours sincerely,

Jackson et al (1987) allude to the notion of social skills training, particularly in assertion, as being the foundation for alternative behaviours to arson. Similarly, Prins' (1994) review of the motivation and management of fire-setting highlights the role of serious 'assertion deficits' which have been identified in the relevant literature. It became clear from the reported observations of staff that Abdul was indeed becoming more assertive and confident in many of his communications. It was also evident, despite the difficulties he has in talking with his father, that he was noted to have been able to state his case about his own future.

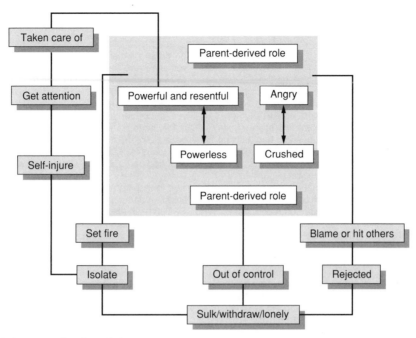

Fig. 7.1 Sequential diagrammatic reformulation.

Goodbye letter

In the last session, a goodbye letter was given to Abdul. It was clear through his responses that he was reluctant to terminate the therapy, making frequent references to previous valued relationships. Perhaps his inability to produce a goodbye letter, despite sufficient literacy skills, was one expression of his sadness. Abdul was able to reflect on this in the session and said that he felt as though he were losing a 'big brother'. The goodbye letter to Abdul was a reflective summary of the therapy and concluded with an 'instillation of hope' (Yalom 1985) in relation to the apparent progress he had made. The goodbye letter is reproduced in Box 7.2.

Reflections on therapy

Through therapy, Abdul was able to develop a much clearer understanding of the procedures and setting events related to his offending behaviour. The reasons for these behaviours were alluded to within the prose reformulation and the SDR. Abdul's self-monitoring was a very productive exercise. First, it gave him greater insight into the repetitive nature of some of his behaviours. Second, it allowed him to express himself in a purposeful way in relation to his past, the present and the future. Ward staff reported a greater sense of Abdul communicating his needs and entering into discussion with others.

Self-injurious behaviour was reduced to occasional veiled threats. With Abdul's permission, staff members were made aware of how to deal with these situations, drawing on information from the SDR and TPPs. Similarly, physical attacks, or blaming of others, declined considerably. Despite the progress in the way Abdul thinks, feels about himself, and how he behaves, it is worth remembering that, in hospital, he is not exposed to the same setting conditions as he was previously.

Conclusions

It would seem that the provision of CAT for people with learning disabilities who have offended, in this case fire-setting, has interesting connotations for future practice. Sadly, the therapeutic literature is rarely inclusive of this client group,

---

Box 7.2   Goodbye letter

Dear Abdul,

Over the past 4 months I feel that you have worked very hard in trying to understand and change the way you think and behave. During our work together you came to realise that some of the experiences in your early life continue to influence you now. You were able to say how you felt less of a person than other members of your family, not seen as a valuable member because you had a social worker. It would seem that your relationships with other people, like your relationships with family members, are extremely important. However, the respect you get from others around you in the hospital might appear more rewarding than those of your family. It is sometimes the sadness of valued relationships coming to an end that makes you feel bad about yourself, leading you to do things that are not useful. This is something you have recognised in our sessions; that the end of a relationship is always sad, but this does not mean it is your fault, or that people do not care.

Perhaps it is the fear of leaving that makes you act the way you do; perhaps the end of our sessions makes you feel as though this is the end of your stay in the hospital, even though you know this is not so. There may be feelings of being left alone, being abandoned and let down, perhaps you could think about this and talk to someone you trust and respect rather than acting in ways that are not useful.

When we started our sessions in April, it seemed as if you were dwelling on the past, and that you felt as though you were powerless and unable to change anything in your life to make you feel better. It was the past that you missed, and you continued to refer to people who were very important to you which made you feel sad and happy at the same time; sad because you miss them, and happy because of the memories that you have of them. I feel that it is useful for you to remember those people from your past and perhaps think about them when you feel upset or angry. In this way you will be able to give yourself some time to stop and think about what you are doing before anything bad happens.

You have also recognised that you do not need to act badly to get attention, but that you can act assertively and get on with people. I feel that this is a very important step, as you have proved to yourself, and others, that you are able to think and behave in ways that are acceptable to all.

I feel that you know and understand what happens to you, and that perhaps you need to change the way you think and behave. You started to do this with me, and are now working on it in group sessions. I believe that you will carry on in your efforts to change for the better.

Goodbye and good luck.

---

despite the positive outcomes described in this case study. It is noteworthy that Abdul has since moved on into a community setting, where his progress is being carefully monitored.

REFERENCES

Jackson H, Glass C, Hope S 1987 A functional analysis of recidivistic arson. British Journal of Clinical Psychology 26: 175–185

Leiman M 1994 The development of Cognitive Analytic Therapy. International Journal of Short Term Psychotherapy, Special Issue, Cognitive Analytic Therapy 9: 2/3

Prins H 1994 Fire-raising: its motivation and management. Routledge, London

Ryle A 1993 Cognitive Analytic Therapy: active participation in change, a new integration in brief psychotherapy. Wiley, Chichester

Ryle A (ed) 1995 Cognitive Analytic Therapy: developments in theory and practice. Wiley, Chichester

Ryle A, Bennett D 1997 Case formulation in cognitive analytic therapy. In: Eells T (ed) Handbook of psychotherapy case formulation. Guilford Press, New York

Yalom I 1985 The theory and practice of group psychotherapy Basic Books, New York

CONTENTS

Group work with women who set fires

Jan Gregoire, Clancy Borastero and Dave Mercer

Introduction

Rather than focus on one individual, this case study outlines the experience of facilitating a therapy group for women who set fires. This was undertaken in the context of a maximum secure psychiatric hospital and represented innovative practice in a number of ways. At an institutional level, it challenged the masculine discourses which have, historically, perpetuated a gender bias in the provision of services and interventions. The disadvantaged and marginal status of women in traditional forensic environments impacted considerably on the process of offence-focused work. Participants were given a 'voice' and many 'stories' emerged to break the collective silence. What in one sense was empowering, in other ways embroiled facilitators in a complex web of interpersonal dynamics, boundary issues and professional dilemmas. Most importantly, though, in the face of structural obstacles and clinical challenges, the survival of the group demonstrated that the most damaged and vulnerable individuals could share their pain and begin to grow stronger.

Theoretical background

Firesetting, or its forensic descriptor arson, embroiled in mythical and biblical symbolism, first attracted the attention of psychiatrists in the early 19th century. Interestingly, these early first attempts to pathologise firesetting, located 'pyromania', as 'the province of pubescent, mentally retarded girls with abnormal psychosexual

181

development and menstrual difficulties' (Geller 1992). If clinical studies of 'female firesetting' have been much neglected since this time (Bourget & Bradford 1989), the theme of sexuality persisted in the domain of secure psychiatry (Tennent et al 1971), though expressed in a male discourse about the 'frigidity' and 'infidelity' of women firesetters.

Deliberate firesetting is one form of aggressive behaviour, which occurs in many different guises and contexts. Though usually an act of indirect aggression against property, firesetting can be directed against people. Perpetrators of this act are normally dealt with severely by the criminal justice system and it is not unusual for the offence of arson to carry a life sentence. Most female offenders appear significantly more traumatised and disturbed and with the diagnosis of borderline personality disorder are more likely to find their way into the Special Hospital system. Many women referred for treatment in Special Hospitals have a history of firesetting. Research (Eaton & Humphries 1996) suggests that regional secure units and other local services are reluctant to accept women with a history of firesetting, and arson is frequently seen as the 'fast track' into indeterminate detention in the high-security sector. Given this, there is a tradition of group treatment for arson in the Special Hospitals. One of the reported findings from this work is the reluctance of women patients to participate with men and their requests for a single sex group (Hall 1995).

Typically, social stereotyping casts women as victims and men as perpetrators, reflected in much of the therapeutic provision in Special Hospitals which is offence-focused and geared towards men (Hemingway 1996). The female offender finds it difficult to be heard, understood or taken seriously. Welldon (1988) makes the point that the idealisation of mothers, prevalent in society, is shadowed by a denigrating counterpart, which falls darkly across those women in Special Hospitals. They have transgressed the limits of socially appropriate and acceptable gender roles, and through the extremity of their behaviours typify the deviant and affirm the

normal (Hutter & Williams 1981). Rehabilitative strategies have often focused on resocialisation underpinned by ideologies of femininity and domesticity (Rowett & Vaughn 1981). If progress has been made in developing, and resourcing, services sensitive to the needs of women, less attention has been paid to challenging the power–knowledge equation which socially constructs their lives (McKeown & Mercer 1998). Talking therapies in secure settings are complicated by the dual role of forensic staff, being both care agents and custodians: 'Say the wrong thing and you might be condemning yourself to more months, maybe even more years, inside' (Lloyd 1995). At the same time, discourse is one way of resisting power by translating the personal into the political. Understood in this sense, and informed by wider concerns than pathology, therapy can offer hope where little exists.

The group work programme presented in this case study comprised two distinct phases, indicative of real clinical need combined with a strong element of therapeutic scepticism. Many of the women had spent considerable lengths of time in institutional care and shared backgrounds of extreme abuse manifested in a range of self-destructive behaviours. Given this deeply rooted damage and vulnerability, there was a good deal of doubt expressed in terms of their ability to sustain the demands of therapeutic intervention, particularly in a group setting. If we were to place the women in this sort of situation, there had to be some guarantee that the experience would not compound the social and emotional privation that had characterised their lives to date. For this reason, an assessment group was organised to allow them the opportunity of making an informed choice about participating. The women were referred by their care teams, but the decision to participate, or not, remained with them. It is hard to describe the courage they showed, the pain they shared or the optimism and humour they managed to hold on to. Working with them has been both a privilege and an emotional trial, which has changed all of our lives. This case study is a tribute to their strength.

CASE STUDY

Assessment group

The development of an assessment group for women who set fires demonstrated some of the difficulties posed when engaging in offence-specific work. Confidentiality, boundary issues, responsibility, trust versus dangerousness, security issues, power relationships, diagnosis and detention under the Mental Health Act 1983 were just some of the contentious issues raised before and during the assessment group.

When interviewed before starting the group, many of the women said they preferred to work in a 'women only' environment, as they felt safer and more at ease. Single-sex groups are often criticised on the basis that they are in some way fundamentally abnormal and likely to distort individual and group processes in an unhelpful way. In our case, however, the treatment process and treatment setting interacted in a powerful and symbolic way. All of the women referred to the assessment group had histories of physical and/or sexual abuse. Price (1988) notes that men often report difficulties in listening sympathetically to women who want to discuss experiences of incest and rape in any depth. In secure psychiatric settings, many of those women who elect to engage in offence-focused, or skills acquisition, groups have little choice but to work with men. As part of a minority, if over-represented, population it is not unusual for a single woman to be placed in a group of 12, where all of the other members are male. Many of these women view the male patients as potential abusers and indeed many of the men are detained in relation to sexual crime. The potential for women to discuss the antecedents of firesetting is, thus, hindered by their inability/unwillingness to disclose sensitive and traumatic events from their childhood in an environment perceived as threatening and abusive.

The assessment group ran for 12 weeks and was a precursor to the development of the longer term women's firesetting treatment group. The aim here was to assess the women's ability to work in a group context, their motivation to attend and willingness to address offences, risk issues and victim empathy. Welldon (1993) expresses the view that in considering forensic patients for group work it is vital to look closely at particular psychopathologies and needs in the selection criteria. Ten patients initially attended the assessment group, out of which number five were eventually felt suitable to engage in a protracted therapeutic programme.

In addition to evaluating the content, themes and issues which emerged from the individual sessions, it was also considered important to evaluate the group as a whole by looking at underlying processes and dynamics. The assessment group provided valuable information about, and insight into, the diverse needs of the women.

The five women who would progress to the firesetting treatment group all shared a diagnosis of either anti-social personality disorder or borderline personality disorder (BPD). All, to a greater or lesser degree, had a history of self-injury which included cutting, burning, swallowing and insertion of foreign bodies under the skin or into the eyes and ears. It was recognised that no single treatment philosophy was appropriate to engage with the range of problems and a multi-modal style of working was adopted. Chiefly, this consisted of a cognitive dimension to highlight and address coping strategies and alternative behaviours to manage trauma, and a psychodynamic perspective to interpret the deeper processes and links to the past. Fineman (1995) lent support to this eclectic model in proposing a dynamic–behavioural formulation to firesetting behaviour. Here, firesetting behaviour is viewed as 'an interaction between dynamic historical factors that predispose the fire setter toward a variety of maladaptive and anti-social acts, historical environmental factors that have taught and reinforced firesetting as acceptable, and immediate environmental contingencies that encourage the firesetting behaviour.'

Treatment group

Goal setting and structure

From the outset, the women were encouraged to be actively involved in negotiating the

---

Box 7.3 Group guidelines

As a member I will:
• Try to attend all sessions
• Take responsibility for being ready for the hospital transport
• Communicate with the group if I am going to be absent
• Attempt to listen to others when they speak, without interrupting
• Offer feedback to other group members
• Talk about feelings, rather than act on them in the session
• Complete homework exercises
• Participate in role plays and other exercises, when possible
• Complete assessment documentation
• Discuss my feelings with my key-worker
• Complete self-reports

---

format and functioning of the group. The opening session was devoted to discussion about the direction and pace of work to be undertaken: for the year ahead, the first 3 months and weekly planning. Each session adhered to a common, and time-limited, structure:

• Review of personal issues
• Group exercise
• Content planning for the future
• Break and tea
• Winding down and relaxation.

In the initial stages, the women and facilitators worked together to establish a contract and set of group rules. Discussion around the need for, and function of, such an agreement produced the guidelines shown in Box 7.3. This was matched by a reciprocal commitment on the part of the facilitators.

Aside from individual responsibilities within the group, the issue of confidentiality was expressly managed. The women agreed to hold private and personal information about other group members in confidence. Facilitators agreed to do likewise, with certain stated exceptions – written feedback to the responsible medical officer (RMO); written assessments to the respective care teams on completion of the 3-monthly modules; and verbal feedback to the ward staff as necessary. In the last case, information given to practitioners outside the group took the form of general concerns rather than specific

details and these were explained to the women before they left the group. It had been anticipated that the sessions might be audio- or video-recorded to enhance understanding and interpretation of the group dynamics. All of the women, though, were uncomfortable with this and the idea was not pursued.

The women and facilitators both recognised the potential for 'anger' to be taken away from the group and the possible implications of this in terms of risk at ward level. Significantly, each of the women said that they felt the need for a support mechanism outside of the group. In response to this they each identified a member of staff with whom they had regular contact and close relationships. This was also a positive step in linking the specific treatment programme with the wider process of care planning.

Immediately after each session, the three facilitators remained together for a de-briefing exercise. This was valuable in a number of ways. Dominant themes, which had emerged in the group, could be identified; the impact of distressing or emotional disclosures could be shared; and issues which needed to be addressed in clinical supervision were explored. A 'group work recording sheet' was completed at this time, with information, observations and interpretations noted under the following headings:

• Aims of the session
• Main themes in the session
• Process and group interactions
• Plan for the next session
• Issues for supervision.

In discussion with the women, a modular framework was constructed, which listed the issues to be explored:

• *Module 1*. Aimed to explore the symbolism and meanings which surround fire; individual firesetting in terms of age, type of fire and context; childhood experiences of firesetting; and, most significant fire.
• *Module 2*. Focused on past and present relationships; sexual and physical abuse; self-injury and the use of illicit substances; depression, anxiety, anger and self-esteem.

- *Module 3.* Addressed victim empathy; coping skills and strategies; education about fire; identification of future areas for therapeutic work.

Process, progress and problems

The original intention had been for the group to run one afternoon a week for 12 to 18 months and focus on specific themes that were highlighted during the assessment period.

However, the group has now been running for over 2 years. Progress has been slow, in part owing to difficulties associated with operating therapeutic groups in large institutions, but also because of the degree of trauma, past and present, with which the women live. Large parts of the sessions have been taken up with 'here and now' issues. The overriding concern of the women is their current situation, feelings of isolation and the desperate attempt to get themselves heard in an institution that does not appear to have the understanding or infrastructure to meet this need. Other therapist colleagues working with women patients in a secure setting have commented that their therapeutic work is dominated, and compromised, by similar problems. Our experience became that the women were reluctant to discuss past events and previous treatment because they could not move away, or separate from, their current situations.

The women often arrive at the group in a distressed state, sometimes after having self-injured or having recently been taken out of seclusion. They speak of the wards being disturbed and regimented, describing their relationships with each other and staff as dysfunctional. Potier (1993) in an article about women patients in high-security services raises this problem by noting that ward staff often represent 'family' for the patients and depict an image of the ward as 'one big happy family'. This is often in direct contrast to the women's backgrounds and experiences outside of hospital. Many relate histories of separation, abuse and chaotic family lives in childhood and beyond.

We often felt, as facilitators, that we became idealised by the women, with an element of splitting between ourselves as 'good parents' and ward staff as 'bad parents'. This dynamic manifested itself, particularly, when almost half of a session was taken up with the women talking about their respective wards. Their main complaint was that the staff ignored them and showed little respect, 'They don't care about us.' They proceeded to talk about feeling valued, and listened to, in the group. They contrasted this with the experience of being separate and alone within their families. Completely out of context to what was being explored, one woman stated that she wished to talk about something as a matter of urgency. She then described a recurring fantasy, which preoccupied her thoughts, about committing suicide by fire. In the fantasy, she would write letters to her doctor, care team, parents and ward staff (not the group) telling them how she despised them. She would then imagine lighting a fire in her room, hiding under the bed and waiting for the staff to respond to the alarm. When other group members pointed out the danger of asphyxiation from the smoke she was matter of fact in retort and unable to connect with the severity of such actions for herself or others. As facilitators we debated whether she was 'testing us out' to measure our care or respect for her, with any rejection consigning us to the flames.

As a group we explored the different roles that staff were placed in, or other significant people, including the group facilitators. This prepared the way for an exploration of difficulties past and present in the formation of lasting relationships and generated intense and overwhelming emotions of fear, isolation, anger, rejection and disempowerment. The possibility that these feelings had, in the past, been externalised in behaviours such as firesetting or self-injury was fed back to the group. Some of the women recalled times of intense distress, which they associated with their offending, self-injury or substance misuse.

There have been numerous group interactions like the ones outlined above, where group dynamics and process have been utilised and worked with in the sessions, or taken to supervision for a clearer perspective and brought back at

---

Box 7.4   Significant issues related to firesetting

- Why is fire fascinating?
- Do you consider firesetting dangerous?
- Is firesetting a grief/loss reaction?
- Is firesetting a need for love, warmth and attention?
- Is firesetting a vengeful act?
- Were you angry at the time you set the fire?
- Did you want to destroy things or people?
- Did firesetting make you feel powerful and in control?
- Is abuse a big issue for women who set fires?
- What is the role of self-image and self-esteem?
- Was substance use an important issue in the firesetting?
- Was firesetting a way of escaping from situations which were awkward, unmanageable or frightening?
- Is firesetting a way of overcoming insecurity and fear?
- Did you want to be caught or punished?
- How do relationships figure in firesetting?
- Were 'others' involved in setting fires with you?
- Did you think about the consequences of your actions?
- Does firesetting stop when external events change?

---

a later stage. The latter support mechanism helped the facilitators to offer feedback to the women and assisted an understanding of what is happening in the group at an unconscious level that typically connects with the women's past relationships.

Part of each session is spent looking at a specific aim or theme. Using a variety of cognitive–behavioural techniques and strategies which have included the keeping of diaries, brainstorming techniques, mapping out individual experiences, homework tasks and problem-solving, we located common themes associated with firesetting. An example is given in Box 7.4 of issues which emerged during one session and the way in which the ideas were reformulated as questions to be explored within the group.

The construction of offence cycles revealed shared experiences around anger, self-esteem, childhood firesetting and accounts of significant fires.

During the early group sessions, it became apparent that communication was a fundamental problem for the women, in terms of opportunity rather than ability. This was demonstrated in different ways, but seemed to be a crucial component in maintaining their frustration and anger and again reflected organisational tensions. This was evidenced when one of the women told how

she had tried to talk to staff on the ward about her urges and fantasies to set fire. Instead of being listened to, she was placed on close observations, which prevented her from attending the group. At a later session, we were able to role play this scenario in the group and explore alternative ways in which she could have managed her fears. Part of this was an encouragement to articulate her desire to light a fire and once this was out in the open she appeared as neither frightened nor frightening.

Conclusions and concerns

It proved difficult to maintain one specific approach to therapy because of the multiplicity of problems the women presented. As facilitators we have grown to appreciate the need to work in partnership with the women, and at a pace which they determine and also the importance of working in close collaboration with the wider care teams.

All the women in the group have spoken about being unsupported, misrepresented and, in some cases, abused by the euphemistically titled 'caring professions'. They all came from families characterised by drug and alcohol use, violence, neglect and sexual abuse. Each member of the group had some experience of foster care or children's homes. One of the women had been raped by a teacher at the age of 14 in an adolescent care facility, where she later set fire to her room. Another who had been in crisis, being systematically sexually abused by her father, was ignored by the social worker and lit a fire to escape her torment.

Multiple motives emerged to account for their firesetting, crystallised in anger, revenge and despair. One of the women had set herself alight in an attempted suicide. Three of the women said they thought of fire when they thought of revenge because it was powerful, made them feel in control and released the tension.

All but one of the women had a fascination with fire at an early age and set their first fire in childhood, the earliest being at 6 years of age. Similarly, they had set multiple fires. All but one of the women had set their fires alone, usually in response to extreme rage, deep unhappiness or utter desperation, and always to signify, or escape, a painful situation in which they felt powerless.

All of the women engaged in self-harming behaviours and attempted suicide frequently. Two had set fires on their wards during the assessment group. Together, they expressed low self-esteem, poor relationship skills and difficulty in articulating their feelings.

Despite the envisaged structure of the treatment group, in reality it was difficult to follow the modular content in sequence. Some of the themes were covered as, and when, they arose in therapy, rather than at a time suggested by the facilitators. The agenda has needed to be framed by the women and we have continually had to return to issues raised in earlier sessions. All of the women have demonstrated a commitment to understand their firesetting. As facilitators, we have found it impossible to address this in isolation given the profound patterns of trauma, deprivation and self-destruction. Therapy, we would suggest, needs to offer a secure base with safe boundaries if we are to enter and explain the complex world of women who set fires.

REFERENCES

Bourget D, Bradford J 1989 Female arsonists: a clinical study. Bulletin of the American Academy of Psychiatry and the Law 17(3): 293–300

Eaton M, Humphries J (eds) 1996 Listening to women in Special Hospitals: the report of a pilot study. St Mary's University College, Strawberry Hill, Twickenham

Fineman K 1995 A model for the qualitative analysis of child and adult fire deviant behavior. American Journal of Forensic Psychology 13(1): 31–59

Geller J 1992 Pathological fire setting in adults. International Journal of Law and Psychiatry 15: 283–302

Hall G 1995 Using group work to understand arsonists. Nursing Standard 9(23): 25–28

Hemingway C 1996 Special women?: the experience of women in the special hospital system. Avebury, Aldershot

Hutter B, Williams G (eds) 1981 Controlling women: the normal and the deviant. Croom Helm, London

Lloyd A (ed) 1995 Doubly deviant, doubly damned: society's treatment of violent women. Penguin, Harmondsworth

McKeown M, Mercer D 1998 Fallen from grace: women, power and knowledge. In: Mason T, Mercer D (eds) Critical perspectives in forensic care: inside out. Macmillan, London

Potier M 1993 Giving evidence: women's lives in Ashworth Maximum Security Psychiatric Hospital. Feminism and Psychology 3(3): 335–347

Price J 1988 Single-sex therapy groups. In: Aveline M, Dryden W (eds) Group therapy in Britain. Open University Press, Milton Keynes

Rowett C, Vaughn P 1981 Women and Broadmoor: treatment and control in a special hospital. In: Hutter B, Williams G (eds) Controlling women: the normal and the deviant. Croom Helm, London

Tennent T, McQuaid A, Loughnane T, Hands A 1971 Female arsonists. British Journal of Psychiatry 119: 497–502

Welldon E 1988 Mother, madonna, whore: the idealisation and denigration of motherhood. Free Association Press, London

Welldon E 1993 Forensic psychotherapy and group analysis. Group Analysis 26(4): 487–502

Problematic substance use

CONTENTS

Substance misuse complicating mental illness

Clare Brabbins and Rob Poole

Introduction

People suffering from severe mental illness are more likely than the rest of the population to have a substance misuse problem (Meuser et al 1990). Whilst many such patients use illegal drugs, it is important to recognise that a larger group misuse alcohol and that a significant group misuse prescribed drugs (Regier et al 1990). The adverse effects of alcohol misuse are, if anything, more far reaching than those for other drug misuse (Hamilton et al 1993).

Substance misuse is a risk factor for violent behaviour in general (Goldstein 1989) and it is not surprising to find that it is one of the few reliable risk factors for aggression amongst the mentally ill (Dyer 1996, Lindqvist & Allebeck 1989, Smith et al 1994, Swanson et al 1990). However, although the problem of substance misuse complicating mental illness is common, it is poorly understood. There is no compelling evidence on the effectiveness of interventions to help people with mental illness to contain substance misuse problems. There is continuing controversy as to whether such patients should be treated within mental health services, substance misuse services or specialist 'dual diagnosis' services (Franey & Quirk 1996, Johnson 1997). The harm-reduction approach draws on recognised good practice in populations suffering from primary substance misuse problems, modified for the mentally ill in the light of clinical experience. It is hoped that interventions will be developed and properly evaluated for 'dual diagnosis' patients. The most promising approaches are based upon cognitive–behaviour therapy (Beck et al 1993, Graham 1998, Liese & Franz 1996) in the context of broader psychosocial interventions (Gournay et al 1996). It certainly seems likely that any effective treatment model will need to take into account the complex reasons for substance misuse. In particular, the behaviour has advantages for the individual, which offset the hazards and adverse effects they experience.

CASE STUDY: MARK

Mark was a 23-year-old single man who was compulsorily detained in a secure unit after being arrested for stabbing a stranger in a pub. He had started using cannabis from the age of 15 and had increasingly misused a variety of substances, mainly amphetamine and cannabis. When he dropped out of school at 17, his parents attributed his changing behaviour to drug use. A few months later, he was arrested for breaking windows at a local shop and in custody was found to be floridly psychotic. He was admitted to a psychiatric unit and diagnosed as suffering from acute paranoid schizophrenia. The presentation was of thought disorder with paranoid delusions that he was being hunted by a criminal gang and auditory hallucinations of the gang threatening him. He made a good recovery on neuroleptic medication and after 6 weeks was discharged to return to his parents' home. They were unable to accept that he was suffering from a mental illness and attributed his psychosis to the effects of drug misuse. Prior to discharge, the clinical team made concerted efforts to help him understand that further drug use was likely to provoke relapse. His undertakings to find new friends and to avoid drugs proved short-lived; within 3 months of discharge, he had discontinued medication and was again using cannabis regularly. An episode when he threatened a neighbour led to assessment at home by the community mental health team (CMHT) and he was re-admitted with similar mental state abnormalities. On this occasion, his recovery was slower and this was believed to be due to the fact that he had fallen in with a group of young patients who used cannabis on the ward.

Over the following 5 years, Mark was followed up in the community by a psychiatrist and a community psychiatric nurse (CPN). He was given depot medication. The CPN attempted to help Mark to find a meaningful daytime occupation, to become more independent of his parents and to gain a better understanding of his illness. Despite this, he was admitted to hospital compulsorily on four further occasions. Each admission was associated with discontinuation of medication and rejection of follow-up. His drug use continued unabated through periods of relapse and remission, but he tended to use more stimulants during periods of relapse. Each admission was precipitated by aggressive behaviour, though this was not serious enough to lead to charges against him. His social circle shrank to a small group of drug users, several of whom also had mental health problems.

His parents continued to support him, though they became increasingly frantic in their efforts to persuade him to change his lifestyle. Their efforts, though well meaning, were counterproductive. Their focus on the single issue of drug use meant that there was a high degree of conflict in the relationship and levels of expressed emotion in the household were high. Mark was unable to cope with this and he tended to experience episodes of hallucinations after rows. His parents' narrow understanding of his illness precluded more helpful strategies to improve his mental health.

At the time of the index offence, Mark had been out of contact with his CPN for 3 months. He had recently started to use amphetamine intravenously for the first time and was paranoid and hallucinated. He had gone to the pub in order to buy drugs, but on entering the crowded bar he had heard a voice telling him he was about to be shot. He noticed a man whom he could tell was a gangster by the way he made eye contact. He stabbed him, later claiming this was in self-defence. Though the victim's injuries were minor, Mark had been rapidly restrained by bystanders and it was unclear whether the assault would have been more severe without their intervention.

Identified problems and planned interventions

After assessment as an in-patient at the secure unit, it was clear that the index offence had occurred as a response to psychotic symptoms. There was a pattern of aggression in the context of relapse. Although Mark was neither intoxicated nor suffering from withdrawal symptoms at the time, his drug use was a major factor in the unstable course that his illness had followed. The multi-disciplinary team (MDT) drew up the following initial problem list and multi-disciplinary action plan:

1. Treat Mark's mental state abnormality

After assessment, the MDT concluded that the risk of aggression was directly related to Mark's mental state abnormality. Previous therapeutic interventions suggested that this was likely to improve satisfactorily on treatment with a depot neuroleptic. Though Mark did not report suffering from marked side effects as a result of this medication, he did not consider it necessary.

2. Help Mark to gain better understanding of his illness

This required psychoeducational work. Although previous similar efforts had been unsuccessful, the seriousness of his situation meant that it was possible that Mark would receive such work more positively. There was also likely to be a longer than usual period of in-patient treatment to allow this work to continue beyond the difficulties of engagement.

3. Help Mark to recognise the problems associated with his drug use

The MDT recognised that there was little purpose in asking the Drug Dependency Service to become involved in Mark's care. He was not physically dependent on opiates so that replacement prescribing was inapplicable. They did not offer a service to cannabis users and were frank over their difficulty in assisting amphetamine users. In any case, Mark did not perceive his drug use as a problem to him.

The first step was for the staff to attempt to understand with Mark why he used drugs. This required the acknowledgement that his drug use brought benefits to him. From his perspective, it was the focus of his social life and intoxication offered him some relief from the anxiety and tedium of his life generally. The routines of drug buying, meeting with friends, preparing and taking drugs, enjoying the effects and recovering provided a structure in his otherwise aimless existence. He felt that drug-taking was the only thing that made life worthwhile.

Not only did the staff need to identify Mark's personal motivations for drug use, they also had to establish their credibility with him. Unless he felt that they understood drug-taking and the problems it solved for him, it would be impossible to help him to identify some of the negative consequences. In an open and non-judgemental relationship it is, over time, possible to help people to make a rational cost–benefit analysis. This need not be led by a service goal of abstinence. A more realistic objective may be to help the person find ways of avoiding the most harmful consequences. This approach has the advantage that it allows the patient to be truthful, acknowledging that prohibition and exhortations to change are rarely effective. Dire warnings of potential health hazards such as developing hepatitis C may have less meaning for drug users than more immediate and tangible hazards such as the drain on finances and the worsening of auditory hallucinations.

4. Assist in developing non-drug-related social activities and daytime occupation

Mark could not be expected to change his behaviour unless his needs were met by satisfying activities to replace drug use. Few drug users would regard activities organised by mental health services as a satisfactory replacement for going to a friend's flat to share a few spliffs. Alternatives have to match the patient's interests. They do not need to be comprehensive; a new activity that engages the patient's interest for a few afternoons a week may be sufficient to reduce (though not eliminate) a heavy cannabis habit. In Mark's case, his interest in painting seemed promising, as there were a number of opportunities within the local community to engage in this activity. Successful involvement in this respect would also have the advantage of extending Mark's social network beyond those accessed through contact with services or drug use.

5. Help Mark's parents to develop more effective and less stressful responses to his behaviour

The parents' response to Mark's drug-taking was understandable. However, the emotional arousal it caused was as damaging to his mental state as the drug-taking itself. It was intended that the staff would engage his parents in psychoeducational work in order to modify communication within the family and to help them to develop problem-solving skills. This had to take into account their preoccupation with drug use, which was unlikely to disappear. The belief that their son had a drug problem rather than a chronic mental illness was unpleasant but more acceptable to them than an acknowledgement that his problems were likely to be lifelong. Even if they came to recognise the nature of his illness, they would be unable to accept or ignore his drug use, which was an affront to their values.

The initial approach would involve an exploration of the relationship between psychotic symptoms and drug use. If his parents were able to identify Mark's wider problems and needs, they might be able to develop a broader problem-solving strategy, which might in turn indirectly curtail his drug intake. They would need help to find ways to honestly communicate their distress and concern over drugs without causing tension and arguments.

Outcomes

Mark's treatment in the secure unit did not proceed smoothly. He made the expected, good, early response to neuroleptics and he displayed no aggression on the unit. However, his visitors brought him cannabis, which he shared with other patients. His mental state fluctuated. Staff could not tolerate drug use on the unit, being particularly concerned about the adverse effects on other, possibly vulnerable, patients. In any case, it is illegal to allow, or even to tacitly acknowledge, drug use within public premises. Hence the staff felt they had no alternative to taking a position of prohibition and control. Immediately, this was incompatible with the harm-reduction strategy and possibly compromised their therapeutic relationship with Mark. However, after several weeks without leave or visitors, other than his parents, his mental state did eventually stabilise.

The second phase of the admission was characterised by a fluctuating level of compliance with conditions of leave. Mark was using cannabis on leave and whilst he showed no aggression, there were periods of recrudescence of hallucinations. There was a major dispute within the MDT over the planned response to this. One group of staff felt that a harm-reduction approach demanded a pragmatic compromise with Mark. If he only used cannabis off the unit, took no amphetamine and restricted his intake to a level that did not provoke psychotic symptoms, then the behaviour would be tolerated. This, they argued, would provide experience that could be examined within the psychoeducational work and would introduce a less damaging pattern of drug use, which would be sustainable on discharge. This position accepted that, regardless of anything the staff could say, Mark would continue to use cannabis when beyond the confines of the ward. The other group of staff felt that this amounted to an unethical collusion with a high-risk and illegal behaviour. They were concerned that the strategy gave a bad message to other patients, with the implication that drug use was acceptable.

The harm-reduction lobby prevailed. The strategy appeared to be successful insofar as Mark continued to have leave and take cannabis without a major exacerbation of his illness. After 6 weeks of increasing and uneventful leave, Mark was returned to the unit by the police, having caused a disturbance at a railway station. He was agitated, thought disordered, paranoid and hallucinated. This state persisted for 48 hours. It emerged that he had taken amphetamine intravenously (IV) on the day of his arrest. It also emerged that he had gradually resumed amphetamine use during recent leaves, concealing this by 'borrowing' other patients' urine for his routine drug tests. He had used the drug intravenously only once, at the suggestion of a friend.

There was another heated debate in the MDT. The prohibition lobby took the event as vindication of their views. The most vehement harm-reductionists wanted Mark to be supplied with clean needles and syringes, but the majority were against this. It was decided to have another period of restriction to the unit, in order to stop IV drug use immediately and to stabilise his mental state and to resume harm reduction thereafter. This compromise pleased no-one. The prohibitionists expressed the view that Mark had been deliberately misleading staff in his apparent co-operation with the harm-reduction strategy. They disclosed that they had confronted him with this view on numerous occasions.

On exploration, it became apparent that the unresolved split in the staff group had sabotaged treatment by establishing a pattern of confused and hostile communication with Mark on the unit. Though different in content to the emotionally arousing communications with his parents, the effects upon Mark were similar, mirroring the singular focus upon drug use as a source of hostility and criticism.

The psychoeducational work with Mark's parents was also difficult. They continued to feel that the most significant task was to control Mark in order to achieve drug abstinence. They disagreed with the harm-reduction strategy and when Mark had leave at home, their behaviour was essentially unchanged. The IV amphetamine use strengthened their frequently expressed opinion that Mark should be detained without leave for a period of several months in the hope that his 'addiction' to drugs would eventually fade.

It did prove possible, however, to lead the parents to the view that their relationship with Mark would improve if he lived in supported accommodation rather than in their home. To achieve this, it was necessary for them to acknowledge that they were powerless to influence his drug use in the short term, not least by arguing with him about it.

Mark was discharged after 9 months. Risk assessment suggested that he was unlikely to behave aggressively provided that:

a. He remained in close contact with the service.
b. His mental state and drug intake could be closely monitored.
c. There was early intervention when risk indicators emerged, such as paranoid delusions or increased drug intake.

Mark went to live in a mental health hostel near to his parents' home. He attended painting classes at a local college four afternoons a week. He formed some friendships there and his work was well regarded. He continued to see his old friends and to take cannabis and, occasionally, amphetamine. He stayed in consistent contact with his CPN and was frank about his drug use. An arrangement was agreed with Mark, whereby his depot was increased during periods of heavy drug use in order to avoid relapse. He continued to suffer from auditory hallucinations from time to time, which he attributed to drug-taking. There were no further episodes of violence. He was re-admitted briefly on two occasions over the subsequent 4 years.

These outcomes were regarded as a significant improvement over the previous pattern of Mark's life. However, his parents remained fearful for him and supplied him with cash on request. This was usually spent on drugs. He remained somewhat feckless and some members of the MDT believed that, by protecting him from the consequences of his drug use, the strategy inhibited his maturation.

Discussion

Within this case study, it is possible to discern a staged approach to harm reduction (see Box 8.1). It is modified by the particular circumstances of risk management in a medium-secure setting. Such adaptations of a systematic approach are usually

> **Box 8.1   Stages in establishing a harm-reduction approach to substance misuse in patients with mental illness**
>
> • Detection of substance misuse
> • Shared recognition with the patient of benefits and hazards of substance misuse
> • Realistic goal-setting
> • Problem-solving aimed at development of alternatives to substance use
> • Planning for responses to relapse and escalations in substance misuse

necessary. This can demand some creativity in dealing with problems. For example, it might have been possible to engage Mark's drug-using friends in the psychoeducational programme or at least in some form of dialogue. If they had understood the dangers to him of particular patterns of drug use, they might have been able to support him in sustaining safer drug usage.

Drug use evokes strong feelings in patients, families and staff. It is difficult to establish a coherent response to it amongst clinical teams. There is invariably a divergence of opinion as to the personal responsibility of patients who take drugs and become more psychotic and aggressive as a consequence. Furthermore, drugs are illegal and there is a very real risk of other patients being recruited into substance misuse by drug users. This forces clinical teams to take an enforcement role which is usually only partially effective, and which is often counter-productive in the long run.

It often takes a long time to achieve even a limited success helping patients to control their drug use. It is frustrating work with frequent setbacks. Nonetheless, the approach set out above does often eventually succeed. Given the lack of more robust and properly evaluated interventions, it is likely to remain the most useful approach for the foreseeable future.

The only alternative is to regard substance misuse as a moral issue. This position suggests that patients should be informed of the relationship between substance misuse, mental illness and aggression and be left to decide whether to stop or continue substance misuse as a lifestyle choice. Patients would then be regarded as fully responsible for their actions if further violence occurs. We do not regard this as a tenable position. Given the importance of substance misuse as a risk factor, it is nonsensical and unethical to neglect it within care planning. The relationship between substance misuse and psychosis is complex and there is some evidence that mental illness leads to substance misuse as well as substance misuse worsening psychosis. These matters cannot be reduced to simple moral issues.

Conclusions

1. Substance misuse commonly complicates mental illness. It is a significant risk factor.
2. A modified harm-reduction strategy appears to be the most fruitful approach to containing the problem.
3. There are complex interactions between mental illness, substance misuse, medication and risk factors such as expressed emotion and social isolation.
4. Substance misuse provokes feelings in people which can be an impediment to a coherent response. These issues must be addressed as part of the overall strategy.
5. There are no properly evaluated interventions available and the subject is likely to remain controversial.

REFERENCES

Beck A, Wright F, Liese B 1993 Cognitive therapy of substance abuse. Guilford Press, New York
Dyer C 1996 Violence may be predicted among psychiatric patients. British Medical Journal 313: 318
Franey C, Quirk A 1996 Dual diagnosis. Executive Summary 51. The Centre for Research on Drugs and Health Behaviour, London

Goldstein P 1989 Drugs and violent crime. In: Weiner N, Wolfgang M (eds) Pathways to criminal violence. Sage, Newbury Park, California
Gournay K, Sandford T, Johnson S, Thornicroft G 1996 Double bind. Nursing Times 92(28): 28–29
Graham H 1998 The role of dysfunctional beliefs in individuals who experience psychosis and use

substances: implications for cognitive therapy and medication adherence. Behavioural and Cognitive Psychotherapy 26: 193–208

Hamilton J, Kopelman M, Maden T, Taylor P, Strang J, Johns A 1993 Addictions and dependencies: their association with offending. In: Gunn J, Taylor P (eds) Forensic psychiatry: clinical, legal, and ethical issues. Butterworth–Heinemann, Oxford, p 435–489

Johnson S 1997 Dual diagnosis of severe mental illness and substance misuse: a case for specialist services? British Journal of Psychiatry 171: 205–208

Liese B, Franz R 1996 Treating substance use disorders with cognitive therapy: lessons learned and implications for the future. In: Salkovskis P (ed) Frontiers of cognitive therapy. Guilford Press, New York

Lindqvist P, Allebeck P 1989 Schizophrenia and assaultive behaviour: the role of alcohol and drug abuse. Acta Psychiatrica Scandinavica 82: 191–195

Meuser K, Yarnold P, Levinson D et al 1990 Prevalence of substance abuse in schizophrenia: demographic and clinical correlates. Schizophrenia Bulletin 16: 31–56

Regier D, Farmer M, Rae D et al 1990 Co-morbidity of mental disorders with alcohol and other drug abuse: Results from the Epidemiological Catchment Area (ECA) study. Journal of the American Medical Association 264: 2511–2518

Smith J, Frazer S, Bower H 1994 Dangerous dual-diagnosis patients. Hospital and Community Psychiatry 45: 280–281

Swanson J, Holzer C, Ganju V 1990 Violence and psychiatric disorder in the community: evidence from the Epidemiological Catchment Area survey. Hospital and Community Psychiatry 41: 761–770

CONTENTS

Use and misuse of prescribed medication

·Dave Harper and Tom Mason

Introduction

This case study presents reflections with hind-sight upon the difficulties for staff in caring for an individual seen to be misusing prescribed medication. The discussion of the case acknowledges the difficulties the staff found themselves in and offers some alternative possibilities for interventions which could have been considered. These draw upon the growing critical literature into the whole issue of medication compliance and incorporates attempts to view such challenging case scenarios from a systems perspective. In this sense, attempts to use more than the prescribed dosage of medication can be seen as an interesting variant on the more typical compliance concerns around the refusal to take medication as prescribed.

The notion of compliance

A recent contribution to discussions in mental health about the concept of compliance (i.e. patients complying with recommended prescriptions of medication) has recommended the use of the term adherence rather than compliance since, it is suggested, the latter term implies passive acceptance whereas the former term implies a more active role for the patient (e.g. McPhillips & Sensky 1998). This seems a little bizarre since, if anything, the dictionary definition of adherence suggests an even firmer notion of sticking to a rule. However, this debate reveals some of the tensions involved in the notion of compliance. The traditional view would be that compliance is

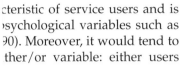

cteristic of service users and is
psychological variables such as
90). Moreover, it would tend to
ther/or variable: either users
were or were not compliant. However, recent
work suggests such a view is simplistic.

First, users' views are not simply pro- or anti-
medication, but, instead, are highly complex, the
result of negotiating between competing priorities in their lives (Day et al 1996). Second, traditional views define compliance from the point of
view of professionals, thus assuming and justify-
ing medical authority (Conrad 1985, Trostle
1988). However, the prescription of medication
could be said to symbolise the nature of the relationship between doctor, other staff and the
service user: is it a collaborative negotiating relationship or a didactic one (Barham & Hayward
1995)? Third, users can be seen as people actively
trying to manage their difficulties with recourse
to a number of strategies. Thus they can be seen
as self-regulating, using prescribed medication
in a more flexible manner than prescribed, perhaps only taking medication when symptoms
arise (e.g. Virji & Britten 1991). Such a view of
self-medication can be taken further to see the
use of non-prescribed and/or illicit substances in
the same way. Further, some have pointed to the
moral status of self-medication and that users
might adopt this position in order to reduce their
feelings of dependence on medication, their feelings of stigmatisation and their wish to assert
control over their problems or their life (Conrad
1987). Fourth, users' choices about medication
can be seen as valid and legitimate, based on a
sensible evaluation of the pros and cons, especially a wish to protect themselves from side
effects (Breggin 1996, Rogers et al 1993).

Of course, compliance is mainly an issue for
users where they have a choice about whether to
take medication. However, where they are
detained and receiving injections of neuroleptics,
compliance per se ceases to be an issue, but other
more complex and subtle problems ensue. A particularly difficult area is that of pro re nata (PRN)
medication, which is prescribed in hospital to be
given when the user requires it, within certain
parameters. This may be administered at the

request of the individual or offered by qualified
nursing staff where the presenting signs and
symptoms indicate a deterioration of physical
or mental health. Effective use of PRN medication can act as a useful form of early intervention
for users, but it is bedevilled by a number of
problems.

First, ward contingencies and practices often
mean that users are not thoroughly or regularly
monitored and thus PRN medication may be
offered in a reactive rather than a proactive manner. Second, the flexibility accorded staff in the
use of PRN medication means a wide range of
influences may determine its use. Although PRN
medication is prescribed by physicians, it is
largely the nurse who initiates the administration
(McLaren et al 1990) and the reasons offered for
dispensing vary widely in the literature (Fishel et
al 1994). Troisi et al (1997), for example, found a
positive correlation between patients' scores on
the paranoid/belligerence cluster of the DSM III-
R Positive and Negative Symptom Scale and
daily dosage of neuroleptic treatment. There is
no reason to assume such variability would not
occur in the administration of PRN medication
too. PRN medication may be given to alleviate
unpleasant side effects or offered in an attempt to
prevent a violent situation occurring. The tension
between focusing on the needs of the individual
and the needs of other users on the ward, and
ward management issues is clear here. Moreover,
there may be wide discrepancies in the way different staff and different shifts administer PRN
medication. In the following case study, we wish
to explore some of the complex issues surrounding compliance, particularly in a setting where
compliance per se is not an issue.

CASE STUDY: DANNY

Danny was from the urban heartland of a major
UK city, born and bred amongst the tenements
and tower blocks of a deprived inner city. He
was from a large family with several siblings,
who experienced marked poverty and his home
life was often chaotic, attracting the attention of
social services around issues of possible emotional neglect. Danny developed 'behavioural

problems' and was described as having a tendency to bully the more vulnerable and manipulate those he perceived to be stronger. Truancy was a typical feature of his schooldays, with the main motivation for attending school said to be easy access to cigarettes, alcohol and soft drugs. Danny engaged in problematic substance use at an early age.

Boredom and petty crime were prominent in Danny's youth which was punctuated by an increasing consumption of alcohol and street drugs. Danny would later state that paid employment, had it even been an option, would not have been sufficient to finance his lifestyle at this time.

Drawing on the survival skills of his early life, Danny identified a particularly vulnerable group of people to rob. He targeted elderly people living alone and eventually murdered an 80-year-old man, going on to ransack his home for money and possessions as the man lay dying. His second murder was more brutal, resulting in the theft of just a few pounds. Increasing levels of violence were evident in Danny's subsequent offences as he went on to commit further murders in similar circumstances before his arrest.

At trial, it was considered that Danny suffered primarily from psychopathic disorder with a degree of psychotic symptoms and required compulsory detention in a maximum security psychiatric facility. Accounts of his behaviour in hospital contained themes reminiscent of descriptions of his earlier life with bullying and manipulativeness predominating. Danny was treated for both his psychiatric problems and a perceived substance withdrawal syndrome. However, unbeknown to staff at the time, he was secreting and using both prescribed and illicit substances. Detained indefinitely under the Mental Health Act 1983, Danny was aware that he was, effectively, serving a natural life sentence. Perhaps because of this he came to be seen as a litigious complainant and was perceived by the staff as a difficult patient.

Danny's illicit drug use, and prescribed treatment, were complicated further by a chronic physical complaint, which required ever stronger pain relief in addition to special dietary foods. He was also viewed as dependent on chloral hydrate, taken for insomnia.

The dynamic of the problem

Through various strategies Danny was seen to cause numerous pressures for professional staff, resulting in difficulties in the day-to-day running of the ward. He was involved in frequent incidents of aggression or assault, including attacks with weapons or attempts at scalding. At other times, staff would report that Danny appeared to be 'playing the game', giving nursing staff an indication that he was improving and then, in their view, delighting in shattering the professional illusion. Danny was seen by staff as having recourse to a number of strategies through which he gained access to a range of medications. For example, he would frequently complain of disturbing nightmares in which he saw the faces of his victims, combining this with a demand for pain relief of some description. On a regular basis, he would require paracetamol for headaches, linctus for a sore throat and kaolin and morphine for his disordered alimentary tract. Similarly, he frequently demanded PRN neuroleptic medication for voices, yet staff often doubted whether these requests were prompted by symptoms. Attempts to suggest alternative interventions would be met with a barrage of complaints and allegations of victimisation and negligent treatment.

Danny came to be seen as an intractable management problem. He was moved between the Special Hospitals, a management strategy not uncommon at the time, with the promise of a new start on each occasion. The law did not allow for a move to prison and Danny appeared to be aware of this. He had many changes of Responsible Medical Officer with each psychiatrist reportedly becoming frustrated and disheartened as every therapeutic attempt appeared to be foiled. At particularly troublesome times, Danny was often moved within the hospital, rotating between wards, each becoming totally disrupted, highly stressed and requiring a period of recovery on completion of his stay. As his journey proceeded, primary nurses were quickly caught up in what they saw as a web of manipulation or complaint, and Danny had numerous changes of key-worker.

Over time, what staff saw as Danny's demanding behaviours were reported to increase and assumed different forms. Danny would place the blame for this on the refusal of staff to give him his medication, thus avoiding censure from his peers. Staff reported that it was not uncommon to see Danny apparently intoxicated by a mixture of drugs, legally prescribed, but illicitly employed. Staff described the unspoken strategy of the multi-disciplinary patient care team meetings held each week as 'keeping the lid on things'. The nursing teams reported that they simply wished to reach the end of the day without incident.

Attempts to establish boundaries were short-lived and staff reported that Danny became expert at breaching parameters. This was accomplished, staff felt, through a variety of means. First, by Danny requesting non-prescription drugs such as paracetamol and then building to requests for stronger ones. Second, he would find a reason to ask for his medication to be given a few minutes early, so that with each occasion the administration was slipping into 'illegal' territory. Third, Danny would often argue that a liquid measure was not up to the mark on the dispenser and attempt to claim more. Fourth, tablets were dropped, to be picked up later and secreted for later use, with Danny reacting aggressively, saying he had not been given the correct number of tablets. Nursing staff were often pressured into giving PRN medication to avert a potentially explosive situation.

Over a 25-year period, despite well-intentioned efforts, the care package in this case can be seen to have drifted into reactive responses to crises, rather than being driven by more sophisticated understandings of the challenges presented to the care team. The strong feeling of staff was that the system had been abused by Danny. He had been seen to invert the therapeutic efforts of professional staff to acquire drugs for his own intoxication and manipulated the hospital, doctors and nursing staff to gratify his own wants. Those who attempted to set boundaries and define limits were seen as being marginalised through Danny's referral of complaints via the hospital's complaints procedures. One view of this situation might be that medication was used inappropriately to stave off criticism and avoid confrontation, rather than for legitimate therapeutic benefit and, as a result, we may well feel that the system failed Danny.

Reflections

Of course, in reflecting on a case such as this we must bear in mind that this is written in hindsight and away from the demanding practical realities of the everyday clinical situation. However, cases like this are far from rare and there can be benefit in thinking through how different professional responses might have been possible. On reading the case, one is struck by the way the account appears to depict a struggle for power between Danny and staff. When a metaphor like this comes to organise the thinking about a situation, it can have a number of unintended consequences. One consequence is that the reasons and motivations of the opposing party are acknowledged minimally and, even then, in fairly negative terms. The opposing party becomes objectified, losing any real sense of subjectivity. What if we were to try to re-introduce Danny's subjectivity in this account? For example, did staff try to see the situation from Danny's point of view? Using principles of motivational interviewing (Miller & Rollnick 1991) staff might try to elucidate from Danny his reasons for using a wide range of prescribed and illicit substances and have a thorough discussion of the pros and cons of their use. For example, it is possible that Danny was attempting to self-medicate psychotic symptoms, physical pain, insomnia and emotional pain as a result of a deprived upbringing.

Once reasons were established, alternative coping strategies could be suggested. Further, staff might try to conduct a thorough and detailed assessment of his psychotic symptoms together with ongoing monitoring (e.g. symptom rating scales) that might provide more objective evidence to consider in deciding whether or not to use PRN medication. Practitioners might also offer counselling since, instead of simply prescribing chloral hydrate, a psychological intervention to enable him to cope better with nightmares might prove beneficial. Such work would be more likely to succeed if it began with goals which Danny himself had set. Detailed assessments might provide enough information on which to base a psychological formulation of Danny's difficulties.

One might wish to identify core beliefs or schemas Danny had gained as a result of his early life experiences. One might be 'the world is hostile and you have to take what you want to survive' and 'the weak have no value' (the latter might also reflect on how he might see himself as weak and as having no value). Such identification might open avenues for therapeutic intervention, for example, helping Danny to counter these beliefs by drawing on less negative experiences in his own and others' lives (e.g. the existence of caring relationships). Thus it might emerge that control and autonomy are important in Danny's life, especially as those involved in criminal activity often have a higher developed sense of autonomy than others.

In the context of detention in a maximum security psychiatric hospital, almost a prototype of the total institution, it may well be that Danny feels his use of medication is the only area in his life over which he has control. An intervention here might be to provide other areas over which he could have control.

Compliance therapy (Kemp et al 1997) has been suggested to encourage users to be more compliant with medication regimes. However, Perkins & Repper (1998) have argued that rather than using a motivational interviewing model,

this therapy has adapted it so much it is simply a disguised form of persuasion. Compliance therapy would not work well in this situation since there is a need to think about staff responses too and also since Danny was not non-compliant in the usual sense, he was over-complying with medication, trying to have more than recommended. Implicit in the presentation of the case are suggestions that Danny aimed at intoxicating himself. We might ask what reasons Danny might have for doing this to himself. Was he so unhappy with everyday life that he needed to cut off from his emotional experiences through substance use?

The provision of a formulation would also be helpful for staff, particularly if it indicated clear practical interventions they could carry out. Some cognitive analytic therapy formulations have been produced which include staff positioning and responses. It might be helpful to interview a wide range of staff to see the different emotional reactions Danny evokes in them: frustration and hostility in many, but perhaps also sympathy in others. A fruitful area for exploration here might be differences within and across shifts. Once staff became aware of the positions Danny invited them to adopt through his behaviour, they could choose to react in alternative ways, for example taking a one-down position rather than acting in a manner which will simply lead to an escalation of a symmetrical conflict. It may well be that further assessment might reveal that there are secondary gains both for Danny and the system in continuing the battle. Systemic thinking can be helpful here in guiding consultation (Harper & Spellman 1994) and in enabling staff to maintain a consistent but thoughtful response rather than one congruent with 'acting out'.

REFERENCES

Barham P, Hayward R 1995 Relocating madness: from the mental patient to the person. Free Associations, London

Breggin P 1996 Should the use of neuroleptics be severely limited? Changes: An International Journal of Psychology and Psychotherapy 14: 62–66

Conrad P 1985 The meaning of medications: another look at compliance. Social Science and Medicine 20: 29–37

Conrad P 1987 The noncomplaint patient in search of autonomy. Hastings Center Report 17: 15–17

David A 1990 Insight and psychosis. British Journal of Psychiatry 156: 798–809

Day J, Bentall R, Warner S 1996 Schizophrenic patients' experiences of neuroleptic medication: a Q-methodological investigation. Acta Psychiatrica Scandinavica 93: 397–402

Fishel A, Ferreiro B, Rynerson B, Nickell M, Jackson B, Hannan B 1994 As-needed psychotropic medications: prevalence, indications, and results. Journal of Psychosocial Nursing 32(8):27–32

Harper D, Spellman D 1994 Consultation to a professional network: reflections of a would-be consultant. Journal of Family Therapy 16: 383–399

Kemp R, Hayward P, David A 1997 Compliance therapy manual. The Maudsley, London

McLaren S, Browne F, Taylor P 1990 A study of psychotropic medication given 'as required' in a regional secure unit. British Journal of Psychiatry 156: 732–735

McPhillips M, Sensky T 1998 Coercion, adherence or collaboration? Influences on compliance with medication. In: Wykes T, Tarrier N, Lewis S (eds) Outcome and innovation in psychological treatment of schizophrenia. Wiley, Chichester

Miller W, Rollnick S 1991 Motivational interviewing: preparing people to change. Guilford Press, New York

Perkins R, Repper J 1998 Viewpoint: softly, softly. Mental Health Care 2(2): 70

Rogers A, Pilgrim D, Lacey R 1993 Experiencing psychiatry: users' views of services. Macmillan/MIND, London

Troisi A, Pasini A, DeAngelis F, Spalletta G 1997 Paranoid/belligerence and neuroleptic dosage in newly admitted schizophrenic patients. Journal of Clinical Psychopharmacology 17: 84–87

Trostle J 1988 Medical compliance as an ideology. Social Science and Medicine 27: 1299–1308

Virji A, Britten N 1991 A study of the relationship between patients' attitudes and doctors' prescribing. Family Practice 8: 314–319

CONTENTS

Relapse prevention for problematic alcohol use

Mick McKeown

This case study describes group work undertaken within a high-security setting aimed at relapse prevention for people with a previous history of substance use problems. Whilst acknowledging differences between substances, a blunt distinction is not drawn between alcohol and other drugs. Rather, the group work addresses problems with drug use generally, and individual's drug-using experiences specifically, for participants who have used various substances. The focus is on an individual, Joe, who had a long history of heavy alcohol consumption prior to admission to a Special Hospital for a serious violent offence. At the start of the intervention, he had been an in-patient for several years and abstinent from alcohol for this time. The relevant assessments, group work and evaluations are described, together with a discussion of the difficulties inherent in such work given the setting in a closed institution.

Drugs and alcohol

Drugs and drug use are exceedingly commonplace in modern society. Indeed, drugs have more than likely been part of human culture throughout history. However, the use of certain drugs, the attendant social consequences and the reactions of governments and the mass media have placed drug use, and its control, firmly to the fore of public consciousness. The 'drugs problem' has escalated to such an extent that the major Western nations now see themselves as engaged in nothing less than a 'war on drugs'.

Such discourse often serves to obscure the adverse social and health impact of substances such as alcohol, which by their relative legitimacy in law and culture can tend to escape the 'drug' label.

There has been much recent public and governmental concern surrounding a perceived growth in illicit substance use and associated societal problems (Parker et al 1995) with a more focused interest in the particular problems of drug-using psychiatric patients (Meuser et al 1992). Reported prevalence rates for co-morbidity of drug use and mental illness vary between 20% and 75% of the samples studied, yet much of this work suffers from methodological inadequacies (Meuser et al 1990). This client group presents a number of difficulties for the provision of services, with problems being particularly acute within in-patient facilities, especially regarding increased levels of violence (Smith & Hucker 1994). Problematic substance use has been implicated in the offending histories of forensic patients (Smith et al 1994), with a positive correlation between drug and alcohol consumption and criminality (Goldstein 1989). Within forensic institutions, drug use remains an under-researched and contentious issue, seen to result in a multitude of undesirable consequences (McKeown & Liebling 1995) and attracting both sensationalist scrutiny in the popular press and more sober deliberations of official inquiries.

Individuals attracting both a mental illness diagnosis and involved in any of the various forms of substance use have been latterly categorised as having a 'dual diagnosis'. This term is rapidly achieving prominence in the practice arenas of mainstream psychiatry and drug treatment services and points to the need for both improved and informed professional training and appropriate research. However, increasing reliance on the language of dual diagnosis has not necessarily been matched by definitional precision (McKeown & Derricott 1996). Some of this reflects broader problems arising from the categorical structuring of psychiatric diagnosis inherent to DSM-IV (APA 1994), particularly the general consideration of co-morbidity (Clark et al 1995). Consequently, the use of the dual

diagnosis descriptor has an homogenising effect when applied to actually quite heterogeneous populations.

Substance use in secure environments

Problematic substance use is a potential problem within any hospital environment. Misuse of illicit drugs can exacerbate behavioural problems such as aggressive outbursts and may cause management problems for staff at ward level. These can be due to behaviours associated with dealing in illicit drugs, including exploitation of more vulnerable patients. Of particular concern in forensic services is the general association between violence, aggression and substance use. The most commonly consumed drug is alcohol, though the emerging dual diagnosis literature tends to emphasise problems around illicit, seemingly more exotic, drugs. Regier et al's (1990) Epidemiological Catchment Area study found 22% of individuals with a lifetime history of any mental disorder also had problems with alcohol use, compared with the 15% who had problems with other substances.

It is usually argued that drug use has an adverse effect upon the course of psychotic illness, with various negative consequences for mental state or relationships. A number of studies have addressed the question of why people with psychotic problems choose to use substances. The reasons for such use are probably as varied and inclusive as, and in many cases identical to, those expressed by the public at large. These might include pleasure, to enhance self-esteem and to expand social networks. However, within the special circumstances of forensic care or general psychiatric services, patients may also turn to drugs to self-medicate symptoms or side effects of neuroleptics, to exaggerate hallucinatory experiences, for excitement, or in a challenge to restrictive or authoritarian hospital environments. These ends may be diverse, inter-related, or contradictory (Dixon et al 1990, Khantzian 1997).

It is difficult to gauge how these issues may affect prescribing decisions or medication adherence. Individuals may be engaged in a range of, perhaps complex, calculations regarding their personal drug use and relative affinity for street drugs, alcohol or prescribed medication. Such decision-making can be accessed, in alliance with drug users, in a cognitive–behavioural framework, towards goals of limiting harmful consequences, relapse prevention or enhancing therapeutic compliance, including adherence to prescribed medication. Readiness to uptake therapeutic intervention and progress in therapy can be enhanced by motivational interviewing techniques (Miller & Rollnick 1991). Advocated strategies include eliciting people's understanding of their drug use and education regarding possibly overlooked negative consequences, including effects on significant others in their social network. Importantly, discussions have to engage with an acknowledgement of positive effects, but also address any interplay between these and the negative effects. This collaborative approach can progress towards agreeing goals around future drug use or abstinence if this is preferred.

Economic modelling of drug use and its control within society as a whole draw attention to issues of supply and demand. Illicit drugs exist as a commodity, albeit an illegal one, within a global market-place. Control strategies are aimed at addressing either the supply of drugs, through the use of police, customs and the legal system or the demand for drugs, through the use of individual treatment programmes or social policy. Wodak (1993) concludes that though supply side measures consume most of the resources in the war on drugs, they are doomed to failure. Hence it has been widely argued for a change of emphasis towards a harm-reduction model, aimed at minimising the problematic consequences of drug use. In the micro worlds of secure hospitals, similar economies exist and even legal substances like tobacco can become a virtual proxy for currency. In the context of a secure psychiatric hospital, alcohol would usually be classified as a prohibited substance entering this semi-closed economic system.

In considering drug use in hospitals, lessons can be drawn from the global economy. First, attempts to control drug use by supply restriction alone will struggle to succeed. Even if this were not the case, such measures would probably have the effect of maximising security at the expense of therapeutic alliances, creating particularly off-putting circumstances for visiting relatives. Second, given a general focus on health, a harm-reduction philosophy makes sense. Within such a philosophy, there need not be any reason why demand-reduction methods, such as active therapy or promotion of alternative social activities, cannot also be pursued.

Assessment

Assessment has to attempt to access the complexity of people's problems and possible interconnections. The usual starting point is a comprehensive history of an individual's drug-taking, including which drugs were used and in what quantities. This might include asking for reasons why this person was using drugs; the reasons which maintain an individual's drug use may be different from those which initiated it. It is important to explore whether a person's offending behaviour is linked to the drug use in any way. We may wish to assess knowledge in particular areas, such as effects of drugs, how different drugs are used, which drugs are illegal, relative harm of different substances and risks associated with different ways of using. This can be accomplished by interview or using a structured questionnaire.

Certain attitudes would be important in either shielding somebody from relapse or placing them more at risk. These might include those concerning self-esteem, realism, hedonism and motivation. Low self-esteem places a person at particular risk of avoiding relapse. Relapse behaviour can be conceived of as occurring in a vicious circle of small failures; generating guilt and a lack of confidence in being able to handle the failure to achieve set goals, leading to further diminished self-esteem and continued drug use or total relapse (Scott 1986). The analogy is of a person attempting to abstain from a 20-a-day cigarette habit; this person has one cigarette, feels terrible about it, states thoughts of failure and an inability to succeed, and this failure, or total relapse, becomes a self-fulfilling prophecy. The Drug Related Attitude Questionnaire (DRAQ) was developed by Scott (1986) to assess salient, dysfunctional, drug-related attitudes. This tool consists of 18 items answered on a seven-point scale of strong agreement to strong disagreement. Sample items include 'If I slip and take drugs it is useless to try and control myself after that', 'I have nothing to look forward to' and so on.

Assessment of some key communication and social skills is also valuable. These may be observed in the course of the assessment interview, during the course of the group interactions, and informed by the observations of key practitioners. One way of identifying which skills may need attention is to elicit individual, high-risk situations, wherein a person would anticipate feeling at risk of relapse. Questioning would focus on what would be done to cope in that situation and how difficult this would be.

Relapse-prevention work

The intervention is based on a cognitive–behavioural approach and is intended to help people avoid future relapse (Jarvis et al 1995, Marlatt & Gordon 1985, Saunders & Allsop 1991, Scott 1986). Relapse in this context would be a failure to achieve personal goals with respect to drug use. Total relapse would be a consistent failure to meet such goals. The group work described needs to be seen as integral to the long-term case management of individuals, supported by other ongoing and subsequent interventions.

What is offered in terms of treatment will depend on an individual's reasons for using, or continuing to use, drugs. Some common patterns may emerge amongst members of a group. An important part of any intervention will be the provision of accurate information aimed at filling gaps in people's knowledge and understanding about drugs.

The drug relapse-prevention group consists of 12 sessions which aim to:

1. Provide accurate information about drug/alcohol use and its risks

2. Develop skills appropriate to prevention of relapse
3. Promote more helpful attitudes.

Referrals include any motivated person identifying drug/alcohol use as problematic in their lifestyle, prior to admission to a secure environment. An individual's drug/alcohol use need not necessarily have been implicated in offending behaviour.

The group work draws on the individual experiences of group members and utilises a range of audio-visual and written material as teaching aids and points of departure for discussions. The range of information covered in the group includes possible effects (pleasurable and unpleasant), legal issues, social myths, safer methods of drug/alcohol use and helping strategies and agencies. The provision of factual and balanced information is geared towards enabling the group members to make real choices about possible future drug-taking. It is recognised that information in itself is not sufficient as part of an effective health promotion package. So the group attempts to work on building the skills necessary to cope with the pressures to relapse. These relate primarily to decision-making, negotiation, assertiveness and problem-solving.

Attitudes to drugs and drug users are explored. Negative attitudes and mythologies are discussed and challenged because the persistence of such views and associated stigma may form potential barriers to uptake of assistance and support within the hospital or the community on discharge. Relationships between attitudes to drug use, social stigma, self-esteem and perceived self-efficacy are addressed in the context of the potential for a vicious circle of guilt, relieved by further drug use. Responses to the DRAQ provide material for use in these particular sessions.

Typically, the group progresses through the following subject areas:

1. Discussion of the concepts of drugs, addiction, dependence, tolerance, withdrawal and relapse
2. Facts about drugs, comparing different substances

3. The benefits and risks of drug use
4. Consequences of drug use for individuals and their social network
5. Factors which influence drug-taking behaviour
6. Drug use as risk-taking behaviour. Cognitive process of taking risks or not
7. Attitudes and stereotypes. Personal attitudes as a factor in relapse
8. A model of harm reduction
9. Alternatives to drug use. Problem-solving techniques
10. Community resources, the utility of a supportive network.

CASE STUDY: JOE

Relevant history

Joe is a 34-year-old man with a history of long-term problem drinking. He stated that, overall, he felt that his drink problems had been more prominent and enduring than those he had experienced from schizophrenia, his eventual diagnosis.

At the age of 17, whilst still living with his parents, Joe started drinking seriously, 'drinking for the sake of getting drunk'. At this time he would drink himself to a stupor on two or three occasions a week. By 18, Joe was brewing his own beer because it was cheaper and was drinking every day. In his early 20s, Joe spent 6 months in psychiatric hospital, diagnosed with psychotic depression. On discharge, he was unemployed with little money. He reports abstaining from drinking for 2 years. He still suffered depressed moods and frequent, but manageable, psychotic symptoms. Joe describes himself at this time as being 'immature and inadequate' without any coping abilities. Faced with many problems, he started drinking again 'for escapism'. For 5 or 6 years his consumption was heavy and progressively increasing up to the time of his admission to the secure hospital.

In Joe's view, his drinking was strongly linked to his offence. He stated that around this time he was drinking heavily because of feelings of depression and was in a cycle of postponing dealing with his problems so that everything was getting worse. He recalls that he was drunk when he committed the offence, a violent and fatal attack with a weapon, and had not felt 'in control' for a long time before. He had previously been remanded to psychiatric hospital for reports following other drink-related incidents.

Importantly, Joe sought out his own referral to this group, indicating a motivation to succeed in avoiding future relapse.

High-risk situations

On initial assessment, Joe had a realistic view of the potential for having any future problems with drink. Considering his lengthy (partly enforced) abstinence from drinking, it was thought that such realism should aid in planning for future events. An important feature of this intervention is the identification of likely social situations wherein the individual would feel particularly at risk of relapse. These would be worked through closely, making connections with expressed attitudes and likely cognitions and behaviours in anticipation of the situation occurring. Both proactive and reactive strategies would be rehearsed in the group, with all group members offering constructive feedback.

Joe stated that a potential high-risk situation for himself would be 'being around pubs, say going for a walk at night, feeling lonely'. He suggested that he would cope with such situations by visiting family and friends. He stated that he would not find such a situation difficult to handle (rated 1 on a five-point scale, where 1 = not at all difficult and 5 = extremely difficult). Given a hypothetical example of a high-risk situation concerning drink, Joe was able to identify appropriate risk factors and suggest potentially beneficial strategies for coping. However, these did not include any spontaneous suggestion of strategies for planning ahead. Formulating such strategies formed a major component of the group work to follow. In this respect, attention is paid to the notion of 'apparently irrelevant' decision-making which might lead a person into a high-risk situation. Participants were also encouraged to think closely about how realistic were their own assessments of anticipated competence in dealing with risky situations. Potentially helpful observations and behaviours are to be positively affirmed, but contradictions can be pointed out.

At assessment for the group, Joe reported that the main reasons he drank were for pleasurable effects, to lose inhibitions and talk more easily in social situations and to 'dampen down' his voices. Other motivations for drinking that he recalled included being bored, depressed or lonely, having no job, to 'escape', not being able to say 'no' and being let down. These issues would be returned to in group discussions and inform the sessions addressing high-risk situations. Group members were also encouraged to contemplate alternative means for achieving some of the needs satisfied previously by substance use or strategies for coping with identified problems.

The assessment interview also inquired about Joe's personal expectations from the planned intervention. He felt that he might benefit from the group work by learning how to communicate better without the use of alcohol. Joe identified a goal of learning skills to cope in situations wherein he might be tempted to drink. His ultimate stated goal was to achieve abstinence with respect to alcohol. Asked if he had any worries about the group work, Joe indicated that he was nervous about performing role plays. However, in practice, this did not deter him from taking part in experiential exercises within the group.

Joe's initial DRAQ assessment indicated various potentially helpful attitudes in 14 of the possible 18 items. However, there was room for improvement as only four of these responses were held with the maximum degree of conviction. Similarly, of the four responses which might indicate potentially detrimental attitudes, none was held with absolute conviction. Joe slightly agreed with the statements 'If you cannot do something well, there is little point in doing it at all', 'To be a good, moral, worthwhile person, I must help everyone who needs it' and 'Being isolated from others is bound to lead to unhappiness'. Such statements intend to elicit problems with self-esteem and views of own resourcefulness. As these were not strongly held, they were

not of major concern, but, nevertheless, were worthy of attention within the group. Of more concern was the fact that Joe agreed very much with the statement 'If I slip and take drugs it is useless to try and control myself after that'. This might indicate problems with ability to avoid relapse in the future.

Within the group sessions, we attempted to deal with the above material. Joe's statements and contributions indicated a resolve not to relapse and realistic assessments of future difficulties. The relationship between attitudes and ability to avoid relapse, and the important role of self-esteem in this, were dealt with in some depth. Joe demonstrated an understanding of the issues involved in this respect. Specific attention was given to the potential impact upon cognitions and decision-making when faced with high-risk situations. Potentially detrimental cognitions, or automatic thoughts, were identified and self-instruction techniques were practised.

Evaluation of progress

Prior to starting the group, Joe's knowledge about alcohol, as measured by a questionnaire, was reasonably good. He was only unsure about the answer to one question. Following completion of the group, this questionnaire was repeated and Joe scored 100% correct answers for those questions appropriate to alcohol. His knowledge of other drugs was patchy, but did improve over the course of the group. However, this is merely of academic value, given Joe's problems being solely confined to alcohol use.

On completion of the relevant portion of the group work, the DRAQ was re-administered. Joe's response to the re-test showed favourable changes in reported attitude, all such change being in the direction of potentially beneficial attitudes. On the re-test, he offered the optimum preferred response in 13 of the 18 items, with four of the remainder within the preferred range. The only potentially detrimental statement with which Joe continued to agree, albeit slightly, was the item 'To be a good, moral, worthwhile person I must help everyone who needs it'. This attitude statement is likely to reflect low self-esteem.

On discussion of this with Joe, it appears that his response with respect to this statement was associated with his religious beliefs.

Joe was a hard-working and conscientious member of this group, consistently demonstrating that he had given some thought to the subjects under consideration. In discussion with Joe, following completion of the group, he was able to describe what he felt he had learnt in some detail. Importantly, Joe was able to describe the model of relapse which had been presented and identify the relevance to himself. Also, he was able to discuss ways in which he might achieve social aims without drinking. He felt he had enjoyed the group and it had helped him in being able to discuss his problems. Joe gives the impression of being genuinely motivated to avoid relapse. He understands the link between his own attitudes, self-esteem and risk of relapse and should be supported by future interventions in maintaining consideration of relevant issues. Further interventions could include a focus on building upon behavioural skills appropriate to coping with his identified high-risk situations. This work would involve some problem-solving techniques, offering Joe an opportunity to enhance his social skills repertoire.

Joe comes across as a quiet, passive individual. Although he managed to overcome this by participating in the group, where he felt comfortable, he would agree that sometimes he would have problems in social situations. It would benefit Joe if he were able to undertake some further work dealing more specifically with assertion.

Reflections

This case study has discussed a relatively successful intervention with an individual having a previous history of alcohol problems and psychosis. However, since a number of factors indicate that this case was relatively less complex than many in this client group, general claims made for the intervention need to be cautious. At the time of the group work, Joe was well motivated, abstinent and relatively symptom-free with respect to his psychosis. Other difficulties,

contingent upon the treatm[e] further grounds for tempering e

The underpinning harm-redu can sit ill at ease with the legitin for security and safety within forensic hospitals, causing various tensions for practitioners. A major area of concern in attempting this sort of work in a secure setting is the removal of individuals from their everyday environment and lifestyle. It is intended that the intervention acts as an 'innoculation' against exposure to risk when it occurs. Difficulties arise in evaluating the success of therapy because the person is not consistently faced with the social situations likely to include a degree of access to drugs. Hence, we cannot know with any degree of certainty whether what is practised in hospital will generalise into the real world experiences of discharged patients. Even if a person is exposed to illicit substance use within the hospital, the secretive nature of such activity may affect the likelihood of that person bringing it to the attention of a therapist. In a more general sense, the whole issue of motivation and treatment uptake in forensic institutions is complex, and practitioners have to strike a balance between positive regard for clients and a healthy scepticism. The links between drug use and offending are not addressed in depth in this group and are worthy of further work.

Despite the given constraints, secure settings may also offer a variety of therapeutic opportunities. Relatively lengthy admissions can help to foster long-term therapeutic relationships with key therapists. With respect to a cycle of change (Prohaska & Di Clemente 1986), there has often been the time for contemplation in conditions where access to the problematic substance is restricted.

Given Joe's ultimate aim of abstinence from drinking, and his past history of psychotic mental health problems, any discharge plan should incorporate adequate community support, assistance and supervision in achieving such ends. Importantly, Joe should be engaged directly in his discharge planning, particularly with respect to detailing strategies for avoiding or coping with potentially hazardous social situations. Importantly, those situations Joe has already identified as risky include times when he is feeling lonely and significant social occasions, such as weddings. These points would indicate a cogent rationale for involving Joe's family and social network in future planning. Thus, all interested stakeholders could be involved in drawing up an individualised relapse-prevention plan, prior to any prospective discharge.

REFERENCES

American Psychiatric Association 1994 Diagnostic and statistical manual of mental disorders. APA, Washington DC

Clark L, Watson D, Reynolds S 1995 Diagnosis and classification of psychopathology: challenges to the current system and future directions. Annual Review of Psychology 46: 121–153

Dixon L, Haas G, Weiden P, Sweeney J, Frances A 1990 Acute effects of drug abuse in schizophrenic patients: clinical observations and patients' self-reports. Schizophrenia Bulletin 16: 69–79

Goldstein P 1989 Drugs and violent crime. In: Weiner N, Wolfgang M (eds) Pathways to criminal violence. Sage, Newbury Park, California

Jarvis T, Tebbutt J, Mattick R 1995 Treatment approaches for alcohol and drug dependence: an introductory guide. Wiley, Chichester

Khantzian E 1997 The self-medication hypothesis of substance use disorders: a reconsideration and recent applications. Harvard Review of Psychiatry 4: 231–243

Marlatt, G, Gordon J (eds) 1985 Relapse prevention: maintenance strategies in the treatment of addictive behaviours. Guilford Press, New York

McKeown M, Derricott J 1996 Muddy waters. Nursing Times 92(28): 30–31

McKeown M, Liebling H 1995 Staff perceptions of illicit drug use within a special hospital. Journal of Psychiatric and Mental Health Nursing 2: 343–350

Meuser K, Yarnold P, Levinson D et al 1990 Prevalence of substance abuse in schizophrenia: demographic and clinical correlates. Schizophrenia Bulletin 16: 31–56

Meuser K, Bellack A, Blanchard J 1992 Comorbidity of schizophrenia and substance abuse: implications for treatment. Journal of Consulting and Clinical Psychology 60: 845–856

Miller W, Rollnick S 1991 Motivational interviewing: preparing people to change addictive behaviour. Guilford Press, New York

Parker H, Measham F, Aldridge J 1995 Drug futures. ISDD, London

Prohaska J, Di Clemente C 1986 Towards a comprehensive model of change. In: Miller W, Heather N (eds) Treating addictive behaviours: processes of change. Plenum Press, New York, p 3–27

Regier D, Farmer M, Rae D et al 1990 Co-morbidity of mental disorders with alcohol and other drug abuse: Results from the Epidemiological Catchment Area (ECA) study. Journal of the American Medical Association 264: 2511–2518

Saunders B, Allsop S 1991 Helping those who relapse. In: Davidson R, Rollnick S, MacEwan I (eds) Counselling problem drinkers. Tavistock/Routledge, London

Scott M 1986 Cognitive–behavioural approach to client problems. Tavistock/Routledge, London

Smith J, Hucker S 1994 Schizophrenia and substance abuse. British Journal of Psychiatry 165: 13–21

Smith J, Frazer S, Bower H 1994 Dangerous dual-diagnosis patients. Hospital and Community Psychiatry 45: 280–281

Wodak A 1993 Taming demons: the reduction of harm resulting from the use of illicit drugs. The International Journal of Drug Policy 4: 72–77

CHAPTER 9

Seemingly intractable problems

CHAPTER CONTENTS

CONTENTS

The silent resistance

Tom Mason and Dave Mercer

Introduction

In his, now seminal, paper on the concept of the dangerous individual in 19th century psychiatry, Michel Foucault (1978) opens with a contemporary scene from a French court in 1977. In depicting the silence of the accused, Foucault shows how the machinery of the court, the law and criminal justice grinds to a halt in the absence of self-explanation. Thus revealing the need for the lubricant of discourse in order to function, Foucault begins:

The accused hardly spoke at all. Questions from the presiding judge:
'Have you tried to reflect upon your case?' – Silence.
'Why, at twenty-two years of age, do such violent urges overtake you? You must make an effort to analyze yourself. You are the one who has the keys to your own actions. Explain yourself.' – Silence.
'Why would you do it again?' – Silence.
Then the juror took over and cried out, 'For heaven's sake, defend yourself.'

In a similar vein, psychiatry too needs the noise of language in order to legitimate the exercise of its power. Just as a court may well condemn a person who refuses to offer any defence, forensic psychiatry can well incarcerate someone who refuses to speak. Yet, both systems lose credence unless the voice of the accused is heard. Only then can the content be deemed untruth or irrational. Once the word is spoken, the 'expertise' of the judge and the psychiatrist can be invoked and, thus, provide a legitimation for the execution of their roles.

Moreover, a singular reliance on observed actions merely produces evidence of behaviour

215

without explanation. To understand behaviour one needs to explore the rationalisations, interpretations and explications mediated through language. Without discourse, it is difficult to assess changes in attitude or thinking which may accompany such behaviour, making problematic any prediction of re-occurrence. The voice is, in effect, an externalised indicator of inner psychic functioning without which psychiatry remains illegitimate.

Theoretical background

Silence is both the lack of communication and a communication in itself. We can outline several examples of this to illustrate the theoretical background of silence.

Ideological silence

History offers many examples of dominant ideologies, where individuals are collectively socialised into an unswerving dogmatic 'faith' that their 'cause' is just and proper. Through this process, members of the 'in-group' become entrenched and blinkered towards their own crusade, often at the expense of others. These systems may well be founded upon religious, political or professional zeal. Our argument pivots on the extent to which any ideological belief system is constructed to absorb its own contradictions. We begin with an extreme example, in which the ideological structures of politics, humanities and morality meshed with the ideological constructs of science, medicine and professionalism to create a monstrous dictatorship in which all opposition and resistance were silenced.

The Nazi holocaust, in which upwards of 11 million people were put to death, occurred during the period of 1939–45. The programme is said to have begun with the killing of a deformed child, at the request of the parents, and was undertaken not in a concentration camp but at the Leipzig University Children's Hospital under the auspices of doctors and nurses (Meyer 1988). It is now well known that the Action T4 programme, the action against handicapped

children, was preceded by almost 5 years (1934–39) of a eugenics policy which involved the compulsory sterilisation of 350 000 persons with hereditary, mostly psychiatric, disorders. Following the outbreak of the war, in 1939, such people were systematically killed. Thus, the early perpetrators of the holocaust were not SS guards but doctors, nurses and midwives. It needs to be acknowledged that while some participated willingly, others co-operated under duress, with a smaller number who refused becoming victims themselves. The end-point, the concentration camps in which millions of Jews, gypsies, homosexuals and political prisoners were exterminated are stark testimony to the march of 'science' in the guise of medical experimentation.

Following the war, many medical personnel faced the Nuremberg courts with a 'rational' explanation; not of shame or guilt, but of conviction. For example, Werner Catel, the Head of the Paediatric Department in Kiel, when on trial for his part in Action T4, claimed: 'complete morons, when considered even from a religious point of view, are not human beings as they have no personality. To exterminate them is neither murder nor killing' (von Schlabrendorff 1979).

What reigned in the immediate post-Nuremberg era, in relation to the (generic) *men* of science and medicine, was silence. The survivors, both victim and perpetrator 'are those who by their prevarication, or abilities, or good luck did not touch bottom' (Levi 1989). This 'bottom', which can only be glimpsed by those who have not touched it themselves, has such significance that it cannot be articulated: 'the best one can do is point to the enormous gap between what is told and what cannot be told, that is, indicate the abyss separating the drowned and the saved' (Lyotard 1990). This silence was complete for nearly two decades. The scientific literature avoided the issue, as victims (survivors), believing themselves to be unworthy narrators of the event, unable to find any worthy listeners, made no sound. The account was finally opened in the 1960s and 1970s with a debate regarding the mass of medical research findings from the holocaust and the ethical implications of such data being utilised by American and Soviet scientists in the 'space race' (Moe 1984). At the same time, personal narratives were beginning to emerge from the writings of Anne Frank and Primo Levi and another strategy of silence materialised. This was encapsulated in the revisionist histories of 'New Right' fascist groups, spawning a denial that the holocaust had ever taken place. Such a denial is the most subtle form of annihilation. They, in effect, completed what the Nazis of the Third Reich could not.

If we transpose for Nazism, not psychiatry in general (as that would be too radical), but certain psychiatric thinkers who fail to see the plight of those drowning in the wake of their propaganda, like the doctors at Nuremberg, we note disturbing similarities. First, we see an ideology considered by professionals as right and proper, yet disregarding the pain and suffering which it creates. Second, we see victims reduced to a silence so profound that no amount of 'white noise' can break it. Third, we see many and varied mechanisms of the will to power in a perpetuation of this system. This brings us to the second level of theory.

Clinical and therapeutic silence

Silence and therapy form a closely interwoven and complex network of coercive strategies adopted at both micro and macro levels. Silence is often used as a strategy by the therapist and the patient alike. Thestrup (1994) outlined the role of silence from the analysts' perspective and shows that with certain group formations, such as incest survivor groups, silence can be used to create a boundary which is reminiscent of, and often connected to, the conflict of speaking out about the original trauma. Martyres (1995) discusses the types of silences encountered in clinical work, believing that although silence is often perceived as uncomfortable, it is an important vehicle for human interaction. Through the therapists' use of silence, she shows how it provides a powerful experiential medium to identify the focus needed with emotional distortions. Taking the notion of Rogerian 'reflective listening', itself based on the Heideggarian concept of 'authentic language',

Sundararajan (1995) claims that this acts 'as a discourse, avoids authorship, prescriptiveness, and self-assertion'. Such therapeutic silence is said to help clients listen to themselves. However, this rather one-sided analysis of silence, created and controlled by the therapist, does not appear to hold the same weight when viewed in relation to a patient's refusal to speak. Such a silence is unlikely to evoke the interpretation that it will enable the therapist to 'listen and reflect'.

From Gendlin's (1990) perspective, 'resistant silence' is one problem that many 'schizophrenic' patients manifest, leaving some therapists frustrated, angry and feeling impotent. However, this can also be the case for patients more generally, not only those with mental health problems. In Silverman's (1987) view, silence can be employed as an adaptive strategy to resist all treatment interventions in the face of the power and dominance of medical systems. The complexity becomes even more profound in relation to 'elective mutism' which is used in attempting to address a perceived imbalance of power, particularly in children (Krolian 1988) who may be in fear of parental forces, or hiding abuse. These avoidance-type interpretations are contrasted with the symbolic representation model of silence as a means of communication (Ehrenhaus 1988) where there may be any number of motivating forces driving the silence as a message medium. When a person rationally chooses silence as a strategy, then its potency is reliant upon someone's need, or desire, to urge the person to speak, for whatever reason, e.g. as a defence strategy in a court of law or to reveal individual thoughts, attitudes and feelings. Before presenting one specific case, we briefly mention the current state of legislation in the UK which deals with the right (or lack of it) of silence in court.

Silence and criminal justice

In the UK, the right of silence when interfacing with the criminal justice system was rescinded in March 1995. This abolition of the right of silence forces the alleged offender to offer a defence, on the basis that failure to do so will permit negative inferences to be drawn by the court.

Furthermore, the right of silence at trial is abandoned and the accused must provide evidence, otherwise the judge and prosecution can comment adversely to the jury about the defendant's refusal. Finally, the suspect must also account for any incriminating circumstances, for failure to do so again attracts adverse interpretations (George 1995). Although the principle that the burden of proof is on the prosecution (i.e. innocent until proven guilty), this policy change undermines the suspect's opportunity of defence. Forced to speak, the individual must reveal, and in revelation resides vulnerability. Ironically, it is the individual's own coerced commentary that condemns an individual. Inverting the chronicle in Foucault's above depiction, the juror no longer shouts 'for heaven's sake *defend* yourself', but now roars 'for heaven's sake *condemn* yourself'. This is uncomfortably close to the notion of 'confession', either religious or psychiatric.

Again, we can see parallels with the compulsorily detained mentally disordered offender and the psychiatric system that coerces the offender's conversation, this forced discourse being used in evidence against the offender and providing a legitimation for the offender's continued detention. The 'mentally ill' are constrained to tell of their 'delusions', 'paranoid schizophrenics' are forced to speak of 'persecutions' and 'sex offenders' are compelled to share their 'fantasies'. The more they confess, the more they are condemned – unless they learn to speak the right words long enough to be convincing. However, when those detained for psychiatric treatment refuse to speak at all, then flaws in the 'therapeutic' alliance become patently obvious and extremely disturbing.

CASE STUDY: VINCENT

Vincent is now a middle-aged man in his mid-50s who has spent over 30 years in a high-security psychiatric hospital.

Early life

The only information that we have of Vincent is either of a secondary nature, from family and friends, or of a hermeneutic quality having observed him for many years. The reason for this is that Vincent has not, to anyone's knowledge, spoken a word for over 30 years, throughout which time he has languished in a Special Hospital. What we know of his childhood is that, according to his relatives, it was relatively uneventful with only the 'usual' prankish behaviour of petty theft, truancy and fighting. He was an only child. His mother was strict and his father was always too busy to give him much attention. He had a strong Catholic upbringing, but this lapsed in his teens. His adolescence was somewhat traumatic as he was a late developer and was teased about this by his peers. His first known sexual encounter was at the age of 17. As a youth he had two court appearances, one for taking and driving away a car and the other for fighting. He enjoyed alcohol, but was not considered a heavy drinker and he is not known to have used any illicit substances.

Vincent had regular girlfriends, but none that lasted for any length of time. One of these women became pregnant and had an abortion, following which the relationship ended. Friends were few and far between, with only one lasting into adulthood. By his early 20s, Vincent had grown into a large man, over 6 feet tall and weighing a good 14 stone. He did not engage in any physical activities, but liked to watch sport on television.

Index offence

In his early 20s, Vincent began to take an interest in weapons and subscribed to several magazines of that genre. He collected an array of knives and imitation guns, but at no time was it perceived as 'unhealthy' or that any untoward incident might take place. Vincent continued to live at home with his parents, but would occasionally stay out overnight which was presumed to be with his girlfriend. One summer evening, in the late 1960s, Vincent abducted an 8-year-old boy and took him to a derelict house where he held him for almost 40 hours. The local news carried headline features concerning the boy's disappearance and the police and neighbourhood residents

---

Box 9.1 Interventive attempts by discipline

- Psychiatric
  Numerous medications and 'cocktails' (often forced), requests to attend group and individual therapies
- Psychological
  Various behavioural programmes including DRO scheduling, systems of reward and punishment and visual flagging of good and bad behaviour
- Nursing
  Primary care and key-worker systems, nursing process and problem-solving approaches and individual

counselling. Many attempts at relationship formation, including buddy systems and advocacy approaches
- Pastoral
  Visits by religious ministers attempted
- Social worker
  Attempts to engage Vincent by use of his family network
- Occupational therapy
  Ward-based attempts

DRO: differential reinforcement of other behaviour (see Mason & Chandley 1999).

were out vigorously searching. Vincent released the boy on the morning of the third day and the police were alerted. He was found at the derelict house, quietly sitting in a chair. On arrest he stated 'I never harmed him', which were the last words spoken by him to the outside world.

There was no evidence of any assault on the boy, either physical or sexual, and Vincent had given him food and fluid throughout the abduction. The boy reported that his captor had not been angry and had spoken to him about a number of things such as football, school, friends and his upbringing. The boy had been very frightened at first and wanted to go home. Vincent sometimes left the room but the boy could neither open the door nor climb up to reach the window.

At his trial, Vincent would not speak or defend himself in any way, refusing to co-operate at psychiatric interview. He had spoken briefly with his lawyer but the content was confidential. The events of the offence were sufficiently 'odd' for two psychiatrists to agree that Vincent was suffering from a psychopathic disorder with a possible mental illness overlay, warranting admission to a Special Hospital on a Hospital Order with restrictions.

Early hospital days

Vincent was very troublesome. He continued his refusal to speak, but would become aggressive towards fellow patients and staff. When

approached with a request, he would either ignore the person and carry on with the task at hand or, sometimes, shake his head to indicate a negative response. If the person pursued the request, Vincent would often attack. He had many periods in intensive care and was heavily sedated at times of extreme violence. He was frequently secluded, but no mechanical restraints were ever used at the hospital. Vincent rejected any direct contact with psychiatrists or psychologists and would not engage with nursing staff. He had no 'friends' amongst his peers and did not accept visits. He wrote letters of complaint in the very early days, but ceased this when they were interpreted within a psychopathological framework. In the first 15 years of his stay, he vacillated between intensive care and a high dependency ward, not attending occupational therapy or in-house social events. Many attempts at a therapeutic enterprise had been made including those in Box 9.1.

Thus, at the 15-year mark, Vincent continued to refuse to speak and the many efforts to engage him in a therapeutic encounter had failed. The main result of this 15-year exercise was the withdrawal of staff and peers from approaching this very difficult and aggressive individual. If you did not bother him, he would not bother you, and the cycle of silence was complete.

Later hospital days

In the mid-1980s Vincent's behaviour changed. Whether this was attributable to the great forensic

Box 9.2 Some relevant questions

- To what extent can we accurately assess the level of dangerousness of the patient?
- What are the ethical considerations of continued detention without treatment?
- Can the patient realistically be released?
- Is psychiatry being illegitimately employed to detain this person?

friend, 'old Father Time', or whether it was more subtly because of changes in the mental health legislation, is difficult to ascertain. However, the alteration in behaviour was significant. Vincent ceased assaulting others and although if pressured he would strike out, it was not with the same vehemence. He would still push his way through groups, or brush individuals aside, but actual fights ceased. He also developed a protectionist approach to weaker patients on the ward and could periodically be seen intervening with a tap on the shoulder and a shake of the head to a bullying peer. His physical size remained commanding. Furthermore, he slowly began to comply with the ward and hospital rules and became a ward worker. This gave him access to more privileges and money and over a 5-year period he settled into a routine which led him to be awarded ground parole, a system of limited access to certain areas of the hospital grounds.

Changes in the Mental Health Act 1983 meant that Tribunals were compulsorily held on the patients' behalf every 3 years, making it necessary to be able to show either a treatment strategy or at least an ability to prevent a deterioration in condition. In the first instance we could do neither because of the silence. A second generation of approaches were made but all to no avail, except that staff were no longer attacked. We are questioned on a number of fronts set out in Box 9.2.

In this second generation of attempts, numerous explanatory frameworks emerged to, in part, answer these questions, or at least salve the conscience and satisfy the Tribunals. For example, it was stated that Vincent was probably suffering from a deep-seated psychosis as no rational person could remain silent for so long. Another

psychoanalytical explanation flippantly observed that it was 'anal retention gone mad'. Others stuck firmly to the psychopathic label proclaiming that Vincent's personality had fragmented and he was socially withdrawn, inwardly hostile and narcissistic. However, as noted earlier, these can all be seen as examples of secondary elaborations of belief adopted to absorb their own contradictions.

Two practical examples

On one occasion, the psychiatrist, under pressure for a Tribunal report, and a patient care team, dissatisfied at the lack of progress in this case, sent a nurse to request that Vincent come and talk to him. Vincent stood tall and shook his head. This was relayed back to the psychiatrist who angrily approached Vincent himself, confronting him with the words 'You will remain here until you do talk to me'. At this point, Vincent gave one of his very rare smiles and clenched his lips tighter. The psychiatrist stormed off in silence!

On another occasion, a flu epidemic had hit the ward population and patients were clamouring for relief of their aches and pains through aspirins and cough linctus. Vincent became a victim and was forced to join the queue at the next drug round. When it was his turn in front of the dispenser of drugs, the nurse enquired 'Yes, Vincent, what would you like?', in the obvious hope of a major breakthrough. Vincent pointed to his streaming eyes, gave a hacking cough and made a humorous pleading gesture of prayer with face and hands, but remained silent. The nurse smiled and dispensed the appropriate medication. Again, this was a rare glimpse of some form of relationship.

Summary

Here, silence is seen in a complex interplay of power sources. At one level, the communication of resistance and at another, the dissipation of psychiatric force. The silence became global in the sense that it was absorbed by the hospital and by the ideology. This was only broken with the emergence of the 'clinical' in relation to the silence of the patient, leaving only questions of morality in relation to the right to be silent.

Over 30 years later, we still do not know what the circumstances of that abduction were about and we do not know if Vincent really is a danger to others. At the time of writing, he remains silent and, although refusing all investigations, it is believed that he has cancer and will shortly die. We also believe that he will die without 'confessing'.

REFERENCES

Ehrenhaus P 1988 Silence and symbolic expression. Communication Monographs 55(1): 41–57

Foucault M 1978 About the concept of the 'dangerous individual' in 19th century legal psychiatry. International Journal of Law and Psychiatry 1(1): 1–18

Gendlin E T 1990 Schizophrenia: problems and methods of psychotherapy. Review of Existential Psychology and Psychiatry, Special Issue 20(1–3): 181–191

George B 1995 The Criminal Justice Act. Gazette 92(1): 1–2

Krolian E B 1988 Speech is silvern, but silence is golden: day hospital treatment of two electively mute children. 16(4): 355–377

Levi P 1989 The drowned and the saved. Vintage Books, New York

Lyotard J F 1990 Heidegger and 'the Jews'. University of Minnesota Press, Minneapolis

Martyres G 1995 On silence: a language for emotional experience. Australian and New Zealand Journal of Psychiatry 29(1): 118–123

Mason T, Chandley M 1999 Managing violence and aggression: a manual for nurses and health care workers. Churchill Livingstone, Edinburgh

Meyer J E 1988 The fate of the mentally ill in Germany during the Third Reich. Psychological Medicine 18: 575–581

Moe K 1984 Should the Nazi research data be cited? Hastings Center Report 14: 5–7

Silverman S 1987 Silence as resistance to medical intervention. General Hospital Psychiatry 9(4): 259–266

Sundararajan L 1995 Echoes after Carl Rogers: 'reflective listening' revisited. Humanistic Psychology, Special issue 23(2): 259–271

Thestrup G 1994 Silence as boundaries and barriers in group analytic focus group (incest). Second congress of the European Federation of Sexology. Nordisk-Sexologi, Special issue 12(2): 146–150

von Schlabrendorff F 1979 Begegnungen in 5 Jahrzehnten. Wunderlich, Tubingen S

CONTENTS

Treatment resistance

Claire Barkley

Introduction

This case study is an account of the treatment of a young male patient chosen to illustrate the medical contribution to the management of treatment-resistant schizophrenia. The case is preceded by an overview of the concept of treatment resistance together with a brief summary of current treatment approaches including the use of clozapine and the newer atypical antipsychotic medications. Their place in forensic cases will be considered.

What is meant by 'treatment resistance'?

In order to understand the basic theoretical background to the pharmacological treatment of schizophrenia, it is necessary to consider the dopamine hypothesis, which has been around for 30 years. It states that antipsychotic drugs owe their therapeutic effects to their ability to block central dopamine receptors. It has been assumed that antipsychotic effects are mediated through actions at dopaminergic receptors in the limbic areas of the brain. If the brain of the person suffering from schizophrenia is exposed to a D_2 dopamine receptor blocker, there will be a significant amelioration of the positive symptoms in around seven out of 10 cases, usually within the first 2 months. A beneficial effect upon the negative features is much less dependable.

Until the 1980s, the concept of treatment resistance was not clearly defined and was usually associated with long-term institutionalisation.

The re-discovery of clozapine as a treatment option for such patients and the development of the newer, atypical, antipsychotic medications has emphasised research-orientated definitions which, of necessity, have been rigidly operationally defined. These criteria have been recognised as too narrow for clinical purposes since functional and psychosocial factors also contribute to the persistent disability of enduring schizophrenia.

Effective treatment of schizophrenia relies upon a clearly thought-out package of multidisciplinary care involving pharmacological, psychosocial and behavioural interventions. The medical treatment must be closely monitored to maximise compliance and check for the emergence of side effects. Failure to respond adequately after 8 weeks of antipsychotic medication should prompt a review of the treatment strategy. Where possible, polypharmacy should be avoided and one change at a time to the drug regimen is advisable to avoid a confused picture.

The standard for what constitutes an unsatisfactory response varies widely and return to best premorbid function should be considered as a standard (Meltzer et al 1990). Treatment-resistant patients will generally have at least moderate positive symptoms, negative or disorganisation symptoms, inappropriate affect and poverty of thought, or one of the above with impaired social function, despite two adequate trials of conventional antipsychotic drugs chosen from different classes of these agents (Kane et al 1988).

Why do some patients fail to respond?

Failure to recover fully on adequate doses of medication may be a result of non-response, poor compliance, illicit drug use, concomitant physical illness or a host of family and social problems. Often it is the emergence of side effects which prevents patient tolerance of conventional doses of neuroleptics which may have been effective if tolerated. The most troublesome side effects seem to be the extrapyramidal side effects (EPSE) (especially akathisia and akinesia) which result from D_2 receptor blockade in the striatum and occur in up to 75% of patients. In forensic practice, where young men are the norm, sexual dysfunction is also a frequent cause for complaint and results from elevated prolactin levels.

Compliance

Poor compliance is a significant factor in the failure of patients to recover. It has also been shown to be linked to a variety of patient, staff, illness and treatment factors including sociopathic personality, impulsiveness, grandiosity, low levels of insight, low socio-economic status, poor supervision and an inflexible approach by the doctor (Buchanan 1998). Clinical experience suggests that a negotiating, collaborative style on the part of the psychiatrist, coupled with a simple drug regimen and assertive follow-up are most likely to succeed. Specific techniques such as compliance therapy, based on the techniques of motivational interviewing have been shown to improve compliance in randomised clinical trials (Kemp et al 1996).

Treatment strategies

There is no current evidence that chronic concurrent prescription of a conventional neuroleptic plus an atypical antipsychotic drug is efficacious, and similar concerns apply to two atypicals together. It is unlikely that a poor response to an atypical drug is likely to improve after 8 weeks although clinical experience with clozapine suggests that there may be continuing gains over months or even years (Mortimer 1998).

The need for high-dose neuroleptics is a controversial topic with no published evidence for the efficacy of high-dose medication as a strategy, either to accelerate therapeutic response or to increase the number of patients who respond satisfactorily to medication (Mackay 1994). High doses are not necessary to block any of the individual receptors currently felt to be important in the therapeutic action of antipsychotic drugs but there is still a relative ignorance of the underlying neurochemical processes involved in the causation and maintenance of the symptoms of schizophrenia. There is evidence for receptor 'cross-talk' and there may well be other important but as yet unknown receptors involved in the process which become significant at higher doses. Currently, however, the generally accepted position is that escalating doses run the risk of serious side effects, including sudden death through hypotension or cardiac dysrhythmia, neuroleptic malignant syndrome, tardive dyskinesia (Mackay 1994) and 'paradoxical' behavioural disturbance (Barnes & Bridges 1980).

Clozapine, the prototypical, atypical antipsychotic, has a relatively low affinity for D_2 receptors, diverse pharmacology and may owe its clinical effectiveness to combined D_2 and $5HT_2$ receptor blockade (Thomas & Lewis 1998). It has been shown to be superior to conventional antipsychotics in the 30% of patients who derive little benefit from conventional therapy (Kane et al 1988). In double blind, randomised controlled trials of clozapine in treatment-resistant schizophrenia, response rates were 30% at 6 weeks (Kane et al 1988), 44% at 10 weeks (Breier et al 1994) and 42% at 29 weeks (Umbricht et al 1997). This compares with response rates with chlorpromazine or haloperidol of 4, 8 and 6% respectively. It remains the drug of choice in the treatment-resistant patient.

Clozapine has the major drawback of causing neutropaenia in 1 in 43 patients. The increased risk of fatal agranulocytosis and the consequent necessity for blood monitoring of white cell counts, together with its liability to induce seizures, hypotension (14%), weight gain, sedation (39%) and hypersalivation (30%) (Baldessarini & Frankenburg 1991) mean that its use is reserved for those who fail to respond to conventional treatment.

Newer, atypical, antipsychotic drugs

Newer, atypical antipsychotics fall into three groups. The first has strong affinities for D_2 receptors and $5HT_2$ receptors and includes risperidone, sertindole and ziprasidone. The second group has a mixed or complex pattern of affinities for numerous receptors, but a relatively poor affinity for D_2 receptors and includes olanzapine, quetiapine and zotepine (clozapine would also be in this category). The third group with D_2 and D_3 receptor affinity contains amisulpride.

To date, atypicals tend to have been reserved, on cost grounds, for patients who have not responded adequately to conventional drugs, but increasingly they are being used as first-line treatments in order to reduce the risk of EPSE and to maximise the potential for recovery by improving compliance. They are as effective as conventional drugs for the acute symptoms of schizophrenia and are superior to placebo in treating negative symptoms (Thomas & Lewis 1998), although the evidence for a direct effect on primary negative symptoms is still unproven. Unfortunately, however, long-acting depot formulations are a long way off, although risperidone and ziprasidone may soon be available in short-acting formulations.

There is a need for good head-to-head comparison studies for the atypicals. One randomised controlled trial (n = 230) of amisulpride versus risperidone suggested slight advantages for amisulpride on the symptom profile, but more adverse effects (Lorex Synthelabo 1997). A randomised controlled trial of olanzapine versus risperidone reported clinically insignificant advantages on negative symptoms for olanzapine and a 50% or greater reduction in total symptoms for 22% of patients on olanzapine as compared to 12% on risperidone. Adverse events, including EPSE, were less frequent on olanzapine (Tran et al 1997).

A double blind study (n=59) by Klieser et al (1995) failed to demonstrate any significant difference in treatment response between risperidone at doses of 4 mg or 8 mg per day and clozapine 400 mg per day over 4 weeks. This suggests that risperidone is at least as effective as an antipsychotic as clozapine over this relatively short period.

More studies are required before firm conclusions can be drawn concerning the relative efficacy and tolerability of the different classes of atypicals. At present, the choice is governed by the side effects already experienced by the individual patient on conventional drugs. For example, a patient who suffered severe EPSE on conventional antipsychotics would not generally be prescribed amisulpride or risperidone, while one who became obese and over-sedated on conventional antipsychotics would do well to avoid olanzapine or quetiapine.

Other pharmacological approaches to the treatment-resistant patient involve augmentation strategies with a variety of drugs including lithium, carbamazepine, benzodiazepines, serotonin agonists or electroconvulsive therapy. Their use is variable across the world and influenced by health policy issues which may limit the use of clozapine in some countries. In the absence of clear data comparing clozapine with augmented conventional treatment, it has been suggested that clozapine be reserved for clear cases of treatment resistance and an augmentation strategy be used for partial responders or those unwilling to take or intolerant to clozapine (Schulz & Buckley 1995).

Approaches to violence and aggression

It has been shown that patients with schizophrenia who manifest violent behaviour frequently have EEG abnormalities in the absence of overt seizures. The use of the anticonvulsant drug carbamazepine in combination with neuroleptics has been shown in double blind studies to confer additional therapeutic benefit in such cases (Neppe 1983). However, it does not seem to possess significant effect when administered alone and is not superior to lithium in its augmenting effect (Schulz & Buckley 1995).

Clozapine has been shown to reduce aggression in schizophrenic patients in forensic settings, with corresponding reductions in the need for restraint or seclusion, although the overall symptomatic response to clozapine in violent and non-violent patients is similar. Buckley et al (1995) postulate a specific treatment response related to its serotonergic effects and point out its potential usefulness in forensic patients who frequently misuse illicit drugs. The response of treatment-resistant patients who have co-morbid substance misuse is comparable

to patients without such abuse and in some cases a reduced craving for drugs has been reported. In a later case-control study of risperidone, Buckley concluded that risperidone was as effective as conventional antipsychotics at moderating aggressive behaviour in schizophrenia and that a direct comparison study with clozapine is required.

CASE STUDY: ALAN

Alan is a 28-year-old, single man with an 8-year history of sporadic contact with general psychiatric services in two different areas. Various diagnostic labels have been applied to date, including various personality disorders, substance misuse, paranoid psychosis, drug-induced psychosis and schizophrenia. He has never been admitted to hospital for longer than a week, has never been detained under the provisions of the Mental Health Act before and has frequently taken his own discharge from hospital.

His employment record is patchy, but he did train as an electrician. Although he did not attain his final qualifications, he coped well with the apprenticeship until the final year, when his attendance became poor. He was forced to leave after failing to turn up for work following claims that his work-mates were 'picking on him'.

He had no history of childhood conduct disorder or developmental problems and had plenty of friends at school where he attained five GCSEs. He had several girlfriends, but none in recent years. He has no children. There were no problems with authority until the age of 22 when he got involved in a drunken fight between two groups of young men outside a city centre pub and was convicted of assault and affray. He served a short custodial sentence. At the time, friends expressed surprise at the intensity of his anger and the degree of violence shown by someone they had previously not considered to be particularly aggressive.

He lived with his parents and sisters until he moved into a bed-sit in a different area at the age of 25 following a family row. The bed-sit was poorly furnished and dirty, in contrast with the family home.

There is a family history of mental health problems in that his maternal aunt spent some years in a psychiatric hospital with a diagnosis of schizophrenia and his mother has been treated by her general practitioner for depression. There is no family history of criminality. His parents have good work records and his two sisters are doing well at school with no obvious problems.

He presented to forensic psychiatric services while remanded in custody on a serious charge of assault against his neighbour, whom he claimed had been deliberately provoking him by spreading rumours about him, playing his music too loudly and emptying rubbish outside the door of the bed-sit.

The index offence occurred late one night as Alan returned from the pub. He met his neighbour, a single man of about the same age, outside the local chip-shop. The neighbour reports that Alan muttered something under his breath and walked past him, then returned and for no apparent reason assaulted him repeatedly with a knife. This attack caused severe injuries which could have proved fatal. There were several witnesses who supported the account of the neighbour and who called an ambulance. Alan fled from the scene and threw the knife into a bin from where it was later retrieved by police.

The police apprehended Alan rapidly following a good description from a bystander. He was arrested while trying to get back into his bed-sit by forcing a window, having dropped his key in the scuffle. He denied all knowledge of the assault and could give no explanation of his movements that night. He was later picked out in an identity parade and forensic evidence from the victim's blood on his clothes linked him with the offence.

He showed no emotion during the police interviews and continued to deny his involvement. He smiled during the interviews, said little and stared menacingly at the interviewers. His general behaviour was not deemed sufficiently out of the ordinary to warrant psychiatric involvement at this stage. However, several of the police officers later commented that he had seemed to have difficulty in hearing or understanding fairly simple questions, frequently asking others to repeat what had been said.

In prison, he appeared to cope reasonably well until he made an unprovoked assault on a fellow inmate. He was seen by the visiting forensic psychiatrist, at the request of staff who noticed he was talking to himself in his cell at night.

On interview, he appeared preoccupied and seemed to have difficulty grasping the thread of the conversation. However, he did volunteer that he believed that fellow prisoners were communicating with his neighbour and family members in spreading rumours about his sexuality, the fact that he was 'the progeny of Satan' and had a special mission related to MI6. He knew these things, he said, because the television was broadcasting news items about him and he could hear voices at night discussing his masturbatory habits. He appeared thought-disordered with a 'woolliness' to his thinking and a belief that those around him could hear his private thoughts. He confessed that he had considered killing himself because of the stress he felt himself to be under in the preceding months. In spite of this, he did not appear depressed. He also admitted to smoking cannabis on a regular basis with occasional use of amphetamines and regular binge drinking. He found it difficult to tolerate the interview and frequently said that he had misheard and requested repetition and clarification. Some of his spontaneous comments seemed unrelated to the conversation and throughout he seemed hostile and edgy with occasional inappropriate smiling. He maintained that he had not committed the index offence and had been provoked by the other prisoner. He had no concern for the condition of either victim, did not consider himself to be ill and could see no need for treatment.

The forensic psychiatrist suspected a psychotic illness and made a presumptive diagnosis of schizophrenia and so Alan was transferred to a medium-secure unit under the provisions of section 48 of the Mental Health Act 1983. The physical examination and routine blood and urine testing were unremarkable apart from a degree of physical neglect and positive urine test for cannabis. He was observed drug-free with close nursing observations but required emergency sedation after 3 days when he became over-aroused and assaulted a nurse by lunging at him with a dinner fork during a meal. He was restrained using approved techniques, but did not settle and appeared to be experiencing paranoid auditory hallucinations.

His old casenotes were studied to establish previous treatment approaches, the police were asked for his full criminal record, his Inmate Medical Record was studied and his family members were approached for a fuller developmental, social and family history and to establish his premorbid social functioning.

It became clear that family members had experienced considerable violence and threats over the years and that they were fearful of him. They felt that they 'had not been listened to' when they had asked for assistance from their general practitioner, mental health services and the police. They reported a subtle and gradual change in his personality and functioning dating back to his late teens and early 20s. He appeared to have lost many of his former friends and mixed with a group known to the police as drug users. This had contributed to his reputation as a troublemaker in the locality. Their comments regarding violent incidents were carefully documented and their views sought on his previous treatment and response to particular strategies.

It appeared that he had previously been treated with oral, conventional, antipsychotic medication on a sporadic basis and his compliance was in doubt. Many of his problems had been attributed to his alcohol and drug misuse.

His treatment at the medium-secure unit was initially with a conventional neuroleptic. Since he had already received zuclopenthixol in the form of Acuphase, he was started on zuclopenthixol in tablet form with a view to establishing him on the depot form of the same drug, subject to his response. However, his symptoms failed to improve sufficiently well to allow him to participate in occupational therapy as he remained acutely assaultive and impulsive. He seemed perplexed and hostile and it was hard to develop a rapport, as he seemed guarded and suspicious of the motives of staff and of other patients. His self-care was poor, he had

little to say and seemed to be responding to hallucinatory voices. He also seemed sedated and became markedly restless and akathisic, pacing the floor and seeming unable to settle. This akathisia did not respond well to a reduction in the dose of antipsychotic medication or to the introduction of small amounts of benzodiazepines, which are sometimes helpful in reducing the sense of inner restlessness. In fact, this made him even less alert and he continued to display both positive and negative features of schizophrenia.

He was then started on olanzapine but complained of difficulty in getting an erection and seemed to be feeling no better. His urine screens were consistently negative for illicit substances after the initial positive test on admission. He had now received two 8-week trials of two different classes of antipsychotic medication, one a conventional drug and the other a novel, antipsychotic agent and he was therefore deemed to be treatment resistant. Following discussion within the team, with him and with the family, he underwent the necessary screening blood tests and was registered with the Clozapine Patient Monitoring Service.

On starting clozapine he was initially very sedated and suffered from hypersalivation. The latter side effect was distressing to him but was helped by a small dose of hyoscine hydrobromide. The sedation gradually improved and the dose of clozapine was gradually increased. These changes were discussed in the team meeting and his progress in occupational therapy and ward-based activities was considered. Hence the prescribing was informed by his day-to-day functioning as reported by himself and as observed by those most closely involved with him so that it did not occur in isolation.

The multi-disciplinary team reviewed the level of nursing observation on a formal basis at least weekly at the team meeting to discuss patient care and far more frequently at ward level in response to or in anticipation of need. This was especially relevant at times of change in his medication.

There were several episodes of assault and property damage averted or minimised by swift nursing intervention. The need for conditions of greater security was kept as a live issue and advice was sought from a Special Hospital. In the event he was safely managed within medium security following the provision of extra nursing staff.

The diagnosis of schizophrenia became clearer, with substance misuse complicating the early picture. Information was gathered to support or refute the previous diagnostic labels attached to the case and the matter was reviewed in preparation for his court appearance.

His response to the medication was slow and seemed to occur over a period of months. The staring subsided and he became warmer and less troubled-looking. He was able to speak to staff in more detail about how he had been feeling and gradually explained that he had felt persecuted by work colleagues, his family and then total strangers. He had experienced third person auditory hallucinations, delusions of reference and passivity phenomena. He had believed that the thoughts of others had influenced him and that he could not resist the external influences upon him to behave in certain ways. He had initially attributed his problems to 'stress' and had consulted his doctor in the community for a range of somatic symptoms. His attempts to find some relief from the voices and paranoid feelings were counter-productive in that he had turned to drugs and alcohol which caused further problems.

He had little insight initially, but once the 3-month period of initial medical treatment against his will was completed, he agreed to continue with the treatment plan as he felt more relaxed and could see some potential benefit to the medication.

When the case came to court he was convicted of the index offence and dealt with by way of a Hospital Order under the provisions of section 37 of the Mental Health Act on the grounds of mental illness. There was an additional Restriction Order under section 41 without limit of time because of the perceived risk of serious harm to the public. He returned to the medium-secure unit to continue with his treatment and rehabilitation. He gradually acknowledged his role in the index offence and moved from a position of total denial to partial acceptance and later a real remorse for the victim of the offence and the later assault in custody.

Following a settled period on clozapine medication and his being nursed on the ward, there was some relaxation of the levels of nursing observation and he was able to participate in individual and group sessions off the ward. These were aimed at addressing his understanding of his illness, the role of drugs and alcohol in his life and his relationships with his family and friends.

Different professional groups led the strands of treatment so that, for example, he attended a substance-awareness group run by occupational therapy and had family meetings facilitated by a social worker and nurse. His personality functioning and strategies to cope with his symptoms were addressed in individual sessions with a psychologist, and his physical complaints, including any necessary investigations, were handled by one particular doctor on the team. The weight gain he experienced on clozapine was tackled at his request with dietary advice and a gradual programme of exercise drawn up by the occupational therapy gym instructor in consultation with the team. Another doctor reviewed all of the available information on Alan's treatment, response to it and violent incidents and charted these for use by the team in its work with Alan.

Alan's parents were also seen on their own for the purpose of information gathering and their contribution to the ongoing risk management strategy.

In addition to the weekly reviews, a detailed Care Programme Approach (CPA) meeting was held on a 3-monthly basis with an opportunity for all parties to be heard and contribute to the process. These meetings were carefully documented with written reports from each discipline submitted to the team before the meeting and a summary of the discussion, overall team aims, risk management strategy and action points for each team member recorded in the case file. These action points were reviewed regularly and revised as necessary. Alan's general practitioner and representatives from his local psychiatric services were invited to the CPA meetings and, if they were unable to attend, they received the relevant documentation in order to be informed of key decisions and of his overall progress.

The medical contribution to the plan of treatment included a general ongoing examination of his health needs including those for neglected physical conditions such as dental problems or other possible contributing factors to his aggression or distress. A regular examination of his mental state, including his views on his treatment and his capacity to consent were documented in his casenotes.

His attitudes to those around him and issues of remorse, judgement, insight and empathy were matters for frequent discussion in his individual sessions. At one stage in his treatment he became quite subdued and low in mood as he appreciated the impact of his offence upon his victim and upon his own future. He was supported through this period without the need for additional medication and was not thought to be clinically depressed, but his need for observations and the possible risk of deliberate self-harm were given more emphasis within his overall treatment.

All members of the team took joint responsibility for the adequate documentation and co-ordination of these plans and updated a multi-disciplinary treatment plan on a weekly basis at the team meeting. At the same time, levels of observation and leave into the garden and later off the ward and into the grounds were agreed and carefully documented. The Home Office Mental Health Unit was approached by the Responsible Medical Officer (RMO) with a detailed plan for escorted community leave with clear aims and objectives for each period of leave.

As his rehabilitation progressed, he was allowed increasing amounts of leave in a variety of different circumstances. He was also assessed for the use of the heavy workshop and continued to use a range of on-site and community resources in order to maintain his skills and provide the opportunities to build on his educational and vocational interests.

He was helped to draw up his own leave plans and to evaluate his own success and any concerns about the progress of leave in collaboration with his primary nurse. Alan also began to participate in a structured programme of self-administration of his medication, starting with his requesting it at the appropriate time and working towards the medication being in his possession. He also co-operated with random screening of his urine for illicit drugs.

The treatment plan was evaluated by monitoring the changes in his mental state, activity levels, social relationships and his response to aggression and incidents on the ward. It was informed by observations of him in a variety of different settings and complemented by formal assessments as part of his risk assessment and psychological and occupational therapy programmes. Emphasis was placed upon the views expressed by Alan himself concerning his own progress and the concerns of his family and those in his social network.

Progress was made steadily to the point where he could have been transferred to local in-patient psychiatric services for further rehabilitation. However, the local service had reservations about its abilities to meet his needs within their existing in-patient facilities, given the lack of high quality rehabilitation services and the predominance of beds for the more acutely ill. Therefore he continued to progress through to the rehabilitation flat, within the secure perimeter of the medium-secure unit until moving to a four-person group house run by a voluntary agency following his conditional discharge from hospital.

He had regular contact with members of the original team, one of whom continued as RMO, with another becoming his Social Supervisor. He was seen in a variety of venues including his house and at the out-patient clinic. Contact was maintained with his family with clear channels of communication to the key professionals. He continued to attend some limited occupational therapy sessions at the medium-secure unit but gradually made the transition to a local college where he started a vocational course, based on his previous work within the medium-secure unit. He rebuilt and resumed his previous good relationship with his family who joined a group for the parents of people who suffer from schizophrenia run by a voluntary agency. His social relationships remained fragile and he was dependent upon benefits.

Alan was seen alone in the out-patient clinic by his RMO in addition to joint meetings when appropriate and was checked in terms of his mental state, compliance, insight, alcohol consumption and any resumption of drug misuse. His perceptions of his general health and any side effects, in particular erectile dysfunction or other sexual side effects, were topics of ongoing enquiry since somatic complaints and sexual problems were relevant features in his background. In addition, any apparent disagreement between him and his house-mates was explored and his community worker from the house was fully involved in CPA meetings. His attitude to his family was explored and also his current attitude to the need to carry weapons.

Medical approaches to the multi-disciplinary management of treatment-resistant schizophrenia

- Ensure that the history is as complete as possible and gathered from a range of sources. Obtain the criminal record, if any, and accounts of incidents of violence and property damage. Consider the risks posed by the patient to self and others and the level of security required for treatment. Review treatment to date including type, duration and dosages of antipsychotic medication and compliance. Note side-effects of previous treatments and especially those which the patient found most troublesome, especially if linked with cessation of treatment.
- Maintain safety while changes in environment and medication are being undertaken. This may necessitate a move to a more secure area and/or increased nursing observations. Ensure adequate incident reporting and review with the need for restraint monitored (where applicable). It may be useful to track this in chart form

against medication changes and other variables such as disturbance on the ward.
- Attempt to clarify the diagnosis and note any secondary disabilities.
- Consider the significance of particular psychopathological phenomena, for example, passivity phenomena, command hallucinations.
- Consider the level of social support and adversity in collaboration with social work colleagues.
- Consider treatment options, discussing these with the patient, carers (if appropriate) and within the multi-disciplinary team.
- Develop a clear treatment strategy with review dates built into the plan. Plan to review on a specific date to avoid 'drifting along'.
- The team should prepare a multi-disciplinary treatment plan with team overall aims and the individual aims of each discipline with a rationale for the particular aims. Involve the team in drawing up the leave programme ensuring that the RMO is aware of, and takes ultimate responsibility for, the programme.
- For the medical plan, ensure adequate documentation of plan, progress, likely side effects of the medication prescribed, for example, fits, falls, etc. (It is beneficial to have pharmacy input to the team so that there is scrutiny and debate about prescribing matters and awareness of possible drug interactions.) Monitor side effects and be alert to continuing substance misuse. This may require random drug screening of urine for illicit substances.
- Consider the impact of changes in medication on the overall treatment plan, for example, performance in therapies and impact on the leave programme, and communicate this to those who may need to know.
- Continue to review issues of consent to treatment and ensure correct recording in the casenotes.
- Take the opportunity of the patient being in hospital to consider screening for other health problems or consequences of neglect, for example, dental problems.

- Monitor level of insight, current strengths and level of motivation and compliance. Consider the need for motivational interviewing to improve compliance.
- Continue to check on the carer perspective as the treatment progresses, noting how the patient reacts to his close family members.
- Support the carers in their own right if necessary and educate them on the implications of the diagnosis. This may involve liaison with other professional teams if there are victims within the family or significant conflicts of interest between the patient and other family members.
- Staff should have continuing training and professional development, access to literature on newer treatments and opportunity to discuss relevant developments within the service, so that newer treatments can be critically evaluated and discussed with the patient and carers where appropriate.
- Assess the general reliability and truthfulness of the patient in preparation for any discharge plans so that this can inform those relying upon the patient for an account of his activities.

Conclusions

This case study illustrates that there is much information to be gathered, collated and evaluated before the team can produce a properly thought-out treatment plan and that incidents sometimes require immediate responses before the whole story is clear. This requires an open-minded approach to previous diagnostic labels and critical evaluation of previous treatment together with a flexible team approach. Given the sort of risks and behaviour presented by Alan and others who become forensic patients, it is not surprising that they are sometimes rejected by generic services at an earlier stage in their illness. Acute services are hard-pressed, but there often seems to be a lack of the longitudinal view of the case in favour of a response to the immediate crisis.

In Alan's case, a close examination of school and work records reveals little data to support a diagnosis of dissocial personality disorder and yet this label was used as a way of rejecting him. His parents and sisters never felt that their account was properly heard and felt tremendous guilt at their rejection of him when they could cope no longer. They could point to an insidious change caused by his severe mental illness, but were encouraged by those who could have helped Alan to view his problems as being related to 'badness' rather than 'madness'. In order to encourage a more constructive working relationship with them, there seemed a clear need for some family intervention by the time he arrived at the medium-secure unit. Their fears that he would once more leave the hospital were allayed by his detention under the Mental Health Act, the close nursing observations and supervision and the security measures common to most medium-secure units. Even if Alan had refused to allow their involvement in his care, there would have been a need to hear their views and give them sufficient information to participate in the risk management strategy, given Alan's threats towards them. Once he was held securely in a therapeutic environment, they were able to speak to staff about their fears and he could begin to tackle his illness and address his offending behaviour so as to rebuild his life within the restrictions imposed by the law.

The quality of the overall service depends largely upon the staff, the degree to which the service operates along multi-disciplinary lines and the leadership provided by those in key roles. However, the correct environment can also play a large part in the recovery process, and for Alan, the provision of personal space, fresh air and a comfortable ward environment, with the opportunity to exercise choices in this limited sphere, were important. He was able to engage in recreational activities, to keep his possessions safe and to retire to his own room for limited periods before he was deemed sufficiently well to go off the ward for therapeutic, educational or vocational activities. He stated that the light, comfortable surroundings made him feel 'less stressed'.

Medication is one part of the overall medical contribution to the multi-disciplinary treatment plan, but can have an impact on the patient's ability to make use of what is on offer from other disciplines, especially if the side effects are disabling. There are obvious drawbacks of supervising a potentially dangerous patient in the community who is taking oral medication, since compliance cannot be assumed and there is less certainty than with depot preparations. It seems appropriate that the choice and rationale for the drug treatment be a matter for discussion with the patient and all concerned in the treatment. Compliance seems likeliest to be improved if everyone can appreciate the need for treatment and underline its importance in the whole package of care. Thus, the pharmacological treatment should be integrated as far as possible with the psychosocial approaches and within the rehabilitative framework.

REFERENCES

Baldessarini R, Frankenburg F 1991 Clozapine: a novel antipsychotic agent. New England Journal of Medicine 324: 746–754

Barnes T, Bridges R 1980 Disturbed behaviour induced with high dose antipsychotic drugs. British Medical Journal 281: 274–275

Breier A, Buchanan R, Kirkpatrick B 1994 Effects of clozapine on positive and negative symptoms in outpatients with schizophrenia. American Journal of Psychiatry 151: 20–26

Buchanan A 1998 Treatment compliance in schizophrenia. Advances in Psychiatric Treatment 4: 227–234

Buckley P, Kausch O, Gardner G 1995 Clozapine treatment of schizophrenia: implications for forensic psychiatry. Journal of Clinical Forensic Medicine 2: 9–16

Kane J, Honigfeld G, Singer J 1988 Clozapine for treatment resistant schizophrenia: a double blind comparison with chlorpromazine. Archives of General Psychiatry 45: 789–796

Kemp R, Hayward P, Applewhaite G 1996 Compliance therapy in psychotic patients: randomised controlled trial. British Medical Journal 312: 345–349

Klieser E, Lehmann E, Kinzler E 1995 Randomised, double blind, controlled trial of risperidone versus clozapine in patients with chronic schizophrenia. Journal of Clinical Psychopharmacology 15 (Suppl 1): 45–51

Lorex Synthelabo 1997 data on file 97-00253-EN-01

Mackay A 1994 High dose antipsychotic medication. Advances in Psychiatric Treatment 1: 16–23

Meltzer H, Burnett S, Bastani B, Ramirez L 1990 Effect of six months of clozapine treatment on the quality of life of chronic schizophrenic patients. Hospital and Community Psychiatry 41: 892–897

Mortimer A 1998 Atypical antipsychotic drugs and their happy place in therapy. Progress in Neurology and Psychiatry 2(3): 41–45

Neppe V 1983 Carbamazepine as adjunctive treatment in non epileptic chronic inpatients with EEG temporal lobe abnormalities. Journal of Clinical Psychiatry 44: 326–330

Schulz S, Buckley P 1995 Treatment resistant schizophrenia. In: Hirsch S, Weinberger D (eds) Schizophrenia. Blackwell Science, Oxford

Thomas C, Lewis S 1998 Which atypical antipsychotic? British Journal of Psychiatry 172: 106–109

Tran P, Hamilton S, Kuntz A 1997 Double blind comparison of olanzapine versus risperidone in the treatment of schizophrenia and other disorders. Journal of Clinical Psychopharmacology 17: 407–418

Umbricht D, Ames D, Wirshing W et al 1997 Predictors of response to clozapine in a long-term double blind treatment study. Schizophrenia Research 24: 189

CONTENTS

The aged offender

Tish Smyer

Introduction

The aging prisoner poses a special challenge to forensic nursing. The care of the elderly psychiatric client requries knowledge of multi-system alterations in physiological functioning and an understanding of the inter-relatedness of these systems. Changes in behaviour and cognition may be the first manifestation of a physiological alteration or may reflect a mental disorder in itself. Add to these changes the unique environment of a correctional institution, with its attendant stressors, and it becomes apparent that there is a need for comprehensive and knowledgeable delivery of care to this population. This study will present background information about the elderly prisoner including a description of the categories of aging prisoners as well as a delineation of the physical and mental health needs of this patient group. This will be followed by a case study of an elderly prisoner with DSM-IV diagnosis of depression and antisocial personality disorder.

Categories of elderly inmates

There are three categories of elderly inmates, based on patterns of criminal activity over time (Aday 1994, Morton 1992):

The initial category is the first-time offender, usually over 60 years of age, who has never been incarcerated (Aday 1994). The crimes usually consist of family violence, fraud, drug sales, sex offences or alcohol-related crimes (Fry 1988). Approximately 50% of the aging prisoners are in this category (Aday 1994). These prisoners are good candidates for community placement because of family ties, however, incarceration in a prison poses special problems as the skills necessary to survive have not been honed over time and these prisoners may be set up for predatory behaviour from other inmates. The health status of these individuals closely mirrors the problems of the elderly in the free world and health problems will be indicative of the normal decrements of aging.

The second category of prisoner is the chronic offender. This prisoner has a history of multiple past incarcerations and he usually adjusts quickly to the prison environment. Alcohol, drug abuse and personality disorders play a large part in this prisoner's life (Morton 1992). Release to the community, while possible, is more problematic because of past employment difficulties and poor family ties. The health status of this individual is usually poor if the chronic use of alcohol and/or illegal substances has taken its toll on the physiological status of the client. Additionally, the sporadic or non-existent follow-up for medical problems may mean a higher level of acuity in existing or chronic health problems.

The third category is the long-term offender or the prisoner who has aged in jail. Sentenced at a young age, this prisoner has few of the landmarks of adult rites of passage and will have undergone irrevocable losses in the traditional life cycle (LaMere et al 1996). These losses pertain particularly to the prisoner's self-concept and sense of autonomy. The lifetime of aging within the prison system makes community release very difficult. The ties to family and friends in the community, lost over time, pose a particular problem for this prisoner and their health status may reflect the level of health care delivery system of the prisons in which he has been incarcerated. The emotional and mental health of this individual is usually of greatest concern because of the lack of free world socialisation and corresponding development of self-concept.

Physical health

Physical decrements associated with the aging process are a problem for the older prisoner.

Because of physiological factors related to lifestyle in prison and the concomitant increased risk factors, approximately 10 years may be added to the chronological age of a prisoner. In the USA, a prisoner 50 years or older is considered to be an older prisoner and may reflect the physiological status of a much older individual.

Annual maintenance with medical costs for the older inmate in the USA is triple that of the younger prison population at approximately $69 000 per year (Clear & Cole 1994). The elderly prisoner has three or more chronic illnesses and is hospitalised more often than younger prisoners (Aday 1994, Glaser et al 1990). Colsher et al (1992) found increased rates of incontinence, sensory impairment and flexibility impairment in a study (n = 119) of aging prisoners. Missing teeth were found in 97%, 42% had gross physical functional impairments and 70% smoked tobacco. 40% of these prisoners had histories of hypertension, 19% with a previous myocardial infarction and 18% with emphysema. The conditions of persistent stress inherent in a correctional setting impose continual wear and tear on individuals and contribute to the aging process (Smyer et al 1997). The decreased adaptive capacity of the aging prisoner makes maintenance of homeostasis more difficult and can contribute to increased mortality and morbidity in this population (Seyle 1978).

Mental health

The elderly are susceptible to mental health problems as with any age group. Frailty and dependence, loss of control and powerlessness all require an emotional and spiritual adjustment (Stanley & Beare 1995). Depression is one of the most common mental health disorders in the elderly and it may be caused by medical illness, chronic pain, polypharmacy, sleep disturbances and selected stressors (Shua-Haim et al 1997). Depressive symptoms may occur in 15 to 20% of the elderly living in the community and up to 30% in the elderly who are institutionalised. Shua-Haim et al (1997) suggest that the morbidity associated with depression relates to decreased quality of life, a worsening medical condition and increased risk for suicide. The lethality index for older adult males is 4:1 (attempts/completion ratio) versus sometimes up to 200:1 in the adolescent population. Depression is also associated with increased use of medical services (Shua-Haim et al 1997).

Presentation of depression differs markedly in the elderly. Sometimes referred to as 'masked depression', the elderly may complain of somatic or cognitive symptoms rather than feelings of sadness. They may present in a 'manic defence' mode and may appear to be cheerful yet overly 'busy'. Significant indicators may be changes in sleep patterns, increased or decreased appetite, physical complaints, psychomotor retardation or agitation, lack of energy, as well as cognitive impairments (Shua-Haim et al 1997).

Cognitive changes caused by dementia may also be a problem with this population. Cognitive changes because of alcohol and substance misuse may present in the younger inmate as well, but dementia of Alzheimer's type (DAT) is more prevalent with increasing age. Vascular dementia as well as amnestic disorder may also present in this population as a result of poor lifestyle choices. Cognitive changes may also be the result of a physiological process and those caring for the elderly prisoner must be alert to the many possible causes of cognitive or behavioural changes and include these in their assessment of the elderly prisoner, as these may reflect a serious medical condition.

CASE STUDY: CHARLIE

Assessment data

Charlie, a 56-year-old convict, has been incarcerated in some type of correctional facility since he was 11 years old. He appears frail and much older than his chronological age. He has tattoos all over his body with the exception of his face. The tattoos were acquired in specific prisons and he uses the tattoos as a road map to historically relate his incarceration experiences. Charlie completed 9 years of school and has a GED (high school equivalency exam). He currently carries a DSM-IV diagnosis of depression and antisocial personality disorder. His medications are Prozac

and lithium. He works as a swamper (cleaner) in the prison when he is able. When interacting with Charlie, the conversation usually remains lively and he is an engaging personality. His affect at times does not match the seriousness, or sadness, of the story he is relating.

Charlie has had a total of 5 years in the free world since his initial confinement with 18 months being the longest time spent out of prison between incarcerations. Charlie began his crime career at the age of 11 after breaking into a house and stealing a gun. He was sent to a reform school at that time. His longest incarceration was for 32 years in a southern US prison for murder. His shortest sentence was for 3 years in a northern US prison for assault. He is currently serving a 10-year sentence for felony assault and has been incarcerated at this prison for 3 years. He will be eligible for parole in the year 2000.

Charlie claims no family interaction or bonds. He states:

I have nothing on the outside. My dad died from alcohol 20 years ago. I went back home when I was 17, the first time I got out of prison, stayed there for 3 weeks then went right back to prison for car theft and burglary. I don't know my family. My mom wrote me in August of this year. I haven't answered. When I got my letter I said this is spooky, I thought she was dead. I thought I didn't have to worry about writing her anymore. It wouldn't hurt me if she died. I don't know her.

Charlie relates that the convicts in the prison system are his family. He describes an earned status as an 'old convict' with much respect for him among the convict population because of his numerous incarcerations. He relates his incarceration history and differentiates between an 'inmate' and a 'convict':

Convicts are stand up dudes who don't take shit from no one. They also don't give it neither. They don't play no games. Inmates are snitches and ass kissers, you know, child molesters or rapists. I'm a convict. I been in some tough prisons. I did 32 years down south in a very dangerous prison. I wish I was there. The guards treat you like a man. They don't play games. 'Yes sir, yes man' or they will kick your ass. Here, why they have T.V. and boom boxes.

Charlie did well in the first year of his incarceration at his current prison. He was assigned to a minimum-security unit with prisoners who were stable and less violent than the general population. Many had chronic illnesses and the prisoners were routinely older. After the first year, Charlie had an episode in which he swallowed razor blades.

As it turned out, this was not the first time he had injured himself. He began when he was 15 years old, beating his head against the wall and cutting himself. This behaviour escalated in severity and he relates that he has had 41 operations, almost all related to swallowing objects or cutting himself. He uses his scars in the same way that he uses the tattoos, as a road map to historically relate different instances of self-injury.

After the incident of swallowing razor blades, he took 200 mg of amiytriptyline and punctured his oesophagus and lungs with a paper clip that he had swallowed. This required close to 2 weeks on life-support systems. He was subsequently moved to a smaller psychiatric unit within the prison for monitoring and was prescribed Prozac. After 6 months in this unit, he swallowed seven nails and was subsequently started on lithium in addition to Prozac. He had another episode of self-injury swallowing needles several weeks later. At this prison, the medical costs for Charlie are approximately $250 000 for the past 2 years. He refuses to sign an advanced directive or 'do not resuscitate' (DNR) order.

Charlie related the following about his state of mind before hurting himself:

I feel things are not going right, nobody gives a damn. I start thinking the hell with it. I don't care. Build up, build up. I'm running into the walls with my hands or my head. I might start thinking about something that happened 20 years ago. I might start punishing myself for what I did to people. Pain I put people through.

Interventions and outcomes

The forensic nurse began a plan of care for Charlie which included an inter-disciplinary approach. The correctional officers were included in this plan of care. For the forensic nurse dealing with Charlie there were specific problems which had to be dealt with directly and immediately.

The first was safety. Owing to the immediate danger of self-harm, Charlie was under surveillance much of his time after discharge from the infirmary and alerting all staff to this possibility limited his capacity to fulfil this. The second effort was directed at the development of a trusting relationship within the correctional environment. His sense of belonging was to the convict culture. He had never learned to trust individuals from outside this culture. The goal of long-term placement in the community for Charlie would be severely compromised by this trust issue.

Charlie was again placed in the psychiatric unit and he was not returned to the general prison population. Charlie became a fixture on this unit. He attended therapeutic groups, began to focus on his art work and began interacting positively with younger mentally disordered offenders. He came to have affection for those with true psychosis, particularly the schizophrenic. He stated:

For the young guys that come in, a lot of them have problems and they need to be watched for, they can get hurt here. They need all the protection they can get. There should be a special building for the young guys. They get taken advantage of, like 'pay me money or you are going to lockup', the bulldoggers mess with these people. They are ashamed to talk about it but a little kid friend of mine, only weighed about 115 pounds. These guys raped him and he is sick. Now he'll never trust anybody never. He's in the state mental hospital and they put him there too. When a guy is really sick, he needs help. I never got that help when I was a kid. Gave me a pill and said, 'See you next month'.

Charlie responded to his medication of Prozac and lithium. He relates that his current medications are the 'best meds I have ever taken'. He stated that the medications 'help me to look inside myself, to look at my problems and helps me not to do the bad things and try to like myself.' He began to develop a trusting relationship with several correctional officers as well as a male psychiatric nurse on the unit. He speaks with affection of these officers as well as the psychiatric nurse.

There are two officers that I really like. If I am having problems, I let them know what is going on. I tell them leave my door closed, I don't need to be around anyone. These officers are my friends. I talk to them all the time. I give the counsellor things that I hurt myself with. There are so many things I can hurt myself with so to be safe, if I am feeling bad I give him these things.

The small unit environment fostered the establishment of trust as well as giving Charlie a role as the older wiser inmate who is 'watching out for these sick kids'. Additionally, this role provided Charlie with a clearly defined purpose which from previous research contributes to self-esteem and ultimately maintenance of mental health (Yurkovich & Smyer 1998). While interacting with correctional officers is not well accepted within the prison culture, Charlie was invested, along with the correctional officers, in keeping these young inmates safe.

Discussion

As the prisoner with antisocial personality disorder ages, the antisocial behaviours may decrease, but he may then exhibit depressive and somatic disorders (Ruegg et al 1997). Studies suggest that antisocial personalities 'burn out' in mid-life (approximately 30 to 40%) and this may provide a window of opportunity to help these individuals. Ruegg et al (1997) report that 30% of patients with antisocial personality disorder get major depression, typically after the age of 30 or 35. These authors relate that the presentation of depressive symptoms is different from the melancholic depressives in that the client can be affectively responsive but will be uncharacteristically passive and will not initiate activity on his own. The suicide risk is 5 to 10% for the antisocial personality and may reflect a high rate of untreated depression (Ruegg et al 1997).

While there is continuing debate about whether to treat or not treat the antisocial personality-disordered client, Ruegg et al (1997: 140) suggest that there are several factors which may be considered to 'weigh in favor of undertaking treatment'. These factors are:

- The presence of Axis I disorder (mood or substance abuse), which is treatable and treatment may decrease antisocial behavior
- Motivation on the patient's part. He is dissatisfied with his life

- External structure that can help monitor behaviour (such as prison)
- History of some positive relationships
- Antisocial behaviour that is impulsive and accompanied by regret, remorse or negative self-judgement
- A desire to live outside jail. The client may be motivated to continue antisocial acts to maintain living in an institution which provides basic life-support.

Charlie meets the above criteria except for the desire to live outside of prison. The opportunity to intervene with Charlie after his last self-injury required a joint effort by all staff involved with him. Taking advantage of this 'window of opportunity' with this aging prisoner required an understanding of the changes that occur as the antisocial personality-disordered prisoner ages.

Charlie received medication which contributed to his ability to function in the prison psychiatric unit. There are no specific medications for antisocial personality disorder, but Ruegg et al (1997: 158) relate that there are some reports that very high doses of Prozac can enhance functioning in the client with antisocial personality disorder. It appears to reduce 'the frequency and severity of mood swings and outbursts of anger, aggression, and reckless impulsiveness'. Lithium, Tegretol and Inderal may also decrease irritable and angry behaviours. Benzodiazepines can seldom be used in these individuals as some get a disinhibiting effect (similar to the feelings they get while using alcohol) and may paradoxically become more agitated (Ruegg et al 1997). Additionally, they relate that doxepine or other sedating antidepressants have the 'reputation among prisoners for turning "hard time" into "easy time".' Chlorpromazine and haloperidol may also be helpful for aggression and irritability.

Conclusions

Charlie is an example of the long-term offender who has essentially aged within the prison system. It is suggested that in the prison environment the prisoner's competency as an adult is compromised and there may be a lack of corresponding graduation of adult responsibilities and self-direction (LaMere et al 1996). These authors further speculate that a prisoner's sense of self-concept as well as sense of autonomy is compromised in the unique culture of the prison. The prisoner may be incapable of managing the daily necessities of life in the free world because so many decisions are made for him. His self-concept, as it relates to loss of traditional adult roles, produces a sense of social disconnection and makes the prisoner view the free world with trepidation. When asked about returning to the outside world, Charlie states:

I don't want to get out. I don't have anything out there. I just start drinking. It won't go well with my meds. I can't work. There is nothing out there for me.

This is my home and the only thing I know. I'll never get out.

Charlie has no wish to leave the world he grew up in and knows well. The predictability of the prison environment provides him with structure and safety in a world he can navigate successfully albeit at times pathologically. It is expected that as his release time comes closer, Charlie will escalate the self-injurious behaviour as a way to deal with his anxiety about coping and adapting to the free world. There is a long history of this coping behaviour working positively for him. The psychological and social needs of Charlie must be understood within the context of the particular sociocultural milieu of the prison environment, for this is Charlie's world.

REFERENCES

Aday R 1994 Aging in prison: a case study of new elderly offenders. International Journal of Offender Therapy and Comparative Criminology 38(1): 79–91

Clear T, Cole G 1994 American corrections. Wadsworth, California

Colsher P, Wallace R, Loeffelholz P, Sales M 1992 Health status of older male prisoners: a comprehensive survey. American Journal of Public Health 82: 881–884

Glaser J, Warchol A, D'Angelo D, Guterman H 1990 Infectious diseases of geriatric inmates. Review of Infectious Diseases 12: 683–692

Fry L 1988 The concerns of older inmates in a minimum security prison setting. In: McCarthy B, Langworthy R (eds) Older offenders perspectives in criminology and criminal justice. Praeger, New York

LaMere S, Smyer T, Gragert M 1996 The aging inmate. Journal of Psychosocial Nursing and Mental Health Services 34(4): 24–29

Morton J 1992 An administrative overview of the older inmate. US Department of Justice and National Institute of Corrections, Washington DC

Ruegg R, Haynes C, Frances A 1997 Assessment and management of antisocial personality disorder. In: Rosenbluth M, Yalom I (eds) Treating difficult personality disorders. Jossey-Bass, San Francisco

Seyle H 1978 The stress of life. McGraw-Hill, New York

Shua-Haim J, Sabo M, Comsti E, Gross J 1997 Depression in the elderly. Hospital Medicine 33(7): 45–58

Smyer T, Gragert M, LaMere S 1997 Stay safe! Stay healthy! Surviving old age in prison. Journal of Psychosocial Nursing and Mental Health Services 35(9): 10–17

Stanley M, Beare P 1995 Gerontological nursing. F A Davis, Philadelphia

Yurkovich E, Smyer T 1998 Strategies used by the chronic mentally ill population to maintain wellness. Perspectives in Psychiatric Care 34: 17–24

CONTENTS

Addressing institutionalisation

Sara Finlayson and Joe Forster

Introduction

This case study describes the care of a young man, Tony, with severe, enduring, treatment-resistant mental health problems. It documents his history and the treatment he has received at a high-dependency unit (HDU), having spent many years in a Special Hospital. A clinical formulation is presented, locating his problems within a psychosocial framework and indicating interventions to improve quality of life and level of functioning. Two specific interventions are outlined: first, graded exposure and modelling; and, second, work with relatives. Progress is described, with a critical evaluation of the case management. There is evidence of a dilemma involved in progressing too quickly as opposed to too slowly; with either provoking negative results. Suggestions for his future care are indicated.

Theoretical background

This case illustrates a psychosocial model of care developed by a multi-disciplinary team. The approach stemmed from a training initiative where all staff were introduced to basic psychosocial interventions for people with severe and enduring mental health problems (see Birchwood & Tarrier 1992). This was grounded in a stress-vulnerability conceptualisation of psychotic problems, viewed as the product of an interaction between intrinsic vulnerability and environmental stress (Neuchterlein & Dawson 1984, Zubin & Spring 1977). The construct of expressed emotion (EE) (Brown et al 1962) was

241

explored, and high levels of EE were seen as important not only in families but also among staff in in-patient settings (Forster 1999). By implication, staff have an important role in modifying ward atmosphere, with the team encouraged to employ a low EE approach to their day-to-day interactions with service users.

To facilitate effective case management, staff were trained in the use of a battery of assessment tools in order to measure symptoms, side effects of medication and social functioning. The training was consolidated by an ongoing series of multi-disciplinary meetings, leading to the development of new documentation and unitary case notes, for use by all disciplines (McKeown et al 1997, Savage & McKeown 1997).

History and context

The negative effects of prolonged institutional care are well documented (Wing 1992), having particular relevance to this case study, describing the care of somebody who has spent many years detained in a high-security hospital. The secure unit where Tony currently resides caters for the needs of people with severe and enduring mental health problems and complex needs; in this case challenging behaviour (aggression and past history of firesetting) and the effects of prolonged institutionalisation. The unit consists of two wards, one of which is permanently locked, staffed by a multi-disciplinary team including a social worker, an occupational therapist, nurses, a clinical psychologist and psychiatrists.

CASE STUDY: TONY

Tony was born in 1961, the youngest of five. His mother describes Tony as a very healthy baby, although he did have a serious respiratory attack when he was 7 weeks old. He is described in reports as 'backward' and slow to learn at school but with no behavioural problems. In contrast, his three older siblings all went on to university. However, another brother now has a diagnosis of manic depression and his mother recalls other relatives who may also have suffered from mental health problems.

Tony's father had strong emotional ties with all his children, particularly Tony. Tony's mother feels that Tony idolised his father. When Tony was 10, his father was diagnosed with leukaemia, sadly dying 4 years later. During this illness, Tony was involved in his father's care, became increasingly isolated from his peers and was teased at school. On the death of his father, Tony became disruptive and aggressive, with little outward expression of grief. He would sit in his father's chair, playing his father's music in the dark with a 'disturbing, self-satisfied grin' on his face. His mother recalls a family holiday some months later, when Tony became increasingly anxious, not wanting to be alone, shouting and threatening to kill his mother. The family did not find their GP to be especially helpful at this time.

Tony's aggressive outbursts continued over the following 2 years and were usually focused on his mother. He was eventually admitted to a large psychiatric hospital. On one occasion, whilst on home leave he refused to return and became increasingly disturbed. His mother called his psychiatrist who came to the house but failed to get Tony to return. Tony then found his father's gun and threatened to shoot his mother. She sought refuge at a neighbour's house and called the police. When an armed response unit arrived, Tony also threatened to shoot a policeman and is fortunate not to have been shot himself. He was arrested and admitted to a remand centre.

Tony's letters to his mother reveal his deteriorating mental state, becoming increasingly irrational in content. Tony was eventually admitted to an interim secure unit under sections 60 and 65 of the Mental Health Act 1959, providing for detention for treatment with restrictions on leave and discharge imposed, and monitored, by the Home Office (superseded by sections 37 and 41 of the Mental Health Act 1983). Here he was diagnosed as having schizophrenia and assessed as functioning at the borderline level of intellectual ability. Various psychotic symptoms were identified involving 'spacemen' and characters from popular television programmes of the time.

Tony improved with medication and was discharged to a hostel at the age of 20. However, he was re-admitted, overtly psychotic, after he seriously assaulted a female resident. Over the subsequent 3 years, Tony's behaviour fluctuated, with calmer periods alternating with periods of verbal and physical hostility. Unfortunately, the latter became more common, and he was frequently involved in incidents, tending to assault female members of staff and weaker patients. He described auditory hallucinations attributed to a fictional television character and in response to these often set off the fire alarms. On two occasions he set fires, once to the bed of a fellow patient. As a result of this, he was transferred to a Special Hospital, where his violence and alarm setting continued.

After 6 years, a trial of a novel antipsychotic, clozapine, was begun which resulted in improvement in his functioning to the extent that he was referred to the HDU 3 years later. However, at the age of 33, having been admitted to the secure ward of the unit, many problems were still evident. These were noted as poor coping in groups, poor personal hygiene, lack of motivation, little or inappropriate interaction with others and strong delusional ideas, though Tony was pleasant and co-operative. Much of his conversation revolved around the same delusional ideas concerning fictional characters now many years out of date, UFOs and religion. Throughout his long history of hospitalisation his mother has kept in touch with him, often travelling fairly long distances. This is despite her visits sometimes being difficult to cope with, in particular when faced with verbal hostility.

Regrettably, his mother feels that she has been let down by the health service in the past, even feeling that over the years she has been treated as 'less than dirt by doctors and psychiatrists'. It was not until Tony was admitted to the Special Hospital that she feels that Tony and herself have been treated with some understanding. She describes herself as having developed a certain toughness over the years and is unwilling to show the distress she feels when thinking about the adversities her family have faced.

Formulation

The system of care developed in the unit places a high priority on framing individuals' problems in terms of a multi-disciplinary formulation, aimed at understanding these difficulties and indicating possible interventions. Obviously, a full formulation takes time to develop, particularly in the case of someone like Tony who has little insight into his problems and with whom it is very hard to build a relationship. Provisional formulations are made and these are tested out and revised as necessary until a better understanding is reached.

Tony appears to have developed schizophrenia at an early age. Indeed, he states that he has felt different since the age of 8 when he had an unusual experience whilst walking under an electricity pylon. He seems to have misinterpreted the sensations he experienced and attributed special significance to these. In terms of a vulnerability to developing problems there may be a genetic component to his illness (given that other family members have experienced mental health problems also, albeit of a different nature). There may also be a physical component to his problems given the respiratory problem he had as a baby and the developmental delay noted as a child. Tony grew up in a family of high intellectual ability and his borderline intellect can only have been highlighted in such a context.

At a crucial stage in his development, his father died and Tony lost the person who he had idolised and who had provided much of his social interaction. This major life event appears to have triggered the prodromal phase of his illness where psychotic symptoms were not in evidence but his behaviour deteriorated and he became increasingly verbally threatening, particularly towards his mother. Thus his adolescence was a time of extreme stress for Tony when he was bullied at school, failed to live up to his older siblings' successes and lost his main role model. All of this is hypothesised to have led to very low self-esteem and a lack of confidence in his ability to cope with everyday tasks.

From the age of 17, he has been cared for in institutions of varying levels of security. This is

Table 9.1

Problem/need	Possible cause(s)
Verbal hostility	Response to hallucinations
Shouting	Frustration at predicament
Punching walls until knuckles bled	Frustration, response to symptoms
Bizarre speech	Response to hallucinations Poor conversational skills
Requesting to return to Special Hospital	Anxiety
Inappropriate social behaviour	Lack of normal social environment at key developmental stages
Problems developing relationships	Lack of opportunity; past behaviour has alienated family; low self-esteem
Poor hygiene	Negative symptoms; low self-esteem

likely to have further reduced his opportunity for social interaction, confidence and esteem. He may well have missed out on achieving basic developmental milestones of adolescence. All reports suggest that Tony has never had a sexual relationship. Many areas of functioning will have been taken out of his control and decisions made for him by carers. His physical freedom has been severely restricted and freedom of choice limited to very minor areas. Firesetting and physical assaults have not been in evidence since he was tried on a novel antipsychotic and it was therefore considered that these were a response to psychotic symptoms. Many of the problem behaviours in evidence at the HDU can be seen in terms of an inability to express his needs in an appropriate manner and as a result of limited exposure to a 'normal' environment. Some are more obviously linked to his diagnosis, for example, his bizarre conversational content; others, for example his poor self-care, may be the result of negative symptoms coupled with low self-esteem.

In the context of a stress-vulnerability model, it was felt important to proceed with change quite slowly. Tony's requests to return to the Special Hospital were seen as indicative of his anxiety, given that he has been protected from the pressures of society all his life. Conversely, it was felt that some of Tony's behaviour was a result of a lack of progress and his frustration

at his predicament sometimes resulted in him punching the wall until his knuckles bled. His inabilities in expressing his feelings appropriately can appear as childish behaviour, which has been described in the past as 'attention seeking'.

Tony's mother is the most important person in his life and he speaks about her as if he were still a child. Clearly it is important to include her in decisions regarding his care, especially regarding parole and possible resettlement. In many ways it is almost as if Tony has been stuck in a 'time warp' and in all aspects, except physically, he has not matured beyond the age of a pre-teenager.

Interventions

Following systematic and ongoing assessment, several problems and needs were identified, and these have been regularly reviewed to ensure progress, or otherwise, is taken into account. Multi-disciplinary meetings focused on Tony's case took place monthly, with in-depth discussion every 6 months. These case reviews also involved risk assessment and management decisions. Over the course of his admission several themes have emerged which form the basis of our interventions. These themes and associated problems can be grouped as shown in Table 9.1.

In addition to targeting these areas, the team also felt that Tony's mother would benefit from support. In particular, she had expressed her fears about Tony being discharged from hospital, given the history of threatening behaviour towards her. She had also stated that she found it difficult to converse with Tony during visits and did not know how to respond to his bizarre speech content. Attempts at involvement of relatives require recognition of the special problems faced by family members of a person in secure care (McCann et al 1996).

Of the range of interventions offered, two will be described in detail. In order to tackle the inappropriate behaviour noted in social situations, a package of measures was designed. These included modelling appropriate behaviour, encouraging exposure to ordinary social situations, and giving positive feedback. The stress-vulnerability model guides staff in adopting a low-EE approach, avoiding criticism and intrusiveness. As all team members had contact with Tony to some degree or another, suitable responses to the typically inappropriate elements in his conversation were discussed in order to ensure a consistent approach by all.

As he was allowed increasing levels of parole, opportunities grew to expose Tony to different social situations in a graded manner. A list was drawn up with Tony, beginning with situations inside the hospital, for example, the cafeteria and workshop, and moving on to situations with which Tony was not familiar, for example, supermarkets. Initially, leave was limited to short periods escorted by staff and the opportunity was taken to encourage structured activity by using this leave to attend other departments within the hospital. Later, as periods of gradually increasing unescorted leave were granted by the Home Office, Tony's mother became a focal point in planning for this. Throughout this leave, inappropriate conversation or behaviour was sensitively pointed out and suitable alternatives suggested and modelled. Appropriate behaviour and conversation were positively reinforced with praise and increased parole. Tony is now able to visit the city on his own and uses public transport with no untoward reports. Integral to

this intervention has been the building of self-esteem; with each small success, his confidence increased, enabling new goals to be agreed. Hence, it was important not to set targets and goals too high, making failure less likely.

The results of ongoing systematic assessment showed broadly positive trends in symptomatology and social functioning. The KGV symptom scale (Krawiecka et al 1977) elicited improvements in scores for delusions and incongruity and the Social Functioning Scale (Birchwood et al 1990) demonstrated improvement in independence, and, to a lesser degree, social relationships. Both scales have been validated and widely used with this client group.

Tony's mother has been kept informed of Tony's progress, especially extensions of parole and reductions in the risk of violence. At first she was frightened that Tony's move to the HDU had brought him considerably nearer home and possibly nearer leaving hospital care altogether. However, over time, she has seen such an improvement in their relationship that she is much less anxious in contemplating the future. She is now keen to see him settle in a group home in the community and has requested unescorted visits to her home for Tony, indicating her growing confidence in Tony and the team. Tony's mother has been an active member of the Relatives' Support Group, led by the clinical psychologist and social worker. Here she played a key role in supporting other relatives, being able to discuss the poor way she has been treated in the past, as well as develop problem-solving strategies for coping with current and future developments. This has been important in building her confidence and developing a trusting relationship with members of the team. More structured family management work is available within the unit should it be indicated. Tony's mother has been involved in the preparation of this case study, finding it a useful exercise in checking some of the 'facts' that repeatedly appear in Tony's case reports.

Outcomes

Tony has made progress in the areas initially identified as priorities. He has been safely maintained on the novel antipsychotic clozapine, continuing to undergo the regular blood testing required. He has gradually increased the time he spends off the unit, from initially being accompanied by staff in the hospital grounds to visiting the nearby city centre, by himself, or with his mother. The Home Office has been involved in these decisions as they have had to grant permission for the leave required. He has moved from the locked to the unlocked ward and been accepted for eventual placement in a community, high-dependency nursing home. Relations with his family have improved.

Tony's tendency to isolate himself and to become aggressive has diminished. Parole has increased in line with his progress and the focus of intervention has moved toward developing social skills appropriate to community living. His behaviour and conversation have become more socially acceptable, although he still sometimes talks in a child-like fashion. The extent to which his conversation revolves around his delusions has diminished and he has more to talk about now. However, he still resorts to those topics of conversation on occasion and is obviously still experiencing psychotic symptoms. Medication has not extinguished them but has, along with psychosocial intervention, reduced the amount of associated challenging behaviour.

Recently, some newer concerns have emerged. There have been a few incidents when Tony has pushed or hit others on the ward. In addition, he has been found to be failing to bathe and change his clothes regularly, to the extent that his odour has been noticeable to others. This particularly distressed Tony's mother on a recent period of leave together. There is a need to review his care plan to take account of the progress made so far and how it would best be consolidated. There is also a need for a detailed risk assessment to enable decisions to be taken about Tony's eventual placement in the community. A risk management plan for such a move would not exist in isolation, but should be an integral part of a comprehensive plan of care.

Discussion

During the time Tony has spent on the HDU, the service has undergone changes. At the time of his arrival, care was provided in a traditional, multi-disciplinary way. The different disciplines regularly met together and discussed progress and planning of care, but tended to work individually on interventions for which separate records were kept. At these meetings, and during informal contact, team members were able to co-ordinate their individual approaches and review progress. About 2 years after Tony's transfer to the HDU, the team began a process of development and training designed to bring about a more responsive pattern of care. The dissatisfaction which led to the demand for this new way of working is evident when looking at Tony's earlier records. On the one hand, there is clarity in the steps put in place to build progress, for example the graded introduction of leave from the unit, the prioritising of areas such as personal hygiene and the careful monitoring of behaviour in order to provide reports to the Home Office. Conversely, problems and interventions were stated in somewhat superficial terms, with little sense of a formulation to place them within the context of psychological or social processes.

With regard to some of the recent difficulties in Tony's care, it is possible to speculate that the introduction of a more systematic, challenging way of working has brought about an increase in tension for him, or, perhaps, that progress has been too rapid and the increased stress has led to an increase in psychotic symptoms. This highlights the dilemmas involved in the care of people with long-standing problems, where change may increase environmental stress, but lack of progress often results in frustration, which can be equally stressful or damaging to self-esteem. Recognising this is important and building safeguards into care plans can help to avoid over-reaction to understandable sequelae.

In dealing with the problem of Tony's transition from conditions of high security to the least restrictive placement which could provide the level of ongoing support he needs, the issue of a graded re-introduction to the community is acknowledged. However, the requirement for the Home Office to grant permission at every stage means that the pace of change can be dictated by factors outside the control of the immediate team.

Conclusions

This case demonstrates the effectiveness of multi-disciplinary case management for a person with a long history of forensic psychiatric care. It highlights the importance of developing and testing out a formulation to account for a person's difficulties and the utility of adopting a psychosocial model of schizophrenia. Of paramount importance has been the development of trusting relationships with Tony and his mother, made all the more difficult by previous experiences of poor quality, unsympathetic psychiatric care.

REFERENCES

Birchwood M, Tarrier N (eds) 1992 Innovations in the psychological management of schizophrenia. Wiley, Chichester

Birchwood M, Smith J, Cochrane R, Wetton S, Copestake S 1990 The social functioning scale: the development and validation of a scale of social adjustment for use in family intervention programmes with schizophrenic patients. British Journal of Psychiatry 157: 853–859

Brown G, Monck E, Carstairs G, Wing J 1962 Influence of family life on the course of schizophrenic illness. British Journal of Preventative and Social Medicine 16: 55–68

Forster J 1999 An investigation into expressed emotion as perceived by psychiatric patients. Unpublished thesis, University of Liverpool

Krawiecka M, Goldberg D, Vaughn M 1977 A standardised psychiatric assessment scale for rating chronic psychiatric patients. Acta Psychiatrica Scandinavica 55: 299–308

McCann G, McKeown M, Porter I 1996 Understanding the needs of relatives of patients within a Special Hospital for mentally disordered offenders: a basis for improved services. Journal of Advanced Nursing 23: 346–352

McKeown M, Finlayson S, Roberts K 1997 Implementing a psychosocial model of practice within a ward environment. Paper presented to the second international conference on psychological treatments for schizophrenia, Oxford, October 2–3

Neuchterlein K, Dawson M (1984) A heuristic vulnerability-stress model of schizophrenic episodes. Schizophrenia Bulletin 10: 300–312

Savage L, McKeown M 1997 Towards a new model of practice for a high dependency unit. Psychiatric Care 4: 182–186

Wing J 1992 Comment on institutionalism and schizophrenia 30 years on. British Journal of Psychiatry 160: 241–243

Zubin J, Spring B 1977 Vulnerability: a new view of schizophrenia. Journal of Abnormal Psychology 86: 260–266

Personality disorders

CHAPTER CONTENTS

CONTENTS

Psychodynamic psychotherapy, personality disorder and offending

Mark Stowell-Smith

Introduction

This case study describes the use of psycho-dynamic psychotherapy carried out in a forensic out-patient clinic with a 48-year-old man who had previous admissions to both prison and Special Hospital. His admission to hospital had been effected under the legal category of psychopathic disorder. The most salient features of his offending history were his violence towards men and his sado-masochism directed at females. In this study, his offending is considered as a dynamic manifestation of underlying personality factors, and I describe the way in which these factors were addressed in therapy.

Psychodynamic forensic psychotherapy

Forensic psychotherapy is the offspring of forensic psychiatry and psychoanalytical psychotherapy and aims to provide a psychodynamic perspective to the understanding, management and treatment of the offender. The overarching aim of forensic psychotherapy is to help the offender understand, and take responsibility for, their actions, in order to reduce the likelihood of re-offending (Cordess et al 1994). In this respect a central focus is maintained on the criminal act, the psychoanalytical understanding of which can be traced at least back to Freud's (1957) hypothesis that certain criminal acts may have an unconscious meaning and motivation, representing, for example, a means of expressing and discharging unresolved guilt.

Within the discipline of forensic psycho-therapy a useful differentiation can be made between careerist criminals, for whom the cost–benefits of the offence may be carefully calculated, and the offender for whom the offence may be the equivalent to a neurotic symptom, the expression of a severe, underlying psychopathology or a defence against an underlying depression (Welldon 1998: 15). Conceptualised in this way, the therapist may address the offence with the patient as, for example, an attempt to gain 'symptom relief' or as an attempt to resolve a conflict arising from a basic primary event.

The case considered here explores therapy undertaken with a 48-year-old man with a long history of sado-masochistic behaviour. In the therapy, this behaviour is considered as a type of perverse solution to a number of psychological problems. The understanding of these problems and the patient's response to them was structured around Glasser's (1979, 1988) notion of the 'core complex'. According to Glasser, this is a psychological configuration comprising a group of inter-related characteristics which have their origin at an early stage of development. The starting point for the complex is the ordinary human need for emotional closeness with the other. However, in certain cases, rather than being enriching this contact threatens to annihilate the self as there is an expectation that contact will result in the self being taken over to the point where it ceases to exist as a separate entity. This distortion may occur, for example, in relation to patients whose early histories have been characterised by abusive, intrusive caregiving. In such individuals a conflict may be set up between both wanting contact and fearing it. One response to this conflict may be withdrawal, but this in turn may activate feelings of abandonment, depression and desolation.

According to Glasser, the 'perverse solution' to this dilemma entails sexualising the aggression elicited by the perceived threat of the other so that the intention to destroy is converted into a desire to hurt and control. This allows the self to retain contact with the other, but at a safe distance – a distance which precludes trust and intimacy (Glasser 1988: 126). This form of relationship is apparent in perversions such as paedophilia, where contact with the other is maintained at the expense of denying the other's individuality. This is chillingly expressed in Glasser's statement that 'One might say his [the paedophile's] "love" for the child is predominantly like that of the dog for the bone' (1990: 744). As we will see, this perverse mode of relating is apparent in the sado-masochism of Steve.

CASE STUDY: STEVE

Background history

Steve was the only child of his parent's marriage. In early childhood, he recalled a lack of parental involvement coupled with acute feelings of being unloved and unwanted. He had vivid memories of his father as a powerful, controlling, figure who was frequently physically abusive to both his mother and Steve. In the absence of parental involvement, much of the practical parenting tasks were undertaken by his paternal grandmother whom Steve described as an unaffectionate disciplinarian. She inculcated him with a number of what were to become enduring beliefs about female sexuality as something that was dirty, contaminating and dangerous.

Although ambivalently attached to his father, Steve's account of his development emphasised difficulties in identifying himself as a separate object from him. He felt controlled, criticised and never able to please his father. This attitude was expressed in his account of his father as 'suffocating and invasive'. He remembered seeing a photograph in which both himself and his father were dressed in the same suits; and he also recalled his father's intrusiveness, describing a number of trivial situations where he would appear and correct Steve's actions. When at home with his father, he felt as though he were 'walking around in the deep end of a swimming pool'; when in prison, he felt liberated and free.

Steve was often bullied in school and he described wanting to pay his victimisers back. As a child, he was able partially to achieve this by eliciting the envy of others, flaunting his family's relative affluence to the other poorer children in his neighbourhood. As an adult, he sought direct confrontation with his male, child-hood, abusers. He described how, in a heavily intoxicated state, he would contrive to meet up with the latter in some of the local bars. He then detailed the pleasure that resulted from the sense of control he felt, adding that bodily trans-formations experienced since puberty meant he was now larger, and more powerful, than his erstwhile aggressors. On occasions when he was able to triumph in these conflicts, he recalled how he would 'swagger' about the bar. His account of this scene incorporated the theme of him transforming the childhood trauma of being small, weak and abused into one of adult triumph in which he was physically and psychologically big, powerful and abusive (Stoller 1986). A similar drama of transformation was enacted in much of his subsequent sexual offending.

Offending history

Steve was charged with a number of offences, the most serious of which included grievous bodily harm, attempted rape and unlawful wounding. Many of his offences were perpe-trated against women and were associated with emergent sadistic fantasies. This formed the basis of his index offence, in which he abducted and sexually assaulted a woman of 25. In dis-cussing this offence he stated that his intention had been to kill the victim, but he was overcome by remorse and phoned the police to give him-self up. Equally disturbing was his account of how he had sought to put his sadistic fantasies into practice on the local prostitutes. Prior to his admission to hospital, he estimated that he had spent approximately £6000 on prostitutes over a 5-month period. In each case the prosti-tute was hired for acts of bondage and sadism. He described how he had been particularly excited by contracting with the prostitute to engage in 'mild' forms of sado-masochism which involved tying the woman up. Having done this he would go beyond the agreed limit, deriving sexual stimulation from the victim's powerlessness and terror.

Intervention

Before therapy commenced, I met with Steve to discuss the terms and conditions under which our sessions would take place. We agreed to meet in a forensic out-patient clinic for weekly sessions of psychodynamic psychotherapy over a 2-year period. When therapy started, he was resident in a probation hostel, having lived there since his conditional discharge from Special Hospital 6 months earlier. He reported to me that he had stopped offending but retained some awareness of his immense hostility towards both men and women. The task for him was to contain and understand this hostility as he was conscious of the extreme acts which these feelings might potentiate.

A theme, which emerged early on in therapy, was his need to regulate his degree of contact with other people. He seemed desperate to con-trol the quantity and quality of social contact with other people in the hostel. These anxieties were expressed in the claustrophobic metaphor of the hostel being like a submarine in which it was impossible to get away from other people. He had to find his own space within this envi-ronment and at times when he could not retreat into his own room, he would hide himself in the toilet. When even this option was denied, he felt most vulnerable and described a feeling of being sucked into the dirty, contaminating hostel. I suggested to him that the anxiety he experienced as he related this struggle to me said much about his own fears of maintaining himself as a separate, boundaried individual.

One of Steve's main defences against engulf-ing emotional contact with others was through the elicitation of either envy or hostility. He described, for example, scenarios in which he would pre-empt the possibility of intimate emotional contact either by behaving in a cold, distant manner or completely ignoring other people. This was taken up with Steve as an example of him both avoiding the possibility of intimate contact with others and re-finding a more familiar type of object relationship in which he was locked in combat with an abusing, paternal object. I suggested to him that this represented a reversal of the childhood situation as it was Steve who was now in control, rejecting others and keeping them at bay. Steve took up this interpretation and was able to identify with the sense of humiliation he felt he had engendered in a person whom he had recently rejected. He reflected upon his compulsion to repeat a type of relationship in which he presented as angry, belligerent and contemptuous of others. He acknowledged how, rather than finding himself the hapless victim in conflict situations with other men, his demeanour played an active, if unconscious, part in setting up these situations. I linked this to the feelings of loss and anxiety he had recently experienced when a resident to whom he had expressed hatred and anger had left the hostel. Steve reflected how hard it was to give up the type of relationship in which he felt threatened and intimidated by a powerful other. He recalled a series of similar relationships dating back to early adulthood and described an emptiness that enveloped him when such a relationship was absent. I suggested to him that this could be linked to his relationship with his father and reflected his childhood dilemma of needing either to relate to an abusing caregiver or risk total abandonment.

A central feature of psychodynamic therapy is an effort to make visible and understand the patient's transference to the therapist. Transference is, in part, the emotional response and 'as if' relationship that the patient brings to the therapy on the basis of past events and the patient's experience of earlier infantile prototypes. For example, despite the therapist's position of therapeutic neutrality the patient may relate to the therapist, as if they were an abusing or abandoning parent. I sensed that Steve's transference to me was influenced by previous history of neglectful or abusive, intrusive caregiving. His response to me seemed at first to be one in which he shut himself down emotionally. This was experienced in my counter-transference (an unconscious reaction to the patient's transference) as being emotionally disconnected or absent from Steve. During many of our sessions, for example, I had a sense that Steve and myself had joined together in talking about a third person, another Steve who was not really with us in the room. This was interpreted as an indication of his need to remain at a safe emotional distance in order to avoid the threat of my intrusiveness.

A further manifestation of his avoidance of emotional contact was to be found in his attempts to impose an implicit agenda upon our sessions. He started many of the sessions by narrating the events of the week to me before settling back into his chair, inviting me to comment. On other occasions, he would ask me directly where he should begin or request an agenda for the session. At these times, my relationship with him felt precarious and it was a struggle to hold therapy together. Again my counter-transference to his lengthy narrations was to disengage from contact with him and long for him not to be in the room with me. This seemed to provide some clue to one of his strategies for being with others and I suggested to him that his attempt to impose a formal structure upon our sessions was something that militated against the possibility of emotional contact in therapy. This was perhaps something that also helped him to deal with negative feelings which he may have held about me, for example, feelings of anger and hostility related to fears that I may despise him or reject him, like his father.

An important feature of Steve's unease with intimate emotional contact was expressed in the sense of disgust experienced at the prospect of another person wanting to be close to him. This was particularly apparent in relation to women. Here he seemed primed to either seek relationships with women in which he could feel directly degraded or, over a period of time, develop the relationship into one in which he could transform this experience into one in which he would become angry and humiliating. His association with prostitutes provided the context in which he could affect this transformation. Here the humiliation at having to pay for sexual attention was, through the sadistic act, transformed into feelings of triumph.

A subtle equivalent to this process became apparent in therapy as Steve acknowledged how, over a period of months, he had courted the attention of a junior member of female staff in the hostel. In discussing the relationship, he described some tender feelings towards the worker and stated that he enjoyed the feeling that he meant something to her. However, he had also developed the relationship by supplying her with money and gifts. Over an 8-month period, he had documented in his diary the type and quantity of gifts given to her. He conveyed a sense of her having become dependent upon him and gave examples of how she had disclosed information regarding her personal difficulties. This had opened up for him a range of powerful emotions. On the one hand, he felt powerful and excited by her dependency but, on the other, felt anger and rage when he considered that she might be exploiting him for her material advantage. This was taken up with Steve as a further example of him setting up a sado-masochistic relationship in which he felt either powerfully in control or humiliated and degraded. This was an important moment in therapy, as although Steve maintained he had ceased actively offending it was important for him to acknowledge how his relationship with the female worker bore many similarities to the type of relationship he had sought to form with prostitutes. For example, his gifts to her had paid for her attention. However, in the knowledge that this constituted professional misconduct on her part, he had then paid her back for the humiliation of having to buy the attention of another, by systematically recording each of these transactions as a weapon which he could then sadistically use upon her at some later date. In discussing these events, Steve recalled a newspaper article which described the rape and murder of a woman 'who had been a nurse by day and prostitute by night'. I suggested that under their conventional, respectable facade, Steve perhaps saw all women as greedy, dirty prostitutes and that he had sought to demonstrate this by transforming his relationship with the residential worker into a 'client–prostitute' relationship.

Reflections on the progress of therapy

As the time approached for therapy to end, we noted Steve's continuing struggle to come to terms with his vulnerability. In therapy, he demonstrated his reluctance to relinquish the need for compensatory, omnipotent control which afforded him a means of maintaining a sense of secure and stable identity. However, the extent of his sadism had reduced and he had reached the point where he was able to share aspects of this vulnerability and continuing struggle with the other professionals involved in his care and support.

Conclusions

This case study has described the use of psychodynamic psychotherapy as a way of treating and managing the offender patient. Psychotherapy with Steve allowed the exploration of a number of important issues that were considered in relation to Glasser's (1979, 1988) notion of the core complex. I considered the different solutions to Steve's core complex anxieties adopted in relation to both women and men. In each case, there was a sense of him wanting to transform the childhood experience of weakness and vulnerability into a feeling of omnipotent control. As therapy progressed, Steve gained some insight and understanding into his propensity for re-enacting this pattern of behaviour. However, whilst therapy sought to engender understanding and insight, in contrast to more conventional versions of psychological therapy, it did not seek to make him feel 'better'. Rather, it sought to enhance his discomfort by making him aware of how dangerous he could be. Arguably, an awareness of these propensities increased his sense of control, thereby reducing his future dangerousness.

REFERENCES

Cordess C, Riley W, Welldon E 1994 Psychodynamic forensic psychotherapy: an account of a day-release course. Psychiatric Bulletin 18: 88–90

Freud S 1957 Some character types met in psychoanalytical work. Standard edition, vol XIV. Hogarth Press, London

Glasser M. 1979 Some aspects of the role of aggression in the perversions. In: Rosen I (ed) Sexual deviations. Oxford University Press, Oxford

Glasser M 1988 Psychodynamic aspects of paedophilia. Psychoanalytic Psychotherapy 3: 121–135

Glasser M 1990 Paedophilia. In: Bluglass R, Bowden M (eds) Principles and practice of forensic psychiatry. Churchill Livingstone, Edinburgh

Stoller I 1986 Perversion: the erotic form of hatred. Maresfield, London

Welldon E 1998 Forensic psychotherapy: The practical approach. In: Welldon E, Van Velsen C (eds) A practical guide to forensic psychotherapy. Jessica Kingsley, London

CONTENTS

Social therapy: a case study in developing a staffing model for work with personality-disordered offenders

Howard Shimmin and Les Storey

Introduction

People with a 'personality disorder', who have offended or are considered to be a danger to themselves or others, have historically presented difficulties for the staff and services who manage their care. Currently, in England, they tend to be managed either within the criminal justice system or within health care by a mixture of professional and semi-professional disciplines, often with acknowledged training deficits in this area (Committee of Inquiry 1992). Difficulties surrounding the definition of personality disorder are well documented elsewhere, and this is compounded in the English justice and health services by the existence of vague and often contentious legal and clinical conceptual definitions and by an often poor interface between the respective systems in practice.

Irrespective of definition, the issues for management, treatment and placement tend to centre around areas of culpability (Zomer 1992) and the many defence mechanisms that are adopted in the name of 'ego protection' by such individuals. In spite of the problems of definition and often unsuitable and ill-equipped service provision, a number of those classified as personality disordered reside in Special Hospitals. Such individuals require an environment which reflects an ability to deal with chaotic effects that such defence mechanisms often produce. In reality, a number end up there as a result of the inability of other services to safely manage or 'treat' them. Hence, the Special Hospitals have been seen as a last resort for this group and the selection

257

of patients has not necessarily been clinically driven.

Background

The Personality Disorder Unit (PDU) was established at Ashworth Hospital in 1994. This was partly as a result of the decision to separate the care of personality-disordered patients from other services within the hospital that focus on those with other diagnoses such as learning difficulties and psychosis. The original staff complement came from services not specifically designed for caring for patients with personality disorders. Within Ashworth, and indeed nationally, little formal training in this work exists for most disciplines and it could be argued that this has contributed to a number of well-publicised and -documented difficulties (Committee of Inquiry 1992, 1999). Additionally, there are undoubtedly less well-publicised effects of this work, such as high staff-turnover rates, increased sickness rates and a low morale amongst staff brought on by burnout and the perceived lack of therapeutic impetus.

One further feature that needed to be addressed is the prediction that recruitment and retention of mental health professionals will become increasingly difficult over the next few years as a result of demographic and economic factors and a decline in recruitment to professional training, especially within nursing. There are traditionally high ratios of qualified to unqualified nursing staff within Special Hospitals and nursing makes up the largest part of the workforce (Health Care Workforce 2000). Changes in nurse education and funding for higher education are issues that have contributed to a downturn in numbers of those entering education programmes or undertaking practice on completion of training. The generic nature of mental health nursing programmes also fails to prepare nurses to work in the specialist field of forensic mental health (Storey & Dale 1998).

Current developments

In 1995, as a response to patient and staff needs, considerable effort was put into the identification and development of core competencies for staff in the PDU. Following this initial work, the need to develop new approaches to the care and management of personality-disordered patients was identified (Melia et al 1999). The High Security Psychiatric Services Commissioning Board (HSPSCB) were approached and they agreed to fund a pilot project for the development of specific training and revised working methods for a new group of workers, namely 'social therapists'. The social therapists were to be employed initially in a new, purpose-built unit, the Wordsworth Project: a four-flat, 16-bed, pre-discharge and pre-transfer facility promoting independent living and enhanced interpersonal skills for male personality-disordered patients using psychosocial models of working.

This initiative has been run in tandem with another HSPSCB funded project to develop occupational standards for the multi-disciplinary staff working across the PDU. The standards project has principally used functional mapping techniques to develop occupational standards which are being used for the definition of competency-based job descriptions for a range of staff, including social therapists. This approach will, additionally, facilitate a training needs analysis and the development of curricula for a range of qualifications at academic levels reflecting the needs of staff, patients and the organisation.

Through the use of functional analysis, we have been able to take an holistic approach to the identification of principles and values and to establish the key purpose of the service. The occupational map reflects the role and function of the multi-disciplinary team from 'hands on' care through to strategic management. The occupational standards can now provide the framework for us to audit the service to personality disordered patients and to introduce a benchmark for the development of service standards and performance review. They have provided us with a tool to measure service outcomes across the whole range of our provision for personality-disordered patients.

Also, through undertaking the functional analysis, we have been able to identify the core curriculum themes that feature in the induction programme for social therapists. These themes include boundaries and interrelatedness, overview and assessment of personality disorder, consistent and coherent therapeutic approaches, management, evidence-based practice, supervision and reflective practice.

The problems

The initial research for this project was taken from a wide range of sources, starting with a very basic set of questions such as:

- What is personality disorder?
- What knowledge base is required?
- What type of environment is required?
- What types of therapies are appropriate for use with personality disorder?
- What are the effects on staff?
- What are the skills required by staff working with this group?
- How can we measure the outcomes of our work?
- What systems and policies are useful?

In short, we were able to design at least part of a service and the workforce skills and qualities from scratch. Initial work was based on existing research, followed by discussion with staff who currently work in the field. Consultation with all disciplines within the PDU, therapeutic communities, other special hospitals and regional secure units (RSUs) and outside agencies including the voluntary and private sectors, was undertaken. Visits were also made to Holland, where a dedicated service has existed for a considerable period of time (the TBS). The resulting framework of practice is an amalgam of ideas and principles from these sources.

The service

The aims of the Wordsworth Project were initially established by the Commissioning Board who took into account the existing PDU structure, that is, as a final part in the process of moving personality-disordered patients into the community or conditions of lesser security. As a pilot, there was no initial intention to

set up a total service, but to slot in with existing services. The focus was on rehabilitation (or in Holland resocialisation) of personality-disordered patients, rather than on initial work such as index offence therapies and the provision of structure to often chaotic patients. The service specification and procedures were simply outlined in order to involve staff and patients (to some extent) in their development to enhance ownership and to determine their workability on the ground.

Recruitment

As we were able to start from basics with the workforce, we identified the best factors from a number of sources based on personal qualities, development potential and existing skills. We were also able to incorporate the initial results from the functional mapping exercise to draw up person specifications and job descriptions. Bearing in mind the needs of the service, we were also able to utilise national demographic and workforce trends and plot possible career pathways for this new group of staff. Other factors that influenced us were the numbers of psychology graduates emerging from colleges and universities with limited opportunities for a career using the degree directly in a practice-based setting, and existing staff with good skills but lacking formal professional qualifications in this field.

The first 10 positions were advertised nationally and attracted over 60 responses for posts that would offer only a modest salary. The short-listing procedure included candidates submitting written submissions on issues relating to personality disorder. 25 people were interviewed and the posts were filled in April 1997, although 20 of the candidates were appointable. We held a number of candidates in reserve to be approached if vacancies occurred or the service expanded.

The candidates came from a range of backgrounds and possessed a range of qualifications, though none came with formal mental health qualifications. There was a predominance of psychology graduates, but social workers, a nursing assistant, drugs counsellors and individuals with social science degrees were also appointed. This range and diversity have proved to be beneficial in developing the team and developing inter-disciplinary working practices within Wordsworth. It also meant that the induction programme had to reflect the variety of needs and experience.

Induction programme

Following recruitment, a training needs analysis was undertaken to ensure that individual needs were matched against the organisational expectation. The induction programme was able to be flexible and was continually reviewed using this and teaching outcome measures.

The induction programme was undertaken in a 3-month block. We were able to do this, on this occasion, because we had no patients within the system and all of the staff were new to the role and most were new to the organisation. Future plans, based on our evaluation of the outcomes of the induction, will ensure that new starters are mentored by experienced social therapists and undertake a planned, individual induction programme over a period of time. This revised induction will include regular reviews and feedback on performance which will contribute to a performance review at the end of 12 months, relating to the standards-based job description developed from the functional mapping exercise.

The revised induction programme has been developed to ensure that there is a consistent and coherent approach to the management of patients. It will include mandatory hospital training comprising the following: child protection, health and safety, security, care and responsibility, breakaway and de-escalation techniques, Care Programme Approach and first aid. In addition, induction for the role of social therapist will include boundaries and inter-relatedness, transference and counter-transference, aetiology of personality disorder, assessment and therapeutic approaches (cognitive psychological, behavioural and psychodynamic approaches), content of programmes, risk assessment and management, teamwork, consistency and supervision.

Assessment methodology

The team within Wordsworth have introduced assessment processes that have evolved from systems used in other areas and from the functional analysis work in the PDU. The current assessment process involves a team approach, involving the social therapists and staff from the originating ward, including the Responsible Medical Officer, nursing staff, therapy staff, psychologists and potential receiving agencies. The approach is a full paper-work search of patient antecedents and interventions, developmental histories, semi-structured interviews with key staff and with the patient, identification of need and the development of a negotiated, therapeutic and behavioural contract. The contract identifies group and individual work, time scales and anticipated outcomes, review processes and patient involvement. In this way, the ground-rules and therapeutic relationship are made explicit. This ultimately forms the basis for a continuing assessment and management package to be available to the receiving agency. The primary focus of any package is on effectively managing change and risk, and passing that information on to receiving agencies effectively.

Teamwork approach

The model of assessment and care that has developed is based on an innovative teamwork approach. This model has evolved from previous work, both within Ashworth and from sources in the UK and Holland, undertaken across a number of disciplines. The principles upon which the model is based are: enhanced team communication, rotating keywork and co-working models; structured reflection on the therapeutic relationships formed by the team members with a patient (including transference and counter-transference issues); the development of a consistent but flexible approach by all staff (who could be new to the patient or who may have had limited previous involvement); the recognition of splitting within teams and between therapists working with a patient; and the development and implementation of a peer supervision model based on constructive criticism, that enables workers to look at the above issues in a safe environment that is conducive to their day-to-day practice.

Review and evaluation

Some of the benefits that have resulted from this approach are diversity of opinion and hypothesis but consistency of approach, lessened splitting or at least acknowledgement of it, with a resultant reduction of the potential for negative dynamic relationships within the team. The team has developed an intrinsic knowledge of individual staff members' weaknesses and limitations, but is able to offer appropriate support and thus compensate in most working situations. We have developed a co-worker inventory to facilitate this process that both provides information on preferred styles of working between staff members and enables us to constantly evaluate any changes as a team, as we neither believe nor wish that this is a fixed phenomena.

So far, there appears to have been the maintenance of greater therapeutic impetus with patients which previous systems of working often considered to be blocked. Through the use of a wide-ranging assessment, and some basic psychodynamic elements relevant to the understanding of therapeutic relationships, we have been able to hypothesise and, to some extent, predict patient defence mechanisms. This has enabled the team to develop a consistent and reflective approach that appears to move patients towards less defended positions.

The core of the system for teamworking is the trained and supervised use of a team debriefing protocol, facilitated by the systematic use of observation of sessions and the subsequent use of the same observers as de-briefers. The methods employed during de-brief are a structured opportunity for venting and an exploration of transference and counter-transference issues, which in turn informs the approach of future sessions. Alongside the evolution of the small team model (four staff at any time), we tried at various points to employ similar methods within the larger team (up to 12 members). This has so far been a failure. There was an initial overemphasis on the role of the large team within the project and the perceived need for it to function in a similarly overtly, critically, constructive manner. This appears to have been far more threatening to staff, in spite of them working in rotation with every individual team member, and the motivation to continue the process collapsed.

Other benefits from this pilot appear to be the recruitment and deployment of workers aimed at a very specific area with rapid learning curves as a result of both individual academic background and experience. Also there was a cumulative team-learning process, enhanced by the establishment of interdependence through small team working methods.

Supervision

As a result of the innovative nature of the project, it was decided that a new supervision model was required and this was developed in part by the workers based on their own needs. Several suggested models were piloted, eventually ending with a mix of individual (reflective practice) and peer group (small team) supervision. The resultant system was written as a series of protocols and practice guides for staff use. The notion of a more flattened hierarchy within the team was taken from the Dutch experience which has led to more effective inter-disciplinary working and support. However, this may not be without problems for the wider organisation as it may be perceived as both a threat to established hierarchies within existing professions and the need of the parenting organisation for traditionally established lines of accountability. This is probably compounded by the prevalence of the medical model within the institution and, to some extent, by current mental health legislation. The model also requires managers to adapt their skills to the needs of the workforce much more than in a traditional model.

Conclusions

At the time of writing, the project outlined has been operational with patients for 10 months.

Although some outcome measures regarding patients are being used, it is too early to infer any great success, as to date the numbers through the project remain small. However, we believe that the methodology that has been established for designing a workforce from scratch, to meet a particular and difficult set of needs, is effective and may be repeated in other situations.

Some particular features appear to be working very well. The small team method maintains a therapeutic impetus with often difficult, vulnerable and neglected patients. At the same time, it affords a suitable degree of protection to staff who in the past have been victims of the cumulated effects of the patients' defence

mechanisms and acting out. The high levels of self-awareness of staff, particularly around boundaries and transference, are of great benefit in this area of work, as is the potential of the workforce to mentor and induct new staff as required.

The project appears to have been able to tap into a previously under-utilised pool of labour, with benefits to individual workers and the organisation. However, the wider implications of this in terms of existing professional and organisational structures are difficult to predict at the present, and the future plans for this model are perhaps dependent on political and legal initiatives within forensic services.

REFERENCES

Committee of Inquiry into Complaints about Ashworth Hospital 1992 Report of the Committee of Inquiry into Complaints about Ashworth Hospital (Blom Cooper Report) Cmnd 2028. HMSO, London

Committee of Inquiry into the Personality Disorder Unit, Ashworth Special Hospital 1999 Report of the Committee of Inquiry into the Personality Disorder Unit, Ashworth Special Hospital (Fallon Report) Cmnd 4194–11. HMSO, London

Melia P, Moran T, Wilkie I 1999 Personality disorder: Ashworth and after. Mental Health Care 2(6): 205–207

Storey L, Dale C 1998 Nursing in secure environments. Psychiatric Care 5(40): 122–123

Zomer M 1992 New practices for old rules. Paper presented at Therapeutic Communities Conference, Windsor, UK, September 1992

CONTENTS

Therapeutic community in a forensic setting

Lawrence Jones

Introduction

The principal concept behind the therapeutic community (TC) approach is to use the whole regime in a treatment setting as a tool for intervention. This is as opposed to having interventions only at certain times of the day, undertaken by various professionals, with the day-to-day management of patients left to nursing and night staff. In a TC, everyday behaviour and interactions with others are seen as an opportunity for learning and personal development, if they are responded to in a creative and questioning way. No event falls outside this general remit. All co-participants in the running of the regime, including patients, cleaning staff, visitors, group therapists, nursing staff and managers are involved in the therapeutic intervention. Learning is achieved through a collective exploration of behaviour to identify the key learning points. Interpersonal problems are seen, as far as possible, as being brought about by the group as a whole not just by the individuals involved. This case study looks at the treatment issues for one member of a TC, John, a young man with a history of drug use and convictions for acquisitive offending and armed robbery.

Theoretical background

Staff in a therapeutic community setting are encouraged to look at the ways in which they might be drawn into a collusive dynamic with patients, for example, behaving in a harsh, punitive, way with a patient group who often come

263

from abusive backgrounds and who treat staff as if they are no different from the adults they have encountered in the past. Or, conversely, treating personality-disordered patients as victims, akin to their presentation, can prevent work on offending behaviour: to 'pussyfoot around the hostility endlessly, because one "feels sorry" for what the patient had endured years earlier, does nothing to check the patient's habitual abuse of others in the here and now' (Stone 1993). Once identified, these collusive processes are explored in small group settings or, when appropriate, in staff and community meetings.

One particular kind of intervention that characterises the TC, but which is not undertaken in the same way in other contexts, is the 'community meeting' which is typically held on a daily basis. This involves all the patients and as many of the staff as possible, sometimes as many as 30 or more people. Used primarily to talk through and collectively problem-solve current issues, the community meeting addresses a variety of issues. Examples might include:

- Why the daily chores are not being done
- How to support a particular patient who is going through a difficult time
- How to help patients face up to their offences, rather than leave the community
- Why some patients, acting as a group, are behaving in a superior way and nobody is talking about it.

Additionally, TCs also have a number of other kinds of therapeutic groups. The greater part of the day is spent in shared activities such as work, education and more specific interventions such as cognitive–behavioural and drama therapy focused on particular areas of need.

There are several different kinds of TC operating in forensic settings, though little attempt has been made to describe them systematically. Typically, two types are distinguished:

Hierarchical Therapeutic Communities were developed in the USA and originated in the substance misuse movement. They tend to emphasise obedience to community rules, which are administered and supervised by community members who are advanced in their therapy.

This is done through a formal hierarchy of community members, with each stage having seniority over junior members. Graduation to higher levels is dependent upon appropriate behaviour. Inappropriate behaviour can lead to demotion and a return to lower status in the hierarchy. For an example of hierarchical TCs and empirical evidence of efficacy, the reader is referred to Wexler (1997).

The Maxwell Jones Style Therapeutic Community tends to lay more emphasis on 'democracy' as a significant educative process. For an account of this model, run in a forensic setting, see Cullen (1997). Typically, many issues, including community membership, are discussed by community members and decisions are made democratically. This decision-making is, however, usually carefully managed by staff who attempt to moderate more extreme malignant group behaviour when it occurs. An attempt is made to allow as much freedom as the community, as a whole, can cope with at any given time.

CASE STUDY: JOHN

Selection

Jones (1997) has highlighted many of the issues that bear on the process of selection for a TC and John is not an untypical referral. John entered therapy ostensibly because he had had a significant history of substance misuse. He had also been given an ultimatum to stop using drugs by his common law wife with whom he had a son, William. John was approaching a parole review panel when he asked his probation officer for help with his drug-taking and offending behaviour. He was also in debt on the wing.

At interview prior to treatment, John had presented as motivated, of reasonable intelligence and showed no signs of mental illness that might make him an unsuitable candidate. It is not uncommon that motivation for treatment is often driven, initially, by extrinsic factors. Thus screening for the risk of drop out is important, in order to reduce the often unacceptably high attrition rate (60%, or more) in TCs.

Intelligence, and the relative absence of serious mental illness, are also significant indicators of capacity to tolerate the TC approach to treatment. In addition, there is a debate in the literature about the treatability of patients meeting the Hare (1991) criteria for psychopathy. Some, such as Hemphill (1991), based on evidence from the now closed Penetanguishene TC in Canada, argue that such environments can make psychopathic offenders 'worse'. Others, for example Dolan & Coid (1993), argue that TCs which adhere to the core tenet of voluntarism can impact significantly on this patient group. They argue that TCs which do not offer the patient a choice of opting in or out of treatment and compulsory regimes such as that at Penetanguishene, may be damaging for the Hare psychopath.

Induction

New arrivals often bring the prison culture with them, distrusting staff and using traditional prisoner strategies to meet their needs. In the early days of his stay in the TC, John was quiet and respectful of others on the unit. However, staff felt that he was treating them as he might those working in a dispersal prison, challenging them every time he felt that he was not getting what he wanted (e.g. phone calls and visits) immediately.

John's behaviour reflects the initial phase of treatment, 'the honeymoon', which often involves disabusing patients of unrealistic thinking where they expect staff to magically 'make them better'. Members may also start off with attempts at impression management, to convince staff that they are likable and suitable for parole or to let other patients know that they cannot be 'walked all over'. Engagement in the therapeutic process takes time and often comes after an initial phase of disillusionment brought about by all of the community members refusing to collude with these behaviours.

Changing

Jones (1997) reports a change process of getting 'worse' before getting 'better'. This can involve offence-related and disordered behaviour re-emerging as stressful issues are encountered

either in day-to-day living or as a consequence of therapy. One aspect of this process can be seen when staff begin to react to conflicting aspects of the individual's behaviour, at times having to resolve these counter-transference issues in the staff group.

In community meetings, John began to treat some of the staff as if they were 'sadistic' torturers, whose main interest was to withhold things from the patients on the unit. Occasionally, these confrontations with staff would feel as if they could become violent. In small group sessions, John was presenting himself as a victim of the 'brutal' system and being challenged by other patients in the group. They explored with him the way that he used perceived injustice to justify his own behaviour. While looking at the notion that 'two wrongs don't make a right', his peers began to link this issue with John's offending behaviour. John did not like what he heard and stormed out of a couple of small groups, making threats to inmates as he left. At this stage, several community meetings were taken up with John's intimidating behaviour. Some people continued to challenge this, others went quiet and a smaller group identified with John who had an ability to 'rabble rouse' and foment anti-staff attitudes.

While describing some staff as 'sadistic', John also talked about his small group therapist in very positive terms. The latter began to identify with some of the issues that John had been raising and took them to the staff group. This generated conflict between those staff who had been portrayed as cruel, who felt that John should be moved off the unit, and the therapist who believed that John had been deliberately provoked and should remain. It was established that both groups were getting drawn into an interpersonal process with John and that this should be explored in the appropriate therapeutic groupings. Eventually, John identified a connection between his perceptions of authority and early life experiences of neglect with his mother and in care.

Whilst at times feeling stretched to their limits, the staff tried to deal with this by not reacting in a retaliatory way. They told John how he was affecting them and asked for help in taking things forward. Occasionally, John showed signs of reflection and began to recognise that his behaviour was incompatible with the unit rules. Nonetheless, his behaviour continued to deteriorate.

Crisis management

Very rarely does therapy progress from 'bad' to 'better' with personality-disordered and offender patients. When this appears to happen, the response is questioned and 'faking good' suspected. A critical feature of working with this client group is crisis management. Within the TC, a crisis is construed as an opportunity to learn and a well-developed 'culture of enquiry' is encouraged to focus on the issues in a collective way.

Crisis 1

John was challenged by another inmate for using drugs on the unit, though he had not apparently been involved in dealing to others. He denied involvement, but, when confronted with the results of a urine test, found it difficult to sustain the denial. John was surprised when, rather than rejection, the majority of the community chose to work with him in establishing what had precipitated the relapse. Initially, he was made a 'scapegoat' by several more senior inmates who wanted him out. After a time, however, the whole community came to see how they had been letting John get away with things over time and consistently failing to challenge this. Others also owned their role in having turned a 'blind eye' to his having had a poster on his wall that portrayed cannabis use in a positive light. How had the community allowed John, who had come into treatment explicitly to address substance misuse problems, to cynically extol the virtues of drug-taking?

John was placed on a contract by the community. This involved a commitment to therapy in order to achieve his core life goals of getting released, being a father and strengthening relations with his family. He also contracted to address his drug-taking more actively, focusing on his relapse process and working up a relapse-prevention plan. On a couple of occasions, feeling cornered, John had stormed out of his group leaving people feeling threatened. Thus, he was also contracted by the community to look at his acting out and therapeutic interference.

During this period, John discussed his 'life story' in group, focusing in particular on his offending behaviour and family background. He talked at length about his mother's 'mental illness' and that for much of his childhood he had felt either frightened of her violence or rejected and unloved. He denied ever feeling any anger towards his mother for this behaviour.

In offence-focused role play, John was encouraged to explore his offence, particularly his victim's experience during it. If these feelings were too strong for him to deal with directly, they were explored in other ways, for example, by imagining what his victim said to her partner after the offence. John became aware that the last time he had experienced this fear of being killed was as a child, when he thought that his mother had tried to kill him. John had locked his victims up in a back room during the robbery, something his mother had done to him for being tearful. Core beliefs about revenge and retribution had been triggered and his offending seemed to have many of the ingredients that were around during abusive childhood traumas.

Offence-paralleling behaviour

Often behaviour in treatment directly parallels aspects of offending behaviour. Jones (1997) explores this issue as essential to risk management and intervention. John's behaviour illustrates aspects of this pattern.

Crisis 2

John would typically challenge the group, threaten it if he did not get his own way and walk out as a way of underscoring his threats. Bank robbery is an offence against a group of people, as was his behaviour towards the larger group, which he appeared to relish 'holding to ransom'.

It was only when Paul, a popular but quiet member of the group, began to say how frightened he was that John began to realise how he was hurting others. He apologised to Paul for his behaviour and asked the community to feedback when he behaved in this way. It was pointed out to John that if he intimidated others, they would be reluctant to give him any kind of positive support. It was some time before John became able to take feedback without retaliating or walking out. Paul, in his turn, was able to use this as a first step towards asserting himself more effectively.

However, John still felt good about the effects which his intimidating behaviour had upon one section of the TC population, the sex offenders. When this was identified, and challenged, John was resistant to an attitude change. In his small group, an exploration of the origins of these aggressive feelings revealed that he had been sexually abused during a period in care and had strong vengeful feelings about this. Later, John disclosed that he had exchanged crack for sexual 'favours' on the street. This was identified as a form of sexual abuse by the group and he was able to examine his role as a perpetrator in this context.

Leaving

The process of leaving therapy is often a difficult and painful business, particularly when the relationship has, of necessity, been a long one. It can be characterised by relapse and triggering of core issues around rejection and abandonment and the dependence issues of seeking premature independence or fear of independence.

After 12 months in the TC, John was elected as chairman by the community. This position enabled him to develop his skills as a leader. In the early stages of the role, he was dogmatic, particularly if others were unwilling to address issues that he had brought to the group. He gradually learned how to be diplomatic and help others with their problems. He developed a greater sense of putting the group interests over and above personal self-interest. He became particularly good at helping others who had similar problems to those that had brought him onto the unit.

Finally, John felt that it was time to move on. Whilst some staff and community members were reluctant to encourage him in this, he was generally convinced that he wanted to 'test out' his resolve, as a changed person in a less protected environment. After lengthy discussion, it was agreed to go along with this. At this stage, John began to challenge staff again and became preoccupied with the same petty grievances that had distracted him in the early days. John indicated that he had done all his changing and that he did not need to do anymore. Through further group work, John recognised the continuous process of change and that therapy was only a first step in the direction of leading a life that did not involve returning to custody. Cognitive–behavioural groups looking at relapse prevention and thinking skills helped him develop strategies for staying out of prison.

Saying goodbye was painful for John and he tried to avoid the final community meeting where he would have to explore these issues. When he did attend, he was able to verbalise what he had learned from the unit and to listen to what others had to say about their feelings concerning his departure. It was an emotional meeting and John was surprised at the feedback he received, particularly from inmates and staff with whom he had not enjoyed the best of terms.

Evaluation and continued contact

Post-treatment evaluation is useful but can be unreliable. Patients often have a vested interest in presenting themselves as having changed and seeing themselves as 'better'. Psychometric assessment following treatment indicated positive changes in personality problems, self-esteem and general offence-related attitudes. He showed good knowledge of his relapse-prevention strategies, but his motivation remained ambivalent, particularly at times of stress.

Whilst re-conviction studies demonstrate how people fare post-therapy (Cullen 1997), such research does not provide qualitative information about the process of community re-integration. What information is gleaned often comes from ex-patients, or professionals, making contact with treatment staff, sometimes under inauspicious circumstances.

After leaving

Six months after discharge, John telephoned the unit to inform staff that he was coping well. The staff member who took this call, interpreted this as a possible cry for help and, on further exploration, was able to ascertain that he had recently relapsed in terms of his drug use. Close work with the probation officer enabled this to be worked with and a return to offending was avoided. A year later, the probation officer contacted the unit about another referral and informed staff that John was still at liberty, but was struggling to keep things going. He had returned to his partner and son and his probation officer felt that this relationship was playing a significant part in his rehabilitation.

Changes brought about in therapy can be enhanced or undermined, depending on the quality of relationships in a person's social network after release. Negative consequences may be more likely if social contact revolves around offending or substance use. Skills developed in a TC setting can help individuals develop the ability to make active choices about who they form relationships with.

REFERENCES

Cullen E 1997 Can a prison be a therapeutic community: the Grendon Template? In: Cullen E, Jones L, Woodward R (eds) Therapeutic communities for offenders. Wiley Chichester

Dolan B, Coid J 1993 Psychopathic and antisocial personality disorders: treatment and research issues. Gaskell, London

Hare R 1991 The Hare Psychopathy Checklist – revised. Multi-Health Systems, Toronto, Ontario

Hemphill J 1991 Recidivism of criminal psychopaths after therapeutic community treatment. Unpublished Masters thesis, Department of Psychology, University of Saskatchewan, Saskatoon, Canada

Jones L 1997 Developing models for managing treatment, integrity and efficacy in a prison based therapeutic community: the Max Glatt Centre. In: Cullen E, Jones L, Woodward R (eds) Therapeutic communities for offenders. Wiley, Chichester

Stone M 1993 Abnormalities of personality: within and beyond the realm of treatment. Norton, New York

Wexler A 1997 Therapeutic communities in American prisons. In: Cullen E, Jones L, Woodward R (eds) Therapeutic communities for offenders. Wiley, Chichester

CONTENTS

Problem-solving training: pilot work with secure hospital patients

James McGuire

Introduction

The concept of 'problem-solving' is one which can be understood on several levels. In a very general sense, most therapeutic endeavours can be considered as having the aim of helping individuals to solve personal problems. Conceptualised in this way, problem-solving could be viewed as a metaphor for almost any form of therapy and the discourse of many therapeutic approaches, employing such words as 'symptom', 'problem', 'obstacle', 'barrier', 'defence' or 'solution' can be construed as instances of it. On a more concrete level, certain actions of therapists, and some features of interactive styles, are described within both counselling and therapy texts and training courses as 'problem' or 'solution oriented'.

However, as applied in the present case study, problem-solving is used at a yet more specific level. It refers here to a designated set of procedures for development or training of selected skills in an individual, which are held to be of potential benefit in assisting him or her. In what follows, there will first of all be an outline of the background to the use of methods and approaches which have been specially developed for this purpose. Pilot work is reported drawing upon these ideas, carried out by a multi-disciplinary staff group in a secure hospital setting.

Problem-solving and adjustment: background

The proposal that the ability to solve interpersonal problems is an important component of adjustment was first explored systematically by Spivack & Levine (1963). These authors worked initially in residential settings for delinquent youths. In their work, they frequently observed incidents in which young people mishandled a variety of everyday situations. They hypothesised that for some young people an accumulation of personal difficulties could be best understood as arising not because of a lack of intelligence in the conventional sense, nor from deep-seated or enduring features of personality, but rather because they may be a product of an absence of, or failure to apply, certain problem-solving abilities. Such problem-solving 'deficits' appeared especially manifest in the interpersonal domain. For example, individuals might repeatedly deal with difficult social encounters in the same rigid way, despite the fact that a chosen course of action had failed in the past. Rather than construing this as a function of underlying psychic conflict, its explanation might lie instead in a lack of ability to think in a flexible way. Similarly, individuals might find it difficult to conceive of a variety of ways in which a problem could be solved; or neglect to look ahead and anticipate the ramifications of a particular decision or course of action. More drastically, when faced with a problem, they might simply not think at all and instead invest energy in action, possibly making the problem worse. The process of satisfactorily solving problems could thus be analysed or broken down into a series of constituent parts, for each of which there might be a specific activity necessary for effective solution of the problem.

This analysis of components of problem-solving skills is by no means unique. Addressing the same question from within a more formal behaviourist framework, D'Zurilla & Goldfried (1971) arrived at a parallel formulation concerning the analysis of problem-solving skills. In a quite different context, similar ideas have also been put forward by the educationalist Feuerstein (1980).

However, the most systematic presentation of these concepts has been that given by Spivack et al (1976) who reported upon an extensive series of investigations with a variety of age groups and of clinical and behavioural problems. Their

work has encompassed comparisons between individuals with a variety of mental health or other problems and non-clinical populations; identification and analysis of specific skills and skill deficits; development of a number of psychometric tools for assessment of levels of such skills; and assembly and testing of a series of training procedures for remediation or enhancement of the skills identified. Collectively, these authors designated the skills as forming a group which were called *interpersonal cognitive problem-solving skills* (ICPS). They further contended that these skills are separate from those assessed by the standard range of 'IQ' or allied psychological tests; and that skills in the interpersonal domain are distinct from those employed in the solving of 'impersonal' problems (e.g. of an arithmetical or mechanical nature) which are associated with manipulation of 'objects'.

It is now well established that a series of quite diverse cognitive operations is involved in solving problems. This means more than the application of formal logical reasoning and cognitive scientists have confirmed that numerous types of thinking are deployed. These include processes of induction, generating ideas, analogical and metaphorical reasoning, deduction and hypothesis-testing (Galotti 1994). This applies even in the solution of problems in the 'impersonal' domain (i.e. connected to manipulation of objects or abstract ideas, as in mathematical, mechanical or practical problem-solving). In the 'interpersonal' domain focused upon interaction with others, and in development and maintenance of relationships, it is likely that an even wider range of operations is required. There are of course, similarities and overlaps and no clear dividing line can be defined between the two.

Research on social problem-solving skills

These hypotheses have been empirically tested in a series of group-comparison studies between psychiatric patient samples and non-patient control samples. In each case, significant differences were discovered between groups in their possession or exercise of component problem-solving skills (Platt & Spivack 1972a,b, Platt et al 1975). Related studies have revealed problem-solving skills deficiencies amongst other groups including adolescent heroin users (Platt et al 1973), adult opiate abusers (Appel & Kaestner 1979), adult prison inmates (Higgins & Thies 1981) and suicidal psychiatric patients (Schotte & Clum 1987).

In the formal model of ICPS put forward by Spivack et al (1976), it was held that failure to acquire or to utilise such skills might lead to failures of adjustment, which if cumulative or enduring might be associated with the emergence of more serious behavioural or mental health syndromes. The underlying skills deficits might occur for a variety of reasons, including the parenting and child-rearing styles to which individuals had been exposed. Some of the latter were found to promote the growth of such skills more effectively than others (Shure & Spivack 1978).

From the standpoint of clinical practice, there is an invaluable corollary to the foregoing set of findings. This is the proposal that it should be feasible to provide therapy or training which by imparting such skills to individuals will enable them to become more effective problem-solvers in everyday life. This has led to efforts to devise methods and exercises which will enable individuals to acquire and develop such skills. More than 30 years ago, Spohn & Wolk (1963) reported a study of in-patients diagnosed as schizophrenic and showing marked withdrawal symptoms. Their work showed that group-based training sessions in which patients jointly worked on 'impersonal' problems reduced their levels of social withdrawal and improved their rates of social contact.

Several later studies reported on the usage of ICPS or similar skills-training exercises with psychiatric patients or clients with learning disabilities. Studies of this kind, reporting positive and encouraging results with in-patient groups, have been conducted by Coché & Flick (1975) and by Edelstein et al (1980). Hansen et al (1985) demonstrated the possible application of the methods as a component of psychiatric after-care following hospitalisation. Employing similar methods, Intagliata (1978) showed that improvements

could be secured in the problem-solving and interactive skills of chronic problem drinkers, while Chaney et al (1978) obtained reductions in alcohol consumption at 1-year follow-up amongst problem drinkers who had participated in an integrated, problem-solving, social skills training programme. More recently, Loumidis & Hill (1997) have described the usage of a problem-solving training package for adults with learning disabilities and obtained significant changes in a number of target problem-solving measures.

Working with offenders in a residential setting intermediate between prison and the community, Platt et al (1980) developed a programme which combined problem-solving training with a focus on a specific style of running a group. This utilised a process called *Guided Group Interaction* with a number of special features: the leader played a highly active role; there was an emphasis on the group and its joint development; a supportive atmosphere was to be created; members were seen as agents of change for others; there was a focus on overt behaviour and on the learning of communication and problem-solving skills in a designated, pre-arranged sequence.

The results of this experiment were very promising. After discharge, at the end of a 2-year follow-up period, those who had been on the programme were significantly better adjusted, as indicated by parole reports and other information. Members of the experimental group had a significantly lower total re-arrest rate (49% as against 66%) and a lower rate of re-commitment to institutions, than the controls; and if arrested, this was likely to be after a significantly longer arrest-free period (238 as compared with 168 days).

Early intervention research has been reviewed in detail by D'Zurilla & Nezu (1982) and by D'Zurilla (1988). Detailed guidelines for construction of sessions and for individual work are given by Bedell & Michael (1985). Coché (1987) has provided guidelines for the application of the methods in practice and reviewed evidence for the usefulness of the approach as '... a valuable short-term group-therapy adjunct to the treatment regimen applied in a hospital setting' (Coché 1987: 101). Platt et al (1988) outlined the ingredients of a combined problem-solving and communication skills programme and forwarded some evaluative evidence.

The question may be raised as to the suitability of interventions of this type with mentally disordered offenders resident in secure hospital settings. The client groups for whom this approach has been employed to date have included psychiatric patients with severe and enduring problems, individuals with long-term alcohol problems and people with learning disabilities. The work to be described here tested the feasibility of using these methods in a secure hospital setting.

Setting and participants

Ashworth Hospital is one of three specially designated, high-security psychiatric hospitals (generally known as the 'Special Hospitals') which receives patients sectioned under the Mental Health Act 1983 in England and Wales. The majority of such patients have committed serious antisocial acts, usually criminal offences including homicide, rape or sexual assaults, other types of personal violence, arson or other serious criminal damage. The majority of patients, approximately 70%, are classified as 'mentally ill' in terms of the Mental Health Act and most are diagnosed as suffering from schizophrenia or other psychotic disorders. The second largest group is classed as suffering from 'psychopathic disorder' (a legal classification, the definition of which remains controversial, roughly contiguous with a psychiatric diagnosis of antisocial personality disorder). A range of other clinical problems including attempted suicide, self-harm and substance abuse is frequently recorded amongst such patients. As patients are sectioned under mental health law, they are not always formally diagnosed in terms of DSM or ICD systems. A smaller proportion are classed as suffering from 'mental impairment' and a few of these patients are admitted to secure hospital under 'civil sections' (authorised by medical staff) as a result of acts of violence or unmanageable behaviour in other residential institutions. As a result of continuing changes in health policies and practices, the proportion of patients admitted under this category has been steadily declining in recent years. Some of the issues facing these hospitals have been summarised by Bingley (1993).

The location for this group was the hospital's Rehabilitation Centre which was a day unit designed for the provision of a range of therapeutic and skills-training activities. These ranged from training sessions conducted individually with patients, designed for assessment or training of 'daily living' and 'survival' skills, to group-based programmes of alcohol and drugs education, social skills training, anger management and empathy training.

Group format and structure

In addition to this 'portfolio' of training and therapy programmes, the possibility was explored that the problem-solving methods could be applied with benefit with mentally disordered offender-patients. A multi-disciplinary professional group was formed as a result of a joint initiative involving psychology, nursing and education staff, with a view to planning and testing the feasibility of a patient training group in social problem-solving.

The programme of activity, when finally assembled, comprised 12 2-hour sessions planned in the following sequence:

Session 1   Introduction
Aims of the course, discussion of the nature of problems, self-assessment of experienced problems.
Session 2   Defining problems I
Knowing when you or another person has a problem; analysing problems into more manageable parts.
Session 3   Defining problems II
Clear versus fuzzy thinking; re-formulating problems in terms of personal goals and objectives.
Session 4   Gathering information
How to identify and collect the information needed to solve a problem.

Session 5   Distinguishing facts from opinions
Evaluating the usefulness of different types of information that might be used in problem-solving.

Session 6   Generating alternative solutions
Producing ideas, use of brainstorming and other methods of listing potential solutions to problems.

Session 7   Means–End thinking
Visualising the steps involved in following a problem through to its solution and recognising obstacles en route.

Session 8   Consequential thinking
Exercises focused on the effects of actions and how to anticipate outcomes and impact on others.

Session 9   Decision-making I
Choosing between different options; assessing advantages and disadvantages of separate courses of action.

Session 10   Decision-making II
Setting personal objectives for the future and analysing them into achievable steps.

Session 11   Perspective-taking
Learning to appreciate a situation from another person's viewpoint; use of role play and role-rotation techniques.

Session 12   Overview and evaluation
Review of areas covered, group members' feedback, discussion of outcomes and future goals.

Sessions occurred weekly and each lasted approximately 2 hours. The sessions were carefully planned in advance and consisted of a series of practical, focused exercises, involving an active and participatory group-learning approach. Brief outlines of the tasks were presented and discussion and review held afterwards. Sessions were designed so that there was a variety of activity, with some individual work, some work in pairs or trios and some in the 'plenary' group. The end-products of the group's work, such as material recorded on flip-chart sheets or copyboard, were displayed on the wall for reference during sessions.

Seven male patients participated in the pilot group. Their mean age was 24.95 years with a range between 22 and 28 years. They were selected at random from a series of 14 applicants for the training (by the simple procedure of placing pieces of paper with each patient's name in a box, and picking out seven names). The remaining seven patients were placed on a waiting-list. The participants were drawn from three separate residential ward areas within the hospital.

All patients taking part were classified under the Mental Health Act 1983 as suffering from psychopathic disorder, '… a permanent disorder or disability of mind … leading to seriously abnormal or aggressive conduct'. This definition is used in a legal sense and is not identical with any single psychiatric diagnostic category. Formal diagnoses were not recorded for most patients, though it is likely most would meet the criteria for inclusion under the category of personality disorders in the DSM system. Their offences included murder, manslaughter, arson, rape, grievous bodily harm and indecent assault. The mean length of time since their admission to Ashworth Hospital was 3.98 years with a range from 3 to over 7 years. Some members of the group had a history of self-harm.

Evaluation

It was planned that there should be a process of evaluation for the group programme, of a fairly elaborate kind. This included the following elements:

- Pre- and post-test assessment and evaluation of change in problem-solving skills by means of specially constructed psychometric tests
- Usage of structured feedback from ward-based staff concerning patients' behaviour and problem-solving skill competencies
- Feedback from participants concerning their experiences of the group, their reactions to it and evaluations of it.

Under the first item, the following measures were employed:

Alternative Thinking Test (Spivack & Platt 1980). A task in which individuals are presented with a series of everyday problems and asked to generate possible solutions to them; the score is the number of distinct solutions produced.

Means–End Problem-Solving (Spivack & Platt 1980). In this procedure, individuals are presented with the beginning and the end of a story, and asked to make up the middle; resultant stories are scored according to the number of steps itemised and obstacles recognised along the way.

Matching Familiar Figures Test (Kagan 1975). This entails presenting individuals with a figure which is shown to them for a short period. They are then asked to find it in an array of eight similar figures. They are scored according to their speed of response (latency) and number of errors made before identifying the correct figure; the test is considered to be a measure of 'cognitive impulsivity'.

Locus of Control Scale (Levenson 1973). This is a self-rating scale to assess the extent to which individuals perceive themselves as being in command of their own lives or alternatively being at the mercy of external forces such as powerful others or of chance events.

In addition to these pre-existing measures, two forms were devised. The first was for obtaining ward-based staff nurse ratings of patients' behaviour on a series of 14 five-point scales, focused on evidence of impulsiveness or of reflection and deliberation in interaction with others. The second was for eliciting feedback from group participants themselves and included a number of five-point rating scales concerning levels of enjoyment, satisfaction with the group and estimation of its usefulness to them in the short and longer term. These were supplemented by several open-ended questions asking patients to list what if anything they had liked about the group experience, what they had disliked and to make suggestions for possible improvements.

Outcomes

Attendance at the group sessions was not consistent, with some sessions missed by patients as a result of difficulties within their ward settings or transport problems within the hospital site. However, it was established by contact with patients that no sessions were missed as a result of group members being unwilling to attend.

One consequence of missed sessions was that pre- and post-test data could not be collected on all measures for all patients. Amongst the data which was obtained there were, however, no significant changes in average score for the group between pre- and post-test on any of the cognitive measures.

Verbal and written feedback from patients themselves by contrast was highly positive. There were many positive comments and ratings showing that group members had enjoyed the sessions, found them useful and wanted to extend the duration of the group. Unfortunately, the number of ward feedback forms returned was insufficient to allow any conclusions to be drawn regarding the effects, if perceptible, of group participation.

In running this group, those involved had the advantages of availability of several potential group leaders and adequate resources for the delivery of the programme itself. This initiative was, however, beset with a number of problems which were primarily organisational in nature. A departure of this kind requires the support of many levels of staff and a shared commitment to a therapeutically-orientated regime; whether this existed in the hospital at that time can be seriously questioned. On a practical level, there also needs to be an adequate flow of referrals in order that appropriate selection and allocation can be made. There is a need for training of other staff and their co-operation to ensure support and continuity of the training/therapy process in other situations. There was no opportunity for this framework to be established in the hospital at that time.

Following completion of this group which was considered relatively valuable by all involved, a second group was run. This, however, proved extremely difficult owing not only to the organisational pressures alluded to above, but also as a result of the selection and mixture of patients. Whilst groups can be run with a small proportion of unsuitable or unwilling referrals, the numbers of each in this case were too large and the combination of personal problems was such that the group became virtually unmanageable.

Despite the limited quantity of positive evaluative information concerning this group, I nevertheless consider the work to have been an example of good practice in a secure mental health setting. The patient participants were enthusiastic about taking part, gave positive feedback and an impression of having genuinely focused on issues and problems of concern to them. With some sessions being cancelled and the learning sequence interrupted thereby, it was difficult to achieve any sustained learning and skill acquisition. Such changes were also not supported across other settings or through consistent efforts on the part of all those involved in patient care. In this light, the absence of observable change in the pre-to-post measures does not seem especially surprising.

Integrated multi-modal programmes containing problem-solving elements

A second reason for expressing more confidence about the methods used than would seem warranted from this pilot work is that the methods form part of effective programmes which have now been used extensively in offender services in a variety of criminal justice settings. Within recent years, problem-solving components isolated within research on ICPS have been incorporated in several 'multi-modal' programmes. To borrow a medical metaphor, the term 'multi-modal' refers to the finding that services which combine a range of educational, therapeutic or training activities yield larger effect sizes in reduction of recidivism than do others which contain a single 'active ingredient' only. Probably the best-known programme of this type for adults is *Reasoning and Rehabilitation* (R&R) which was developed on the basis of research indicating differences between persistent offenders and other groups in a number of problem-solving skills (Ross & Fabiano 1985). This programme, which consists of 35 2-hour sessions, was first extensively site-tested within Canadian correctional services and subsequently in the USA, but is also currently in use in a number of countries outside North America (Ross & Ross 1995). Evaluations of the use of this programme with adult offenders in probation settings (Ross et al 1988) and in prisons (Robinson 1995) have given evidence of its effectiveness, especially in relation to reduction in rates of violent and sexual offending. In work with juvenile offenders, the use of social problem-solving training has been explicitly recommended for inclusion in a 'multi-systemic' approach, for which there is now mounting evidence of outcome effectiveness (Henggeler et al 1998).

Large-scale research reviews have indicated that such multi-modal cognitive–behavioural programmes have achieved the most consistent success in reducing rates of criminal recidivism (Harland 1996, McGuire 1995, Ross et al 1995). At the time of writing, the findings of that research are leading to a steady expansion of interest in the use of programmes along these lines, and in some instances to an investment in staff training and organisational change to allow delivery of such work in penal settings. The introduction by HM Prison Service in 1996 of a *Key Performance Indicator* (KPI-7) linked to the provision of programmes designed to reduce recidivism has been a notable innovation in this respect. Conjoined with this the prison service has also devised and published a set of *Accreditation Criteria* for judging the acceptability and monitoring of the delivery of such programmes (HM Prison Service 1998). Probation services are currently being encouraged by their inspectorate to follow a similar direction (Underdown 1998).

Conclusion

The problem-solving sessions described in this case study have been assimilated into a multi-modal programme in which offence behaviour is itself included as a problem alongside others identified by participants. The programme *Problem-Solving Training and Offence Behaviour* (McGuire 1996) exists in separate versions for prison and probation contexts and has been accredited by HM Prison Service under KPI-7 and also nominated as a *Pathfinder* project by HM Probation Inspectorate.

Interventions which make use of problem-solving-training ingredients are thus now playing a significant part in services provided for high-risk offenders both in prison establishments and in the community. There has not, regrettably, been a corresponding growth of interest in such activities within forensic mental health services. It has been pointed out that in follow-up studies of discharged secure hospital patients, the most commonly favoured dependent variable is criminal recidivism (Eastman 1993). However, when research findings on the follow-up of mentally disordered offenders are reviewed, it is rarely possible even to identify 'treatment' as an independent variable (McGuire 1998). It must be hoped that these circumstances will alter such that the coming years may yield a number of treatment–outcome studies from secure hospital settings.

Acknowledgements

I wish to thank a number of colleagues who contributed to the development and running of the pilot problem-solving training groups described in this chapter: Ann Baldwin, Kathy Chapman, Hazel Chipchase, Stuart Guy, Howard Jackson, Helen Liebling, Aisling O'Kane and Celia Vishnick.

REFERENCES

Appel P, Kaestner E 1979 Interpersonal and emotional problem solving among narcotic drug abusers. Journal of Consulting and Clinical Psychology 47: 1125–1127

Bedell J, Michael D 1985 Teaching problem-solving skills to chronic psychiatric patients. In: Upper D, Ross S (eds) Handbook of behavioral group therapy. Plenum Press, New York

Bingley W 1993 Broadmoor, Rampton and Ashworth: Can good practice prevent potential future disasters in high-security hospitals? Criminal Behaviour and Mental Health 3: 465–471

Chaney E, O'Leary M, Marlatt G 1978 Skill training with alcoholics. Journal of Consulting and Clinical Psychology 46: 1092–1104

Coché E 1987 Problem-solving training: a cognitive group therapy modality. In: Freeman A, Greenwood V (eds) Cognitive therapy: applications in psychiatric and medical settings. Human Sciences Press, New York

Coché E, Flick A 1975 Problem-solving training groups for hospitalised psychiatric patients. Journal of Psychology 91: 19–29

D'Zurilla T 1988 Problem-solving therapies. In: Dobson K (ed) Handbook of cognitive behavioral therapies. Guilford Press, New York

D'Zurilla T, Goldfried M 1971 Problem-solving and behavior modification. Journal of Abnormal Psychology 78: 104–126

D'Zurilla T, Nezu A 1982 Social problem solving in adults. Advances in Cognitive–Behavioral Research and Therapy 1: 201–274

Eastman N 1993 Forensic psychiatric services in Britain. International Journal of Law and Psychiatry 16: 1–26

Edelstein B, Couture E, Cray M, Dickens P, Lusebrink N 1980 Group training of problem-solving with psychiatric patients. In: Upper D, Ross S (eds) Behavioral group therapy: an annual review. Research Press, Champaign, Illinois, p 85–102

Feuerstein R 1980 Instrumental enrichment. UPP, Baltimore

Galotti K 1994 Cognitive psychology in and out of the laboratory. Brooks-Cole, Pacific Grove, California

Hansen D, St Lawrence J, Christoff K 1985 Effects of interpersonal problem-solving training with chronic aftercare patients on problem-solving component skills and effectiveness of solutions. Journal of Consulting and Clinical Psychology 53: 167–174

Harland A (ed) 1996 Choosing correctional options that work: defining the demand and evaluating the supply. Sage, Thousand Oaks

Henggeler S, Schoenwald S, Borduin C, Rowland M, Cunningham P 1998 Multisystemic treatment of antisocial behavior in children and adolescents. Guilford Press, New York

Higgins J, Thies A 1981 Social effectiveness and problem-solving thinking of reformatory inmates. Journal of Offender Counseling, Services and Rehabilitation 5: 93–98

HM Prison Service 1998 Criteria for accreditation of programmes 1998/99. Offending Behaviour Programmes Unit, London

Intagliata J 1978 Increasing the interpersonal problem-solving skills of an alcoholic population. Journal of Consulting and Clinical Psychology 46: 489–498

Kagan J 1975 Manual for the matching familiar figures test. Department of Psychology, Harvard University

Levenson H 1973 Multidimensional locus of control in psychiatric patients. Journal of Consulting and Clinical Psychology 41: 397–404

Loumidis K, Hill A 1997 Social problem-solving groups for adults with learning disabilities. In: Stenfert Kroese B, Dagnan D, Loumidis K (eds) Cognitive–behaviour therapy for people with learning disabilities. Routledge, London

McGuire J (ed) 1995 What works: reducing re-offending: guidelines from research and practice. Wiley, Chichester

McGuire J 1996 Problem-solving training and offence behaviour. (Programme manuals, user guide and supplements.) Unpublished. Department of Clinical Psychology, University of Liverpool

McGuire J 1998 Follow-up of mentally disordered offenders: implications for future research and service provision.

Paper presented at the XXIII International Congress on Law and Mental Health, University René Déscartes, Paris

Platt J, Spivack G 1972a Problem-solving thinking of psychiatric patients. Journal of Consulting and Clinical Psychology 39: 148–151

Platt J, Spivack G 1972b Social competence and effective problem-solving thinking in psychiatric patients. Journal of Clinical Psychology 28: 3–5

Platt J, Scura W, Hannon J 1973 Problem-solving thinking of youthful incarcerated heroin addicts. Journal of Community Psychology 1: 278–291

Platt J, Siegel J, Spivack G 1975 Do psychiatric patients and normals see the same solutions as effective in solving interpersonal problems? Journal of Consulting and Clinical Psychology 43: 279

Platt J, Perry G, Metzger D 1980 The evaluation of a heroin addiction treatment program within a correctional environment. In: Gendreau P, Ross R (eds) Effective correctional treatment. Butterworth, Toronto

Platt J, Taube D, Metzger D, Duome M 1988 Training in interpersonal problem solving (TIPS). Journal of Cognitive Psychotherapy 2: 5–34

Robinson D 1995 The impact of cognitive skills training on post-release recidivism among Canadian federal offenders. Correctional Services of Canada, Ottawa

Ross R, Fabiano E 1985 Time to think: a cognitive model of delinquency prevention and offender rehabilitation. Air Training and Publications, Ottawa

Ross R, Ross R (eds) 1995 Thinking straight: the reasoning and rehabilitation program for delinquency prevention and offender rehabilitation. Air Training and Publications, Ottawa

Ross R, Fabiano E, Ewles C 1988 Reasoning and rehabilitation. International Journal of Offender Therapy and Comparative Criminology 20: 165–173

Ross R, Antanowicz D, Dhaliwal G (eds) 1995 Going straight: effective delinquency prevention and offender rehabilitation. Air Training and Publications, Ottawa

Schotte D, Clum G 1987 Problem-solving skills in suicidal psychiatric patients. Journal of Consulting and Clinical Psychology 55: 49–54

Shure M, Spivack G 1978 Problem-solving techniques in childrearing. Jossey-Bass, San Francisco

Spivack G, Levine M 1963 Self-regulation in acting-out and normal adolescents. Report No. M-4531. National Institute of Health, Washington DC

Spivack G, Platt J 1980 Measures of social problem-solving for adolescents and adults: manual. Preventive Intervention Research Center, Hahnemann University, Philadelphia

Spivack G, Platt J, Shure M 1976 The problem-solving approach to adjustment. Jossey-Bass, San Francisco

Spohn H, Wolk W 1963 Effect of group problem solving experience upon social withdrawal in chronic schizophrenics. Journal of Abnormal and Social Psychology 66: 187–190

Underdown A 1998 Strategies for effective offender supervision: report of the HMIP what works project. Home Office, London

CONTENTS

Relating neurological and neuropsychological deficits to antisocial personality and offending behaviour

Howard Jackson and Joseph Martin III

Historical beginnings

Perhaps the most interesting historical example of the relationship between acquired brain injury and offending behaviour is that of James Hadfield. Despite pre-dating the more famous and widely cited case of Phineas Gage, the case of James Hadfield has gone largely uncited in neuropsychological literature. Prior to his injuries, Hadfield had been a silversmith and family man of good repute. He joined the King's footsoldiers and fought at the Battle of Fraymar in 1793 where he received sword wounds to his head. So severe were his injuries that he was left for dead on the battlefield. However, he survived and little was heard of him thereafter, although reports indicate that he 'fell in with a bad lot', until he made an attempt on George III's life with a pistol aimed at the King in Drury Lane Theatre. He was admitted to Bethlam Royal Hospital where he killed a fellow patient. Not only does Hadfield provide an excellent example of the potential relationship between head injury and antisocial behaviour, but he was also the catalyst for the development of special provision in England for mentally abnormal offenders. He eventually died from tuberculosis in 1841 whilst resident in Broadmoor Special Hospital. Post-mortem examination revealed two frontal lesions 'the size of hen's eggs'.

Although this and other cases point to the usefulness of examining the direct effects of brain injury/pathology and subsequent neuropsychological dysfunction on personality and emotional behaviour, it may also be prudent to consider the brain function of individuals with disorders of personality. One may suspect that there would be some fundamental differences in the processes involved between those who suffered personality change because of a brain injury and those who suffer from personality disorder because of experiential or genetic causes. However, any similarities found are likely to be of considerable interest to an overall understanding of personality and emotional disorder in neuropsychological terms.

At a phenomenological level, there are considerable similarities between the symptoms of psychopathy and the personality disorders seen in many traumatically brain-injured survivors. Impulsiveness, shallow processing of emotions, low tolerance for frustration, egocentricity, lack of self-insight, an apparent absence of anxiety, apathy/loss of interest, perseveration, difficulties in learning from experience and predisposition to immediate gratification are all characteristics which have been associated with psychopathic personality disorder (Cleckley 1976, Millon 1981, Vaillant 1975) which have also been observed in personality-disordered, traumatically brain-injured victims.

Biological perspectives

There is a longstanding literature regarding the relationship between neurological dysfunction (EEG and brain-imaging abnormalities and temporal lobe epilepsy (TLE)) and aggressive/violent behaviours. Associations between EEG abnormalities and habitual aggressors were stressed in early works by Hill & Watterson (1942) and Jenkins & Pacella (1943). Krynicki (1978) reported that paroxysmal activity, particularly in the frontal lobes, appeared to be the most important EEG feature related to assaultative offending adolescents. Interesting findings have also been produced in the brain imaging of repetitively violent offenders, demonstrating, albeit in a small sample of four, blood flow and metabolic abnormalities in the left temporal lobe (Volkow & Tancredi 1987). Two of the four patients also showed abnormalities within the frontal cortex. Examining the relationship

through individuals with known head injuries, Hill & Watterson (1942) concluded that head injury contributed little to habitually aggressive behaviour. Other reports, however, (Fromm-Auch et al 1980, Yeudall 1978) cite a high incidence of head injury in juvenile delinquents.

Woods & Eames (1981) have argued for both epileptic and learning components to aggressive behaviour in which the combined treatment with anticonvulsants and behaviour modification procedures prove effective where either one alone is insufficient. Abnormal EEG recordings do not necessarily indicate seizure activity but may represent dysfunctioning areas of the brain and a longstanding question is whether the abnormal EEG recording indicates the effects of cerebral dysfunction or the direct impact of epileptoid discharges.

The relationship between TLE and aggressive behaviour is now firmly established (Monroe 1986) and numerous studies have found links between TLE and aggression, violence and psychopathy (Betts et al 1976, Delgado-Escueta et al 1981, Ferguson et al 1986, Hermann et al 1980, Jackson et al 1987). The research, however, into the connections between neural substrates and aggression and violence has been equivocal, with some critics finding no evidence for the relationship in their studies (Rodin 1973, Small et al 1962, 1966). Other studies have noted that aggression occurs in only a sub-set of those with TLE (Ounstead et al 1987), with higher probabilities occurring with psychiatric disorders, early age of onset and low IQ. These findings have supported previous studies relating aggressive behaviour to early onset (James 1960).

The research undertaken in the relationship between TLE and aggression points to several conclusions. First, there are no specific neural structures that can be unequivocally identified as the cause of aggression in TLE. It is perhaps more appropriate to consider specific neural sites, such as the hypothalamus and amygdala, as part of a larger information-processing system rather than attempting to assign emotion-functions to the sites. Second, violence associated with temporal lobe disorders may be seen as an artefact of a more general dyscontrol than as an emotional outburst, such that the dyscontrol is reflected in the individual's current state, behavioural dispositions and situational circumstances. The more general concept of episodic dyscontrol (which may include many different aetiologies than TLE) allows for inclusion of many other often complex actions in which the circumstances play an important role. Indeed, it has been reported that individual patients with seizure-related dyscontrol will exhibit a whole variety of dyscontrol acts (Monroe 1986). Finally, the early onset of TLE and its relationship to violence may suggest that other inhibiting factors, socialisation or more sophisticated coping strategies may serve to mitigate against the emergence of interpersonal violence.

Of course, the additional cognitive and psychosocial problems associated with severe acquired brain injury may restrict compensatory mechanisms and further induce the emotional states and situational circumstances which would lead to a disinhibition and provocation of episodic, seizure-related violence in cases where TLE is also a sequelae of the injury, thereby mimicking the effects of early onset. If the dyscontrol provoked by TLE is dependent upon the individual's socio-cognitive processing abilities or tendencies, then both socio-cognitive development and disturbed informational processing brought about by traumatic brain injury are likely to be important variables. Although this hypothesis remains to be tested, Matthews et al (1977) reported that emotional disturbances as measured by MMPI were more related to cognitive impairment and psychometric variables than to age of onset.

The situational and state-dependent responses to temporal lobe activity also lead to a potential confusion between premeditated violent acts and unpremeditated or autonomic acts often seen in violent offenders with TLE. The result is often the misdiagnosis of the disorder and inappropriate treatment. Furthermore, the complex interaction between localisation of epileptic activity, pre-morbid characteristics and development, situational circumstances and cognitive ability may also account for the number of

negative findings between aggressive propensities and TLE (Rodin 1973, Small et al 1966). Again, we are led to conclude the neural factors are neither necessary nor sufficient to promote aggressive personality and the underlying determinants of epileptic-related aggression are likely to be socio-cognitive in nature.

Neuropsychological dysfunction and information-processing deficits

The hypothesis that dysfunction of the left hemisphere (Flor-Henry 1976), the right hemisphere (Yeudall et al 1982) and the frontal lobes (Gorenstein 1982) are particularly involved in some forms of psychopathic personality disorder and also in some severe and repetitive delinquents raises the question of the functional relationship between organic dysfunction, information-processing deficit and antisocial personality disorder. There are a number of possible relationships which together may impose upon the sufferer a view of the world and self such that psychopathic personality disorder and/or offending behaviour would be likely to result.

Bias towards negative affective reactions

Perhaps the most simple hypothesis of the functional relationship between left-hemisphere impairment and psychopathic personality is in the suggestion that the right hemisphere is involved with 'lower', involuntary and subconscious forms of organisation of mental activity whereas the left hemisphere provides higher order organisation functions (Luria & Simernitskaya 1975). This interpretation would suggest that a left-hemisphere-injured patient would necessarily be operating at a more 'primitive' social level without the social concepts necessary to inhibit antisocial behaviour or maintain moral standards.

Zenkov (1976) has suggested that a dominant lobe dysfunction effectively renders a situation as being difficult to verbalise or to understand. This impoverished analysis may lead to the sufferer perceiving the world as frightening, unpleasant and emotionally negative. Given a tendency towards perceiving the world negatively, it is easy to hypothesise that a dominant-hemisphere dysfunction may result in a number of defensive strategies based on self-preservation, including social withdrawal (and hence impoverished social skills and social perception), impulsive aggression, over-responsiveness to criticism, reduced ability to respond to positive social reinforcement and problems of self-esteem.

This perceptual problem is exaggerated further if one considers the left hemisphere to be biased towards the processing of positive emotions (Gainotti 1969). Clearly, a disruption of the ability to attend to the positive affective components of the environment may further exaggerate a bias towards a negative and frightening perspective of the world and thus, antisocial or aggressive behaviour.

Verbal regulation

A rather simplistic interpretation of the relative deficiencies in verbal intellectual functioning is that social behaviour is regulated by verbal means. Thus, a relative deficit in verbal information processes may result in a tendency to respond more impulsively (Flor-Henry 1976). In line with the philosopher Vitgosky (1962), Joseph (1982) considered thinking as the left-hemisphere internalisation of language. This internal language structure allows for the use of complex symbols and concepts, self-evaluation and self-regulation. Cleckley (1976) has argued that psychopaths present with a dissociation between language and emotion such that they have difficulty verbalising their own feelings to the extent that he proposed that the term 'psychopathy' should be replaced by the term 'semantic dementia'. Meichenbaum (1975) stressed the importance of verbal mediation to the development of self-control. Similarly, Camp (1977) concluded that both learning and behaviour problems in aggressive boys may be the result of ineffective linguistic control systems. Luria (1980) reported evidence based on his study of patients with mediobasal lesions that these regions of the frontal lobe operate higher forms of regulation

through associations with the language centres. Such verbal regulation offers the subject more stable and complex levels of voluntary attention which over-ride immediate demands. A disruption in frontal lobe functioning associated with such verbal regulation is likely to severely impair 'the intimate relationship between verbal behaviour and socially relevant aspects of social attention' (Miller 1987:133).

There is an obvious disagreement between the relative importance to offending behaviour, with some researchers advocating left-hemisphere dysfunction (e.g. Flor-Henry 1976) and some advocating right-hemisphere dysfunction (Yeudall et al 1982). It is possible that both forms of dysfunction will provoke violent or antisocial behaviour. The left hemisphere may provide a form of verbal regulation in the control of behaviour, evaluating consequences and relating future behaviour to moral rules of conduct. Several investigators (Day 1977, Hines 1976) have pointed to the advantage of the left hemisphere in processing abstract words. In contrast, Semmes (1968) argues that the right hemisphere processes information more diffusely, in a holistic manner, and is able to accommodate only concrete verbal information. Similarly, Myslobodsky & Rattok (1977) suggested that the right hemisphere reacts to impeding stimulation in an undifferentiated way and is therefore suitable for mediating the emotion-laden fight or flight response. Under conditions of threat, a dysfunctioning right hemisphere may provoke an over-reaction to the affective components of the 'threat', thereby initiating an impulsive and extreme reaction. Equally, a dysfunctioning left hemisphere may result in a failure to inhibit the impulsive violent response, may misjudge the moral course of action or the potential consequences of that action or misinterpret the 'threat' in a concrete, simplistic manner.

Prediction and planning

Siminov (1986) has pointed out that the right hemisphere (especially the frontal and temporal lobes) is particularly involved in the initiation of 'goal formation'. In this sense, the non-dominant hemisphere initiates and generates needs which the individual wishes to fulfil. In contrast, the dominant hemisphere plays a more significant role in objectivising the need. In this sense, the left hemisphere provides the means by which to satisfy the need. An individual who suffers from a dominant-hemisphere dysfunction, then, is in the unfortunate position of experiencing many needs but with little ability to satisfy them (or perhaps even define what the needs are). Under these circumstances, it is understandable that behaviour may be non-directive, agitated, impulsive and aggressive in response to the frustration derived from an ill-defined and unmet sense of need.

Another potential functional relationship between an impairment of the left hemisphere and psychopathic personality disorder is the involvement of the left hemisphere in the formation of abstract concepts which are not temporally bound. In contrast, damage to the right hemisphere results in disruption to the perception of time and space. Siminov (1986) suggested that the right hemisphere is connected with the past and the present whereas the left hemisphere is concerned with the future. It is possible that psychopaths with a left-hemisphere dysfunction suffer from considerable difficulty with 'what if' predictions of likely consequences and as a result are 'stimulus bound' to the immediate environment. Ross & Fabiano (1985) have pointed out that many repetitive offenders suffer from highly concrete thinking and exhibit particular difficulty making predictions concerning the likely outcome of their actions. When the ability to hypothesise and analyse future events is impaired, the individual is 'trapped' in the here and now. Over-dependence on here and now circumstances may well lead to extreme emotional and behavioural responses because of a relative paucity of perspective and context within which events can be cognitively framed.

More support for an 'organic-like' cognitive dysfunction in psychopaths without a medical history of organic injury has come from the work of Birkett (1988). He found that they performed as poorly as brain-injured psychopaths and brain-injured non-psychopaths on both the

Benton Verbal Fluency test (BVF) (a 'left frontal lobe' test of word generation) and the Digit Span sub-test of the Wechsler Adult Intelligence Scale. Problems in the generation of alternatives may be explicitly and directly involved in the processes leading to poor, social, problem-solving abilities and impulsive behaviour. The performance of at least some psychopathic patients on the BVF may suggest that many psychopathic personality types have considerable difficulty generating possible alternative courses of action and thereby appear to respond impulsively.

Equally, the impaired performance of some offenders on a test of alternating attention such as the Trail Making Test (B) and on the Wisconsin Card Sort Test (Berman & Seigal 1976) suggests that cognitively-impaired offenders have difficulties of perseveration which is unresponsive to feedback. To some degree, this may account for the often cited characteristic of psychopaths in that they fail to learn from experience. In addition, such cognitive rigidity may have particularly profound effects on social problem-solving in that it inhibits the generation of alternative solutions or courses of actions.

Judgement

An interesting finding by Buchtel et al (1976) suggested that the right hemisphere surpassed the left hemisphere on a classification task where the stimuli to be classified were unequivocal. However, the left hemisphere was more effective under circumstances where the stimuli were ambivalent. Thus, the dominance of the left hemisphere in conflicting situations permits a greater tolerance of ambiguity. When this function is impaired, it is likely that extreme judgements will result in ambiguous or complex situations, confirmed in our own studies (Jackson et al 1987). On a questionnaire requiring a true or false reply to items testing 'moral anxiety', it was found that significantly more psychopathic offenders reported at the extremes (either very morally anxious or very unanxious) than normals whose rating hovered round the combined group mean. Similarly, Thomas-Peter (1988) reported that psychopathic offenders provided extreme responses on a sliding scale compared to matched non-offender controls. At a clinical level, it is noticeable that many psychopaths and severely brain-injured patients have considerable difficulty tolerating uncertainty and ambiguity such that their social and moral judgements appear absolute.

This type of 'bipolar' thinking may have several major effects. It results in either feelings of persecution or demands for punishment, since individuals will make an absolute judgement about personal innocence or guilt. Such judgements are likely to provoke 'absolute' responses that are impulsive, disinhibited and extreme. Consider the situation where an individual with a dominant-lobe dysfunction makes an extreme and absolute judgement that he has been wronged by another. Since his perception is that he has been 'absolutely and severely wronged', then his response to this wrong-doing can be equally extreme and severe. The left-hemisphere-impaired individual is likely to suffer considerably from situations which invoke cognitive dissonance. Take the situation where it was discovered that a good friend (who will have been perceived as a close and 'perfect' friend) somehow betrays that friendship in a relatively minor way. The exaggeration of both the level of friendship and the seriousness of the betrayal creates major contradictions for the sufferer that can only be resolved by an abandonment of the friendship or a total dismissal of the 'offence'. It is noticeable how many psychopaths tend to dismiss their own offences as being minor incidents or overemphasise the severity of their misdemeanours.

Self-monitoring

Of course, not all psychopaths suffer from a dominant-hemisphere dysfunction and it is possible for antisocial behaviour to develop in respect to other loci of injury. In particular, an attentional deficit normally attributed to the non-dominant hemisphere is attention to one internal state. A diminished ability to interpret internal states has been reported in the case of H.M. who underwent bilateral medial temporal resection (Hebben et al 1985). Siminov (1986) notes that when there is a defect in the medial section of the right frontal lobe, the emotional component of recognising one's own emotional states is disrupted. The general emotional consequence of such injury is towards indifference or positive emotion. However, in certain circumstances such a dysfunction may provoke offending behaviour.

This problem was noted in a repetitive sex-offender, D.P., who under most circumstances was socially skilled, good-humoured, well liked, co-operative and emotionally stable. Neuropsychological examination revealed mild, bilateral, frontal lobe dysfunction and moderate amnesic disturbance. However, most striking was that he never complained of being hungry or of being hot or cold. He also could not remember having these experiences. However, his eating and drinking behaviour was normal. D.P. did have an alcohol problem in that outside a controlling environment he would frequently get drunk, although he did not suffer from withdrawal effects or excessive desire for alcohol. Penile plethysmograph showed normal sexual arousal, but his cognitive awareness of this was severely impaired. A dysfunction of awareness of internal state makes the control of arousal difficult because of poor ongoing feedback to consciousness. If awareness only becomes available at high arousal levels, then the chances of inhibiting that arousal (and the consequent motivation and behaviour) are severely reduced.

In other cases, anosognosic or insight problems may militate against psychopathic personality disorder in that they serve to protect the individual from problems of self-esteem and social identity. In this sense, the preponderance of dominant-hemisphere dysfunctioning in psychopaths can be considered to result, not from the specific effects of this dysfunction, but because brain dysfunction in general predisposes the individual towards psychopathic behaviour and right lateralisation of dysfunction masks these tendencies. The right-hemisphere-dysfunctioning individual may be irresponsible and socially inept, but does not evidence the extremes of aggressive behaviour found in most psychopathic offenders. An obvious exception to this interpretation is where there is a degree of provocation, which, together with the greater impulsiveness of non-dominant hemisphere patients, results in a dyscontrol syndrome and potentially violent outbursts.

Of course, poor self-awareness may result from factors other than neuro-cognitive deficits, such as a conscious or unconscious defensive mechanism. However, poor self-monitoring may go some way to account for the apparent lack of concern or anxiety amongst some psychopaths and recidivistic delinquents.

Empathy and emotional recognition

The importance of empathy to personality is implicit to the personality theories of Mead (1934) in the form of role-taking and Kelly (1955) in the form of role-construction. Both emphasise the ability to appreciate the emotional reactions of others. A basic component of empathic appreciation is the ability to process and decipher socio-emotional interaction cues. There has been research to suggest that psychopathic individuals are impaired in such abilities. On a test of emotional recognition from faces in which the subjects were required to rate each expression on each of six emotions (happy, sad, angry, disgusted, fearful and surprised), Ashcroft (1989) found that psychopathic offenders rated more towards the extremes of the scale than controls regardless of the type of emotion being rated or the category of the emotion stimuli. Most striking was the psychopaths' tendencies to rate expressions as being very highly representative of a particular emotion. Impaired emotional recognition has also been suggested among other groups such as schizophrenics (Bannister & Salmon 1966, Williams 1974), traumatic brain injured (Borod et al 1985, Jackson & Moffat 1987), sex offenders (Lipton et al 1987) and violent offenders (Pollack 1980). Coupled with other cognitive deficits reported in mentally abnormal offenders such as impaired social problem-solving skills (Ross & Fabiano 1985) and extreme and rapid biases in social judgement (Howells 1981, Thomas-Peter 1988), these basic social

perception deficits may invoke emotional responses which are incongruent with environmental events or circumstances, both in terms of type and size. Furthermore, such emotional recognition deficits may go some way to explaining the low levels of social competence observed in many such offenders (Stermac & Quinsey 1986).

Although poor empathy skills are frequently alleged in psychopaths and delinquents (Hogan 1975), there has been little empirical investigation to test these assertions. Heilbrun (1982) emphasised the importance of the lack of empathy as a major diagnostic criteria for two of his three psychopathic sub-categories. Similarly, Cleckley (1976) describes the psychopath's apparent inability to relate his emotions and his verbalisations, and Schacter & Latane (1964) postulated that psychopathy was in part caused by a failure of some individuals to apply emotion labels to their arousal states. The potential importance of accurate emotional perception with respect to psychopathy has some face validity considering Hare's *Checklist for Psychopathy* which includes lack of concern for others, egocentricity and shallow emotional expression (Hare 1980). Emotional reactions of others serve to stabilise and maintain accurate social communication. Emotion signals provide the primary feedback for the development of social behaviour both in terms of direct and vicarious learning. In addition, they provide the primary discriminative stimuli for appropriate social interaction. Plutchik (1980) has argued that personality differences are largely habitual tendencies to feel or show particular emotions in response to environmental events. Since the 'felt and expressed emotion' is partly determined by the individual's perception of the emotional responses of others, a bias or an impairment in emotional recognition is likely to have corresponding results on social behaviour and personality. Thus, a deficiency in the processing of the emotional signals of others is likely to have profound effects both progressively (i.e. the development of personality) and immediately (i.e. cueing and reinforcing socially appropriate and congruent behaviour). Despite, however, the obvious importance of emotional perception to personality disorder and offending behaviour, it has received relatively little attention in the research literature.

Disinhibition

The concept of disinhibition is poorly defined but has clear implications for offending behaviour. In a general sense, it infers an impaired ability to inhibit responses. This may result as a consequence of increased activation or as an impairment of constraining functions. There are a host of potential dysfunctions of inhibitory mechanisms following acquired brain injury including:

1. Perseveration (usually resulting from injury to the frontal lobes of the brain, involving the impairment of cognitive functions that allow for the modification of behaviour or thoughts in response to conflicting information or external stimuli). The perseverative brain-injured person will often demonstrate a failure to learn from previous experience which may arise from an impaired ability to perceive and process the associations between previous experience and current situation. Such individuals have a rigidity of thought and behaviour.

2. Impaired evaluation of the consequences of actions. Again this is a characteristic of patients with brain injury to the frontal lobes. Impaired 'consequential thinking' may arise because of an impairment in the ability:

   - to sequence information into logical order
   - to hold in mind two pieces of information at the same time
   - to compare and contrast different possible outcomes
   - to estimate probability or likelihood
   - to generate possible outcomes.

3. Misperception of social or emotional cues. As mentioned above, impaired emotional perception may create a number of severe psychosocial problems. Accurate processing of social/emotional cues in terms of category and intensity is important for:

   - appropriate emotional and social responding
   - acquisition of social and emotional skills
   - stability of mood and behaviour.

4. Impaired appreciation of moral and social rules and habitual prosocial behaviours.

5. Impaired abstract thinking. Much of human communication involves abstract ideas, innuendos, inferences and analogies. Perception of social behaviour, verbal communication and attributions such as 'intent', 'context' and 'perspective' become difficult for individuals whose abstract abilities have been impaired.

Individuals presenting with impaired information processing cannot utilise previous experience or the projection of likely consequences to guide current behaviour. Hence, individuals are overly reliant on immediate stimuli and information, becoming highly impulsive, unaware of the longer-term consequences or the abstract morality of their behaviour. The sufferer is 'stuck in the *here and now*', overly reactive to the immediate situation. Obviously, dinsinhibition and excessively impulsive behaviour is not only likely to result, but, owing to the failure to learn from experience, will be difficult to modify. In this sense, disinhibition can be appreciated as not necessarily a simple cause and effect relationship between localised neurological injury and behaviour, but rather a reflection of the combined neuropsychological impacts of injury upon the information-processing mechanisms needed to control and modify potential behavioural responses.

Self-concept

Miller (1987) offers a more developmental aspect to information-processing deficiencies, such as impoverished verbal processing, poor self-insight and abstract thinking, observed in mentally abnormal offenders. These combine to inhibit the development of a mature self and social identity. He reports two major ways in which impoverished self-concept may be related to offending behaviour. The first involves the failure to adequately communicate feelings, needs or wishes either to others or to the self, resulting in increased frustration and anxiety. The second involves the lack of sophistication of self-concept and the limited number of (situationally responsive) self-schemas which could have developed in information-processing-impaired individuals. Thus, under situations of stress, ambiguity or frustration, the absence of a sophisticated or appropriate self-schema which could prompt prosocial responses may provoke a regression to lower order coping mechanisms and thereby offending. Similarly, an overly rigid self-concept which is unresponsive to the idiosyncratic demands of a social situation may provoke a stereotypic form of responding when other more effective and prosocial responses were indicated. Many psychopathic patients, for example, will explain their offending in terms of their rigid self-concept with responses such as 'That's just the way I am.' Such a self-concept will inevitably provoke internal inconsistencies which will threaten the integrity of the self, perhaps provoking a variety of internal conflicts which will seek expression and resolution in irrational offending behaviour. We have noted in patients in a maximum security hospital that neurological and neuropsychological problems appear to have their onset in the early stages of development. If social, emotional and moral development is impeded at these stages, then self-concept is also likely to be affected. It is interesting to postulate that the pre-existing self-concept for moral and social behaviour developed in adult head injury victims may be preserved after injury and serve to defend against severe antisocial behaviour.

Summary

Considering the heterogeneity of offender populations, neurological and neuropsychological deficits are to be found in only a sub-set of offenders. However, it would be reasonable to conclude that the same may also be said of environmental determinants of offending. Thus, whilst offending behaviour and antisocial personality may be related to poor socio-economic or cultural factors, it is by no means certain that antisocial personality will result. One may expect an additive effect of both neuropsychological and social deficiencies in the promotion of antisocial personality. Of course, the tendency for initial neuropsychological deficits to lead the sufferer to impoverished and amoral social circumstances, either through poor judgement or by inevitability, has yet to be adequately demonstrated, but remains a plausible hypothesis.

The varying importance of different informational processes to offending behaviour is evident, with those associated with social functioning and executive control being most prominently deficient in antisocial personality groups. There is currently a paucity of adequate assessment procedures for evaluating such socio-cognitive deficits and an over-reliance on descriptive personality assessment.

Research studies have tended to concentrate on identifying factors which promote offending. A serious omission from the literature concerns those factors which protect the neurologically impaired individual from the emergence of antisocial personality disorder and offending behaviour. Such factors may not only be important to a fuller understanding of antisocial personality disorder, but may be essential to the successful treatment of such disorders. For example, Matthews et al (1977) found TLE patients with a high IQ to show a lower psychopathic deviate score on the MMPI than TLE patients with a low IQ. Work of our own (Jackson et al 1987) suggests such psychologically prohibitive mechanisms presenting arson as an option for resolving conflict or changing undesirable circumstances. 'Protective' variables may include social, pre-morbid, other intact cognitive functions, self-concept or learning history.

CASE STUDY: ROB

This case study illustrates some of the complex interplay between neurological, neuropsychological and social/environmental forces in producing offending behaviour. It is worth noting that a continuum of offending behaviours may result from traumatic head injury and even serious incidents may go unreported because they occur within hospitals, rehabilitation units, prisons and other institutional settings. Even within the community, many lesser incidents of offending behaviours may go unreported until such time that a serious offence is committed, necessitating the intervention of law enforcement. The totality of the local environment is an integral, and perhaps underestimated, consideration in predicting and controlling the likelihood of engagement in offending behaviour. Although an individual may not display the behaviours or commits lesser acts within secure, structured or closely controlled environments, or where community location does not allow access to provocative influences, placement within unstructured, unmonitored, ambiguous or inappropriate settings may result in the emergence and possible escalation of antisocial acts.

Rob sustained a severe brain injury, including both brain stem and cortical involvement, following a road traffic accident at the age of 18. Following the accident, he experienced a prolonged coma and then an extended period of post-traumatic amnesia. He had left school at the age of 16 without sitting any exams, working as a butcher and within a plastics manufacturing plant. He enjoyed physical activity and would participate in swimming and working out as leisure interests. His socialisation was adequate, including friendships and relationships and he had no pre-morbid involvement with the police. There was no previous history of neurological illness, psychiatric complaints or possible head trauma. As a result of the accident, he had been left with a left-sided hemiplegia, mild dysarthria, ataxic gait and impairment of fine-motor co-ordination. Though these physical impairments were relatively minor, he experienced profound behavioural changes. He became socially disinhibited, often making provocative sexual and other offensive remarks in public places to relative strangers. He experienced explosive outbursts of temper, including physical assault, usually directed towards family members. Rob had been banned from numerous places in his local community, including hairdressers, public houses, shops and café bars.

However, he showed no insight into the connections between his own actions and these consequences. Law enforcement became involved following a claim of indecent assault against a minor while in a swimming pool.

Nearly 10 years after his injury, Rob was assessed for admission to a residential brain-injury rehabilitation unit. At the time he was residing in a psychiatric hospital, sharing a dormitory with 15 others. His medications included the anti-convulsant carbamazepine, the anti-Parkinsonian procyclidine, the anti-psychotic droperidol and the sexual drive-reducing cyproterone. During the interview, he admitted to assaulting his mother's boyfriend but stated that the incident of indecent assault had been accidental. He displayed limited awareness of his deficits other than his physical impairments and came across as overly flippant and joking. He also showed an inability to follow the rapid presentation of ideas in conversation and his self-generated conversation topics were generally egocentric.

Formal testing revealed a Wechsler Adult Intelligence Scale-Revised Full Scale IQ of 68. Rob's pre-morbid IQ as estimated by the National Adult Reading Test was 90. His performance on the Williams Delayed Recall Test was grossly impaired, indicating a severe memory deficit. On tests of frontal lobe functioning, Rob performed within the low-average range on the Benton Verbal Fluency Test, but was slow and perseverative on the Tapping Test (Andrew 1978). The Cognitive Estimations Test showed evidence of extreme misjudgement (e.g. he responded that a milk bottle weighed 7 lb). Rob also demonstrated impairments in both alternating and divided attention and his overall speed of cognitive processing was noticeably slowed.

Following his admission to a non-secure, residential brain-injury rehabilitation programme, he displayed a variety of challenging behaviours. In any other context, these would have constituted offending behaviours. There were episodes of violence against property and assaults against staff members, including several incidents where, in response to immediate frustration, he threw scalding drinks on staff members. Verbal abuse towards both staff and residents occurred, together with unwanted sexual comments and advances towards female staff, residents and members of the community. On one occasion, Rob attempted to kiss a female resident against her wishes in her room. When she attempted to shout, he placed a pillow over her face. The resident escaped from the room and the police were notified, although she declined to press charges. This particular incident illustrates the way in which one offending act may lead, through impairments of judgement and decision-making, to the possible unintentional commission of a more serious offence. After these incidents, Rob denied or minimised responsibility for his actions, often claiming that he was provoked.

It is possible to view these incidents within a global picture of Rob's difficulties, including impairment of the normal internal and external feedback mechanisms by which most individuals plan, evaluate and modify their behaviours. In addition to the critical behaviours, Rob's general social interaction skills were gauche and disinhibited, particularly with women. He was socially imperceptive and unresponsive to most subtle social cues and hence persistent in unsuccessful approaches. Upon meeting women during periods of access to the community, he would immediately ask them for their addresses and phone numbers. Sometimes he would be successful in obtaining an address and would write the woman a letter. Even though he never received a reply, he would continue the behaviour. At times when more direct feedback was provided about his behaviour from staff, or the rejection of any advances, Rob would quickly attribute the rejection to the personality of the person providing the feedback. This was often expressed in a variety of gender and sexually-based insults, allowing for the behaviours to be maintained rather than modified.

Rob's overall ability to manage frustration and criticism was poor and his primary coping strategy was to avoid potentially anxiety-provoking situations (he would often lock or barricade himself in his room). As a result of limitations of memory, sequencing and abstraction,

he could not maintain plans or organise himself, leading to impulsive decisions without consideration of limitations or possible consequences. These cognitive impairments also meant that he could not recall information given to him, or he would only recall selected pieces and add confabulatory elements, leading to decisions based upon misperceptions. Periodically, Rob experienced periods of paranoia and delusional thought processes. He would believe that staff members or family were impostors, that there was a motorcycle gang out to kill him, or that specific events in the present had been predicted by the friend who had died in the accident. However, his medication also had the effect of reducing his arousal levels, thus increasing his attentional and cognitive impairments. He also displayed a fragile sense of self-esteem and would often boast of his present abilities and perseverate in conversations about his pre-morbid capabilities.

Rob's treatment recognised the importance of integrating medical, psychological, neuropsychological, social and vocational interventions. A trans-disciplinary professional team including expertise in clinical psychology, clinical neuropsychology, physiotherapy, occupational therapy and medicine managed his rehabilitation. Elements of his treatment included the introduction of planning and organisational aids on both a daily and weekly basis to assist Rob in structuring his time and reducing impulsive decisions. Attention-training and teaching in the use of a notebook and methods for structuring and clarifying incoming information were used both to improve attention and reduce the impairments caused by slowed speed of processing. Behavioural modification principles, including
• participation in a token economy, were utilised to functionally analyse challenging behaviours and motivational problems to provide for the differential reinforcement of alternatives. Prior to activities where difficulties could be anticipated, priming and saturation cueing was utilised to provide errorless learning of appropriate responses. Compensatory systems were integrated to encourage Rob to begin to increase his self-awareness of the discrepancies between his

perceptions of his actions and those of the individuals around him. Participation in group and individual sessions and repetitive role-playing were stressed to teach appropriate social interactions and conflict resolution skills. Medications were carefully adjusted and changed to balance their behavioural stabilising effects with the adverse effects upon cognition.

Rob's progress was gradual and characterised by periods of improvement followed by periods of deterioration. At one time during treatment, the possible transfer to a secure psychiatric unit was considered. Complicating the rehabilitation picture was the gradual development of progressive orthopaedic difficulties which reduced his ability to walk and further exaggerated and confused motivational problems, learned helplessness and authentic pain and mobility complaints. Over the course of 4 years and multiple changes and modifications in treatment goals and priorities, overall reductions in both the frequency and intensity of offending behaviours were obtained. These improvements were in conjunction with an improved and more consistent use of compensatory systems (e.g. planners, notebooks, self-monitoring aids) to manage the information-processing aspects of his brain injury, along with placement in an appropriate vocational setting, providing tangible evidence of success and responsibility and the provision of supervised access to the community. Progress was assisted, approximately 2 years into treatment, as a consequence of medication changes.

A combination of lithium and a different antipsychotic (sertindole) was prescribed. The cyproterone was discontinued owing to concerns over the possible long-term effects, particularly its potential contribution to the orthopaedic difficulties (e.g. increased weight and calcium depletion), the psychological impacts of body alterations (e.g. breast enlargement) and possible exacerbation of cognitive deficits through increased fatigue.

At the time of writing, Rob has had no episodes of violence against either persons or property for approximately 1 year. Social perception difficulties and disinhibited comments and remarks continue to require the intervention of staff members, but within the rehabilitation environment these have become less frequent. There have been no episodes of grossly inappropriate sexual behaviour for over 2 years. Interestingly, Rob's insight into his behaviours and ability to accept responsibility for his actions have not improved as much as expected, though he now shows a greater willingness to accept feedback. It is not expected that Rob will be able to return successfully to independent accommodation within the community, but that he will be capable of managing within a small group home with moderate levels of supervision. It is likely, however, that Rob will always require supervision when interacting in the community because of continued social disinhibition, particularly when he is in the presence of unfamiliar women.

REFERENCES

Andrew J 1978 Laterality and the tapping test among legal offenders. Journal of Clinical Child Psychology 7: 149–150

Ashcroft J 1989 Emotional recognition in mentally abnormal offenders. Unpublished PhD thesis, University of Liverpool

Bannister D, Salmon P 1966 Schizophrenic thought disorder: specific or diffuse? British Journal of Medical Psychology 39: 215–219

Berman A, Seigal A 1976 Adaptive and learning skills in juvenile delinquents: a neuropsychological analysis. Journal of Learning Disability 9: 583–590

Betts T, Mersky H, Pond D 1976 Psychiatry. In: Laidlaw J, Richens A (eds) A textbook of epilepsy. Churchill Livingstone, Edinburgh, p 145–184

Birkett J 1988 Attentional deficits in brain injured psychopaths, non brain injured psychopaths and non offending head injury victims. Unpublished Masters dissertation, University of Liverpool

Borod J, Koff E, Perlman M, Nicholas M 1985 Channels of emotional expression in patients with unilateral brain. Archives of Neurology 42: 345–348

Buchtel H, Campari F, DeRisio C, Rota R 1976 Hemispheric differences in discriminative reaction time to facial expressions: preliminary observations. Bolletino–Societa Italiana Biologia Sperimentate 52: 1447–1452

Camp B 1977 Verbal mediation in young aggressive boys. Journal of Abnormal Psychology 86: 145–153

Cleckley H 1976 The mask of sanity, 5th edn. Mosby, St Louis

Day J 1977 Right hemisphere language processing in normal right handers. Journal of Experimental Psychology: Human Perception and Memory 3: 518–528

Delgada-Escueta A, Mattson R, King, L 1981 The nature of aggression during epileptic seizures. New England Journal of Medicine 305: 711–716

Ferguson S, Raport M, Corrie W 1986 Brain correlates of aggressive behaviour in temporal lobe epilepsy. In: Doane B, Livingstone K (eds) The limbic system. Raven Press, New York, p 251–266

Flor-Henry P 1976 Lateralized temporal–limbic dysfunction and psychopathology. Annals of the New York Academy of Sciences 280: 777–797

Fromm-Auch D, Yeudall L, Davies P, Fedora O 1980 Assessment of juvenile delinquents: neuropsychological, psychophysiological, neurological, EEG, and reading test findings. Unpublished manuscript, Alberta Hospital, Edmonton, Canada

Gainotti G 1969 Reactions 'catastrophiques' et manifestation d'indifference au cours des atteintes cerebrales. Neuropsychologia 7: 195–204

Gorenstein E 1982 Frontal lobe functions in psychopaths. Journal of Abnormal Psychology 91(5): 368–379

Hare R 1980 A research scale for the assessment of psychopathy in criminal populations. Personality and Individual Differences 1: 111–117

Hebben N, Corkin S, Eichenbaum H, Shedlack K 1985 Diminished ability to interpret and report internal states after bilateral medial temporal resection: case H.M. Behavioral Neurosciences 99: 1031–1039

Heilbrun A 1982 Cognitive models of criminal violence based upon intelligence and psychopathy levels. Journal of Consulting and Clinical Psychology 50: 546–557

Hermann B, Schwartz M, Karnes W 1980 Psychopathology in epilepsy: relationship of seizure type to age of onset. Epilepsia 21: 15–23

Hill D, Watterson D 1942 Electro-encephalographic studies of psychopathic personalities. Journal of Neurology and Psychiatry 5: 47–65

Hines D 1976 Recognition of verbs, abstract nouns and concrete nouns from left and right visual fields. Neuropsychologia 14: 211–216

Hogan R 1975 Empathy: a conceptual analysis and psychometric analysis. The Counselling Psychologist 5: 14–18

Howells K 1981 Social relationships in violent offenders. In: Duck S, Gilmour R (eds) Personal relationships in disorder. Academic Press, London

Jackson H, Moffat N 1987 Impaired emotional recognition following head injury. Cortex 23: 293–300

Jackson H, Glass C, Hope S 1987 A functional analysis of recidivistic arson. British Journal of Clinical Psychology 26: 175–185

James I 1960 Temporal lobectomy for psychomotor epilepsy. Journal of Mental Science 106: 543–558

Jenkins R, Pacella B 1943 Electroencephalographic studies of delinquent boys. American Journal of Orthopsychiatry 13: 107–120

Joseph R 1982 The neuropsychology of development: hemispheric laterality, limbic language and origin of thought. Journal of Clinical Psychology 38: 4–33

Kelly G 1955 A theory of personality. Norton, New York

Krynicki V 1978 Cerebral dysfunction in repetitively assaultive adolescents. Journal of Nervous and Mental Disease 166: 59–67

Lipton D, McDonel E, McFall R 1987 Heterosocial perception in rapists. Journal of Consulting and Clinical Psychology 55: 17–21

Luria A 1980 Higher cortical functions in man. Basic Books, New York

Luria A, Simernitskaya E 1975 Function interaction of the hemispheres of the brain in the organization of verbal-mimetic functions. Fiziologiia Cheloveka 1: 411

Matthews C, Dikmen S, Harley J 1977 Age at onset of seizures and psychometric correlates of MMPI profiles in major motor epilepsy. Diseases of the Nervous System 38: 173–176

Mead G 1934 Mind, self and society. Chicago University Press, Chicago

Meichenbaum D 1975 Theoretical and treatment implications of development research on verbal control of behaviour. Canadian Psychological Review 16: 22–27

Miller L 1987 Neuropsychology of the aggressive psychopath: an integrated review. Aggressive Behaviour 13: 119–140

Millon T 1981 Disorders of personality: DSM III, Axis II. Wiley, New York

Monroe R 1986 Episodic behavioral disorders and limbic ictus. In: Doane B, Livingstone, K (eds) The limbic system. Raven Press, New York, p 251–266

Myslobodsky M, Rattok J 1977 Bilateral electrodermal activity in waking man. Acta Psychologica 41: 273–282

Ounstead C, Lindsay J, Richards P 1987 Temporal lobe epilepsy 1948–1986: a biographical study. MacKeith Press, Oxford

Plutchik R 1980 Emotion: a psychoevolutionary synthesis. Harper, New York

Pollack N 1980 The relationship between criminal behaviour and constricted role-taking activity. PhD thesis, University of Toronto

Rodin E 1973 Psychomotor epilepsy and aggressive behaviour. Archives of General Psychiatry 28: 210–213

Ross R, Fabiano E 1985 Time to think: a cognitive model of crime and delinquency prevention and rehabilitation. Academic Arts and Sciences, Johnson City

Schacter S, Latane B 1964 Crime, cognition, and the autonomic nervous system. In: Levine D (ed) Nebraska symposium on motivation. University of Nebraska Press, Lincoln

Semmes J 1968 Hemispheric specialisation: a clue to mechanisms. Neuropsychology 6: 11–27

Siminov P 1986 The emotional brain. Plenum, London

Small J, Milstein V, Stevens J 1962 Are psychomotor epileptics different? Archives of Neurology 7: 187–194

Small J, Small I, Hayden M 1966 Further psychiatric investigations of patients with temporal and non-temporal lobe epilepsy. American Journal of Psychiatry 123: 303–310

Stermac L, Quinsey V 1986 Social competence amongst rapists. Behavioural Assessment 8: 171–185

Thomas-Peter B 1988 Construct theory and cognitive style in personality disordered offenders. Paper presented to a conference on PCP, deviancy and social work, London

Vaillant G 1975 Sociopathy as a human process: a viewpoint. Archives of General Psychiatry 32: 178–183

Vitgosky L 1962 Thought and language. MIT Press, Cambridge, Massachusetts

Volkow N, Tancredi L 1987 Neural substrates of violent behaviour. British Journal of Psychiatry 151: 668–673

Williams E 1974 An analysis of gaze in schizophrenics. British Journal of Clinical Psychology 39: 246–252

Woods R, Eames P 1981 Application of behaviour modification to the rehabilitation of traumatically brain-injured adults. In: Davey G (ed) Application of conditioning theory. Methuen, London

Yeudall L 1978 The neuropsychology of aggression. Clarence M Hinks Memorial Lecture: Psychological approaches to aggression in mental illness and mental retardation. Alberta Hospital, Edmonton, Canada

Yeudall L, Fromm-Auch D, Davies P 1982 Neuropsychological impairment of persistent delinquency. Journal of Nervous and Mental Disease 170: 257–265

Zenkov L 1976 Some aspects of the semiotic structure and functional organization of 'right-hemisphere thinking'. In: Unconsciousness, vol. 1 [in Russian]. Metsniereba, Tbilia, p 740

Community care

Primary care, probation and risk management

Michael Pavlovic

Introduction

This case study examines the case of Mark, a 33-year-old man, who spent 10 years at a Special Hospital. It aims to consider the difficulties the probation service has in acting as the lead agency in monitoring potentially dangerous offenders in the community, examines the importance of accurate risk assessment in the light of insufficient background material and concludes that, unless a multi-agency approach is taken, some offenders will remain dangerous whatever policies are put in place to manage risk.

Probation

The probation service, in common with many other agencies, has been in a process of re-examining the emphasis it has given to the assessment and management of risk. In the last decade, a succession of new laws has led to a root and branch reform of the institutional response to criminal behaviour in England and Wales. This has, in turn, led to a change of emphasis in terms of how best to manage those individuals who pose a significant level of risk to the public. Arguably, this process began with the Children's Act 1989, proceeded with the Criminal Justice Acts of 1991 and 1993, and continues unabated, as evidenced by new sex offender laws in 1998. These legislative instruments have resulted in protection of the public being at the forefront of the work of the probation service.

Safeguarding society from all those who wish to commit harm is an admirable aim, but, unfortunately, is not completely possible, even if unlimited resources and the blessing of hindsight were available. The best we can achieve is to highlight risk accurately, more often than not, and, where risk does exist, to take measures to contain or reduce it. To accomplish this, the probation service has had to confront a number of difficulties. These include tensions arising from a historical professional focus on the interests of the offender (still typically referred to as clients) and notions of autonomy held by medical services, where an emphasis on patient confidentiality can hamper the sharing of information between agencies.

In one sense, the outcome for Mark could be said to have been relatively unsuccessful, given that he recently returned to prison, albeit for a shorter than usual sentence. However, the reflections on the case, whilst not playing down the problems in practice, highlight ways in which co-operation between criminal justice and mental health agencies can move forward.

CASE STUDY: MARK

History

Medical records, only recently accessed, indicate that Mark's early development was characterised by behaviour that was both destructive and disruptive. Studies have suggested that such early behaviour may indicate an already developing personality disorder, which can lead to 'a stubborn persistence into adult life' (Gunn et al 1991). An early example was an attempt by Mark to set fire to his younger brother's pram. At the age of 6, his parents requested that Mark be taken into care because of their inability to cope with his behaviour. He spent the next 9 years in a variety of children's homes, interspersed by short periods at the family home. These times always seemed to break down quickly owing to Mark's continuing disruptive behaviour, which included one allegation of sexual abuse against his 8-year-old brother when Mark was only 11 years old. After this alleged incident, contact with his family ceased for some years.

During his time in care, Mark began to commit offences, mainly involving theft and taking a vehicle without the owner's consent, which were dealt with by local Magistrates' courts. He was, around this time, also becoming increasingly violent, both towards staff and other child residents. Eventually, at the age of 15, Mark assaulted another resident at his children's home and was brought before the crown court. A psychiatric assessment for this hearing diagnosed psychopathic disorder and Mark was ordered to be detained under section 60 of the Mental Health Act 1959, together with an order under section 65 restricting discharge without limit of time. The Mental Health Act 1983 re-classified his detention, under sections 37 and 41 of the new Act.

As a result, Mark was detained at one of the Special Hospitals where he remained for 5 years. A transfer to a medium-secure unit was made as a prelude to his eventual discharge. He remained there for 18 months, until recalled to the more secure hospital because of difficulties with his behaviour. A clinical report at this time stated:

This patient suffers from a psychopathic disorder of such a nature which requires treatment in hospital. He had extensive rehabilitation at [name of hospital] for 18 months but failed to demonstrate he is able to control his emotions, especially sexual feelings, which could have been dangerous to a female staff member he became attached to at the unit ... He is unfit for discharge due to his social skill deficits, emotional immaturity and potential to violence.

In the light of this report by his psychiatrist and knowledge of Mark's subsequent behaviour, which I would argue was predicted and predictable, he remains an ongoing risk to the public. This makes his subsequent lack of medical support all the more concerning.

Mark enjoyed one further period at the rehabilitation unit and was then conditionally discharged back to his parents' care at the age of 22. He had spent most of his life from the age of 6 in institutional care and the past 7 years in secure conditions. He was, therefore, totally unprepared for independent living and had little positive experience of family life. Soon after his discharge, Mark and another man were the chief suspects in an alleged rape, where the victim was

Mark's brother's girlfriend. The woman was apparently too traumatised by the events to take the matter further and, although the police and Mark's social worker investigated the allegation, no further action was taken. At this time, Mark was subject to out-patient appointments with a local psychiatrist in addition to contact with his social worker. Although the probation service was not involved at this stage, medical records suggest that Mark quickly dropped out of contact with those statutory bodies responsible for his care. He then committed serious offences of theft and arson and as a result was recalled to the Special Hospital for another 2 years.

At the time of Mark's ultimate discharge from hospital, the medical opinion was that he was no longer treatable in secure conditions, although the original diagnosis of psychopathic disorder remained. He had however been hospitalised between the ages of 15 to 24 on the basis of his amenability to treatment. This highlights just one of the areas of concern when trying to monitor those who potentially pose a risk to the public. At what point does someone stop being treatable? The perception of those whose involvement continues, after doctors appear to wash their hands of these potentially dangerous clients, is that it is resource implications which are paramount. This is despite the continuing behaviour that resulted in hospitalisation originally. The practicalities of managing and supervising psychopathic offenders are acknowledged as posing 'one of the most difficult challenges for those purchasing or providing mental health services' (Department of Health 1992).

When the debate amongst psychiatrists over diagnosis is combined with the question of what services to offer and how to fund them, those who work solely in the field of criminal justice are left not only bemused, but frequently frustrated and angry. The Butler Committee, as long ago as 1975, commented on the lack of medical agreement about diagnosis and treatability, while the Mental Health Act 1983 unhelpfully states that compulsory treatment can only be applied if that treatment is, 'likely to alleviate or prevent a deterioration of that condition' (Mental Health Act 1983).

Whatever the situation regarding Mark's treatability or otherwise, 1990 saw the end of his formal contact with mental health services. What followed was an example of several agencies working together to assess and minimise Mark's potential to harm others, yet hamstrung by the lack of assistance and support from health services, who refused until 1998 to even allow the viewing of relevant medical records, citing patient confidentiality.

Within a few months of his discharge from hospital, Mark committed a night-time house burglary. Having disturbed the elderly occupier, Mark proceeded to beat him severely. On this occasion, it seems that a return to hospital was no longer an issue, given that no psychiatric assessment was requested, though he had been discharged for only 3 months at this time. For this offence of aggravated burglary, Mark received a sentence of 6 years imprisonment.

It is well documented that psychopaths can demonstrate an ability to manipulate and to convince those in authority that they have reformed. Hare (1995) states:

> they had learned enough … jargon to convince therapists, counsellors and parole boards that they were making remarkable progress, but they used that knowledge (of how to 'play the game') only to develop … better ways to manipulate and deceive.

Demonstrating his own abilities in this respect, Mark quickly moved down the risk categories within the prison service and eventually was housed at a category C jail. Such was his perceived lack of risk that he was allowed out of the prison to present a charity cheque, having raised the money, along with other inmates, by making soft toys. Although escorted by two officers, Mark managed to escape. Though his period at large was short-lived, it highlights what can happen without adequate sharing of information between different agencies.

Despite his apparent compliance and progress within the prison, Mark was unable or unwilling to gauge the implications of escaping at a time when approaching eligibility for parole. As a result of this, Mark was refused parole and served his complete sentence. Had the prison governor been fully aware of Mark's psychiatric background when considering granting his leave, it is inconceivable that such a risk would have been taken. Following his release from prison, Mark began formal contact with the probation service. Although his supervising officer was obviously aware that he had a diagnosis of psychopathy and a pre-sentence report had been prepared for his court appearance on the burglary offence, little more information was available other than that already in the public domain. Mark had been allocated a field probation officer who visited him in prison and helped him plan for release.

An integral part of every long-term prisoner's discharge plan is accommodation. Correspondence and discussions with mental health managers took place regarding whether Mark could be maintained in supported accommodation on his release. Unfortunately this was rejected and it became clear that local authority or private landlorded accommodation was the only option. Mark was therefore released with no settled accommodation, quickly dropped contact with his supervising officer and re-offended (burglary and handling) almost immediately. He was remanded in custody prior to receiving another custodial sentence. This pattern remained for another two sentences of imprisonment.

During his most recent sentence, it was decided to review the way Mark was being managed in the community. The previous 8 years had seen Mark in the community for no more than 4 months at any one time before being locked up again, Mark's recidivism resulting in very short periods at liberty in the community, interspersed with extended spells in prison. While there he is contained, perhaps resulting in a sense of 'out of sight, out of mind'. However, if effective risk management is to be achieved, both the needs of Mark and the needs of society as a whole have to be reassessed.

Risk management

The quest for a foolproof method for assessing risk, and effectively managing that risk in all cases, is akin to searching for the Holy Grail. The best we can hope for is that we ask the right questions:

- What is the likelihood of serious harm and its extent?
- To whom might this harm be directed?
- What triggers might make an incident more likely?
- What can be done to reduce the likelihood of the harm occurring?

These questions are outlined in the Home Office guidelines for the probation service (Home Office 1995). Of fundamental importance is knowledge and, particularly, knowledge of an individual's offending:

To obtain as much information as possible about past offending in considerable detail, since this may afford useful diagnostic clues … A mere list of previous convictions devoid of elaboration provides no real information upon which to make even the most tentative predictions.

Prins 1988

Mark had, for many years, been considered a high risk by the probation service, both regarding the likelihood of his re-offending and his relative dangerousness. He had proved that he was at significant risk of committing further offences but he had not (to our knowledge) been involved in violent offending since 1990. Although those who have studied psychopathy suggest that the propensity for violence continues to be higher than in offenders who are not suffering from this disorder, Hare argues that criminal activity decreases with age. Mark was now in his 30s and had been exhibiting criminal behaviour for over 20 years.

The difficulties in gaining access to Mark's clinical records have led to an over-reliance on the basic diagnosis last used over 9 years ago, possibly leading to inaccurate evaluation of risk posed. In certain situations, lack of a comprehensive social history does not amount to an insurmountable problem, as the offender can fill in the gaps during the course of interviews. Mark, however, has never been prepared to discuss his background and his family has moved away from contact. His early life, the period of hospitalisation, or his offending history, are also closed books; Mark only discusses events superficially, if at all. Additionally, staff changes mean that officers who may have had anecdotal background knowledge of Mark are unavailable for consultation. The lack of medical notes was eventually solved by contacting C3 Division at the Home Office, as Mark had been detained under criminal sections 37/41. Although having initially misplaced them, the records were eventually located and forwarded. It was from these papers that the background described earlier in this case study was gleaned. It is this kind of seemingly pointless red tape and obstruction that frustrates those trying to work with potentially high-risk offenders, particularly as this is an issue that has been highlighted as a barrier to good practice:

...risk assessment and the sharing of information between probation, health and social services were often arbitrary, leading to gaps in service.
Department of Health 1997

While the information contained in Mark's records has undoubtedly been useful, this knowledge has to be used appropriately. Prins has pointed out that with detailed background information, we may be able to spot potential danger signals and therefore be in a better position to make a judgement call should similar situations arise again, given that past behaviour is the best indicator of future behaviour. However, it is also important not to get carried away by the past and constantly be seeking signs that a client is about to run amok. It is also necessary to take account of new triggers, as Kemshall (1996) points out:

...there is often an over emphasis upon known existing problems to the exclusion of learning about new ones ... the tendency for services to focus on known 'dangerousness' rather than to consider the nature of the risks presently before them.

Mark's previous offending, at least in recent years, involved property crime and he had not been involved in violent offending for about 8 years. If it had not been for the diagnosis of psychopathy, and the time in a Special Hospital, would Mark be subject to the same level of concern? There would seem to be numerous recidivistic burglars who are not considered

'dangerous'. One might question the extent that Mark's behaviour remained suggestive of psychopathy, especially since he had not been psychiatrically assessed for almost 8 years. From the limited contact the probation service had been able to maintain before 1997 and the end of his at that time most recent custodial sentence, he remained a man who appeared to be self-centred and demanding of others, to obtain what he perceived to be 'his rights'. Attempts to engage Mark in considering victims, particularly in the aggravated burglary, proved pointless. He had an inability to either empathise with the suffering he had caused, or even acknowledge that he had done anything wrong. He repeatedly stated he had 'just pushed him out of the way'. In fact, he had assaulted an elderly man in order to escape from his house, using force which was, by any criteria, excessive. Should he be confronted again, there is no reason to believe that he would act differently. His behaviour corresponds closely to the accepted presentation for psychopathy, so he remains a potentially violent man.

Although trying to determine the likelihood of violence is a fundamental issue in risk assessment, making a prediction of re-offending is also important. Previous convictions have highlighted the fact that Mark burgles houses in his immediate neighbourhood. If he could live in settled accommodation then, at the very least, the police would be aware of the risk of burglary to that area. Previous attempts to find Mark accommodation had proved unsuccessful. It was, therefore, a priority to obtain a commitment from the local authority to house him on release. The local authority have a statutory obligation to find accommodation for the vulnerable. Though Mark could be regarded as a predatory and dangerous man, liaison with the local housing department produced assurances that, given his mental disorder, a flat would be found on release. Although he distrusts probation officers almost as much as psychiatrists, Mark could see the benefit in agreeing to a new assessment, allowing the re-involvement of health services in his case. As anticipated, the diagnosis from a forensic psychiatrist, new to the area, was of 'severe antisocial personality disorder'. He also made clear that he was not willing to offer any treatment other than to suggest that Mark consider HMP Grendon with its treatment centre for his next sentence!

While the lack of input from health services was obviously disappointing for the other agencies involved, one positive feature of the assessment was that on his release Mark was offered a flat in a block of 12. For the first time in his life, he had the opportunity to have a settled base and a generous community care grant from the Department of Social Security gave him the start that he had asked for. The incongruity is obvious. It appears that the psychiatrist was prepared to assess Mark as ill enough to warrant priority housing, but not ill enough for psychiatric treatment.

While the mental health services were unwilling to entertain the idea of offering even outpatient care, the other agencies, including housing and the police, met regularly to share information and concerns. Given Mark had previously followed a predictable pattern of offending, committing burglaries in the immediate vicinity of where he was living, the local police were anxious that he remained in one place. They decided that for the first few weeks they would keep a visible presence, to ensure Mark knew he was under surveillance. Mark found this irritating, particularly when he was stopped for driving whilst disqualified. This led to his appearance in court and being placed on probation, with the result that even when his post-custody licence period ended, statutory contact would continue.

Mark had been at liberty for over 8 months before further offences led to a prison sentence and the revocation of the probation order. While this was double the length of time he had previously been able to maintain in the community, and his rate of offending slowed, the situation is that on his release he will not be subject to statutory supervision. He has also been assessed as intentionally homeless, which allows the local authority to withdraw their offer of accommodation. He will therefore be homeless, without money, and probably very angry, on his release. Furthermore, he faces court proceedings for a

burglary in the vicinity of his flat, although it was committed during daylight hours, whilst the house was unoccupied.

Mark's reporting with his probation officer had been good, initially attending weekly, then every fortnight. This enabled high levels of monitoring and surveillance. He was also a little more prepared to engage in the relationship with his officer and a sense of trust was, perhaps, beginning to develop. Certainly, he was prepared to discuss his day-to-day worries, without ever disclosing incidents from the past. With time, the barriers to more open communication may have further diminished. If, as seems likely, further contact is made with Mark, then this relationship could be developed. In this respect, despite continued offending, risk management could be said to have been moderately successful.

An alternative view might be that nothing positive was achieved evidenced by other incidents. Mark was unused to social living and his behaviour toward his neighbours, many of whom are elderly, left them terrified of him. Loud music, abusive language and criminal friends visiting at all hours of the day and night created problems. On one occasion, which the police are currently investigating, friends of Mark brought another man to the flat and proceeded to torture him regarding a supposed drug debt. The victim of this assault was then alleged to have murdered one of those present. Mark discovered the body of his friend and contacted the police. It may be that Mark was simply unfortunate in being involved on the periphery of these very serious offences, or it may be that he is more deeply involved. Whatever happened, over the following weeks before his imprisonment, Mark's flat was broken into and ransacked on several occasions, and he bought himself a large dog.

Conclusion

Can any one organisation take responsibility for people like Mark? Does the very nature of psychopathy make such individuals too dangerous to manage in open society, no matter what strategy is implemented to minimise the risk? Sutton (1997) believes:

Psychopaths are rational and aware of what they are doing and why. Their behaviour is as a result of choice.

If this is so, then must we endure Mark until he becomes too old to offend or commits an offence so serious that he goes to prison for many years? If an answer is to be found, then the organisations at the forefront of assessing risk, criminal justice and health have to take on mutually supportive roles. Both can learn from each other:

Health services may benefit where good local probation practice has been identified in such areas as skills of assessment and case management; decision making support structures; crisis management and rapid reaction. Equally the probation service may

benefit from local NHS expertise such as that developed in forensic psychology assessments.

Department of Health 1997

A policy of containment cannot be the only solution. An alternative must be found and, by including practitioners such as forensic community psychiatric nurses to liaise closely with criminal justice organisations, the gaps in provision for those with personality disorders can begin to be addressed. It still seems strange that, at the age of 15, a child can be labelled a psychopath and hospitalised for the best part of 10 years, fail to conform to the treatment regime, be declared untreatable and inflicted onto society without a backward glance. This tacit avoidance of any moral responsibility for future care and social survival is, in my opinion, plainly wrong.

REFERENCES

Children Act 1989. HMSO, London, ch 41

Criminal Justice Act 1991. HMSO, London, ch 53

Criminal Justice Act 1993. HMSO, London, ch 36

Department of Health and Welsh Office 1983 Code of practice. Mental Health Act, 2nd edn. HMSO, London

Department of Health and Home Office 1992 Review of health and social services for mentally disordered offenders and others requiring similar services (Reed Report). HMSO, London

Department of Health 1997 Probation and health. A guidance document aimed at promoting effective working between the health and probation services. HMSO, London

Gunn J, Madden T, Swinton M 1991 Mentally disordered prisoners. Home Office, HMSO, London

Hare R 1995 Psychopaths. New trends in research. Harvard Mental Health Letter. September 1995

Mental Health Act 1959. HMSO, London

Mental Health Act 1983. HMSO, London

Home Office 1995 National standards for the supervision of offenders in the community. Home Office Probation Division, HMSO, London

Kemshall J 1996 Risk assessment. Fuzzy thinking or decisions in action? Probation Journal (September)

Prins H 1988 Will they do it again? The problem of the assessment of dangerousness. In: McKay R, Russell K (eds) Psychiatric disorders and the criminal process. Leicester Polytechnic Law School Monograph 25(3): 88

Sex Offender Act 1997. HMSO, London, ch 51

Sutton D 1997 Dangerous offenders and public safety. unpublished presentation at Cognitive Centre Foundation Conference

Diversion from custody

Simon Jones

Introduction

This case study shows how the process of diverting mentally disordered offenders from custody is implemented in a local Magistrates' court. An examination of the historical treatment by the criminal justice system and psychiatry of mentally disordered offenders is described together with an overview of current service provision. Methods of data collection are described together with a detailed picture of the models used in the assessment procedure utilised in the case of Paul, a young man suffering from schizophrenia. The results of this process and the subsequent interventions are outlined culminating in the multi-agency discussion on the disposal of the case.

Mentally disordered offenders and diversion from custody

Mentally disordered offenders have historically been remanded in custody to enable reports and recommendations for treatment to be completed by psychiatrists. This has often been the start of an extended period of remand that has not always led to successful and appropriate health outcomes (Bowden 1978, Coid 1988). Conditions in remand prisons are, in general, not compatible with providing suitable care for mentally disordered offenders (Fennel 1991) as the treatment provisions of the Mental Health Act do not apply, except under common law. Regimes have frequently been criticised and the increased number of suicides blamed on inappropriate detention

(Herbs & Gunn 1990, Home Office 1990a). Mentally disordered offenders remanded for reports included both individuals who required immediate hospitalisation and those who needed only out-patient care and reconnection with local generic services (Bowden 1978, Faulk & Trafford 1975). Often the main reason for the remand in custody was the inability on the part of the offender to provide evidence of residence (Joseph & Potter 1993).

Traditionally, the system of collecting psychiatric reports was rather cumbersome. If a mental disorder was suspected, a request would be made to the prison medical officer to arrange psychiatric opinions. There would be a delay in organising the assessment followed by further delays in the disposal of the case at court. If, following the psychiatric assessment, a disposal under the Mental Health Act was recommended, there was a further delay whilst a bed was found. Generally, these factors combined to make a mentally disordered offender more likely to be diverted into custody than out of it.

Home Office circulars 66/90 and 12/95 (Home Office 1990b, 1995) highlight provision for keeping mentally disordered offenders out of remand prisons by encouraging strategies such as multi-agency working and diversion from custody schemes. Reed endorsed this and suggested that assessment schemes should feature at all Magistrates' courts (Department of Health and Home Office 1991). These schemes should be planned as part of the overall local community psychiatric provision and should reflect local need and availability of health and social care (Henderson & Field 1996, Hudson et al 1995). The aims are to intervene at an early stage in the criminal justice system, by providing the courts with a mental health assessment that would suggest alternatives to custody via treatment or support in more appropriate settings.

Establishing the court diversion scheme

The local court diversion scheme, featured in this case study, was established between the local NHS Trust, social services and the Magistrates' courts at Northallerton and Richmond, North Yorkshire. The forensic community psychiatric nurse (FCPN) attended the Magistrates' courts two mornings per week to offer assessments and advice to all court users. Those individuals appearing on days when the FCPN was unavailable were remanded until the next available visiting day. Protocols have been established to facilitate the sharing of information between agencies and easy access was arranged to Crown Prosecution Service (CPS) files, defence solicitors and probation officers. In addition, further health information was available via the Trust's patient information system, to which the FCPN had access. Referrals were taken from any court service user.

CASE STUDY: PAUL
Referral

Paul was referred to me, the FCPN, by the duty probation officer who had seen him at the court the previous day. Following concerns he was remanded in custody to re-appear the following day when the FCPN would be in attendance. Bail was refused because of the nature of the charge and concerns over Paul's vulnerability. It was reported that he had made statements containing evidence of persecutory and delusional thoughts, and was very agitated at interview with the probation officer. The CPS informed me that he was charged with assault occasioning actual bodily harm. The incident arose when Paul was standing on the platform at the local railway station when he approached a group of five youths. A conversation took place during which Paul accused the youths of 'staring him out'. The youths found the whole incident rather bizarre and, according to their statements, he just lunged at them, assaulting two of the party, causing minor cuts and bruises. The station attendant called the police who attended and arrested Paul. At subsequent interview, Paul claimed that his actions were in self-defence as he thought that the youths were about to assault him.

History

Reviewing Paul's psychiatric history through the patient information system, and eliciting further details from his case notes over the telephone, I was able to build up a picture of Paul's mental health. The CPS furnished details of Paul's previous convictions, which consisted of six minor public order offences for which he received non-custodial sentences.

He had first come to the notice of health services in 1993, when his parents reported that he would not leave his bedroom, exhibiting physical and verbal aggression whenever his family approached him. This led to an admission to hospital, initially under section 2 of the Mental Health Act 1983, later converted to section 3. He was diagnosed as having a schizophrenic illness, prescribed depot neuroleptic medication and discharged with follow-up care provided by a community psychiatric nurse (CPN). He also attended the local day hospital. 3 years later he had another brief admission, relapsing after refusing his medication. Since being discharged this time, the periods between appointments with his CPN have lengthened and he is only being seen at 6-monthly intervals.

Assessment interview

My initial goal was to build a rapport with Paul as quickly as possible owing to the time and environmental constraints of conducting assessments in the cell area. This was achieved using skills of engagement, reflection, paraphrasing and reassurance, identified as being of particular importance when in the initial stages of relationship-building (Egan 1990, Hawton et al 1989). In order that Paul confided in me, I had to communicate my understanding of his predicament and my commitment to help him find the most appropriate outcome. The assessment process consisted of a semi-structured interview, aimed at securing socio-demographic data and a detailed psychiatric history. The Brief Psychiatric Rating Scale (BPRS) (Overall & Gorham 1962) was also employed in assessing mental state and the overall severity of the psychiatric disturbance. The Global Assessment Scale (GAS) (Endicott 1976) was also used. These two scales were chosen primarily for their brevity, as speed of completion is of particular importance when interviewing in custody. I was able to both relax Paul, making him feel less threatened and observe his levels of functioning and behaviour. I also completed a risk assessment using a weighted risk indicator.

Paul presented as a casually dressed and fairly fit-looking young man. His eye contact was reasonable, assisting in the engagement process. I explained the purpose of the assessment, whilst at the same time observing his behaviour. He appeared somewhat distant on occasion and was easily distracted by the noises common to the cell areas of courts. The immediate striking feature about Paul was his disorganised and occasionally incomprehensible speech patterns, lacking in logical structure. This was more prominent when I enquired about his thoughts and feelings or asked him to describe events in detail. Paul also told me that he heard external, background voices, talking about him and his sister. He claimed that he was unable to control these voices and it was these phenomena that were present when he assaulted the youths. I was able to identify positive symptoms of thought disorder and a certain amount of emotional withdrawal. Following the structured assessment, there was time to discuss wider issues. Paul related that he was taking prescribed medication (Olanzapine 10 mg bd) but admitted to missing occasional doses.

He described an isolated existence, living alone in a bedsit, only occasionally enjoying socialising in local pubs. He denied illicit drug use but admitted drinking between 40 and 50 units of alcohol per week. He was in receipt of benefits totalling £90 per week so claimed he had no financial worries.

Interventions

Having completed the initial interview and obtained information from other sources, I now felt able to discuss Paul's case with other agencies likely to be involved and to make certain recommendations. My impression of Paul was that he was suffering from a psychotic illness and this was probably connected in some way to the offence for which he had been charged. His social functioning appeared adequate, although I was concerned that this would deteriorate if his symptoms became worse (Bellack 1990).

I felt that Paul needed a much more comprehensive assessment of his mental state and a complete review of his treatment plan. However, I did not feel that Paul's symptoms necessitated admission to hospital, as the assessment and review could be completed on an out-patient basis. I was able to discuss my assessment with Paul's psychiatrist, who agreed to review him as an out-patient, in conjunction with the community mental health team (CMHT). I produced a brief report outlining the events leading up to the incident, the current situation regarding Paul's mental health, including comments on the level of risk that he posed, and the recommended interventions to enable Paul to receive the most appropriate input into his health care needs.

The interventions recommended included the necessity for a more thorough and immediate assessment by the CMHT, attendance at the psychiatric out-patients department and request for a comprehensive report detailing a subsequent plan of care. All relevant agencies then discussed the case. Although the Crown Prosecution Service (CPS) were not willing to discontinue the legal process without speaking to the victims, they were willing to accept a 6-week adjournment to enable the psychiatric services to complete their assessment. This plan was put to the magistrates who readily agreed, and bailed Paul to re-attend the court 6 weeks later.

Subsequently, Paul saw a psychiatrist and other members of the CMHT. They reviewed his medication, arranged both structured and drop-in day care and produced a much more robust care plan which monitored Paul at more frequent intervals. Effectively, the four main elements of the care programme approach (CPA) were satisfied (Department of Health 1996). First, an assessment of Paul's health and social needs had been carried out. Second, a care plan was formulated which addressed these needs. Third,

a key-worker was appointed to monitor the delivery and effectiveness of care. Finally, regular dates for review were established and circulated to all concerned parties.

The psychiatrist provided a report detailing the above information for all agencies involved in the case, to enable a full discussion to take place and a decision to be made as to how we should proceed. The issue of confidentiality was addressed and in this case Paul gave his permission for all details of his health and background to be passed to the agencies concerned. Sharing information in these cases is sensitive but vital if effective multi-agency working is to be achieved (Ritchie et al 1994).

The CPS had spoken to the victims and acting as their advocate accepted that there was nothing to gain in proceeding with the charges. All agencies felt that the fact that Paul had been re-engaged with the psychiatric services was a positive outcome to the case.

Conclusion

This study highlights the importance of early intervention in the care and treatment of mentally disordered offenders and demonstrates the benefits of inter-agency co-operation. If Paul's mental health problems had not been identified at an early stage, he would undoubtedly have spent a considerable period of time in custody, at risk of further deterioration. This in turn could have led to his admission to hospital and a prolonged, and costly, spell as an in-patient. Instead he was identified early by court staff, who are becoming increasingly aware of mental health issues, thanks to the multi-agency initiatives and effective liaison in operation. Rapid and efficient assessment followed, leading to inclusive multi-agency discussion and care planning, effecting Paul's re-integration back into mainstream community psychiatric services. He now has a package of care that includes both medical and psychosocial interventions, and systems are in place to monitor any relapses in his mental health which could lead him to come into contact with the criminal justice system again.

REFERENCES

Bellack A 1990 An analysis of social competence in schizophrenia. British Journal of Psychiatry 156: 809–818

Bowden P 1978 Men remanded into custody for medical reports: the selection for treatment. British Journal of Psychiatry 133: 320–331

Coid J 1988 Mentally abnormal prisoners on remand: rejected or accepted by the NHS? British Medical Journal 296: 1779–1782

Department of Health 1996 Building bridges. HMSO, London

Department of Health and Home Office 1991 Review of health and social services for mentally disordered offenders and others requiring similar services. Report of the Community Advisory Group (Reed). Department of Health and Home Office, London

Egan G 1990 The skilled helper, 4th edn. Brooks/Cole, California

Endicott J 1976 The Global Assessment Scale. Archives of General Psychiatry 33: 766–771

Faulk M, Trafford P 1975 Efficacy of medical remands. Medicine Science and Law 15: 276–279

Fennel P 1991 Diversion of mentally disordered offenders from custody. Criminal Law Review: 333–348

Hawton K, Salkovskis P, Kirk J 1989 Cognitive behavioural therapy for psychiatric problems. Oxford Medical Publications, Oxford

Henderson G, Field V 1996 Overview of the commissioning and provision of services for people with mental health problems who come into contact with the criminal justice system. Mental Health Review 1(2): 11

Herbs K, Gunn J (eds) 1990 Mentally disordered offenders. Butterworth Heinemann, London

Home Office 1990a HMP Brixton: report by HM Chief Inspector of Prisons. Home Office, London

Home Office 1990b Provision for mentally disordered offenders. Circular 66/90. Home Office, London

Home Office 1995 Mentally disordered offenders – inter-agency working. Home Office, London

Hudson D, James D, Harlow P 1995 Psychiatric court liaison to Central London. Riverside Mental Health Trust, London

Joseph P, Potter M 1993 Mentally disordered homeless offenders: diversion from custody. Health Trends 22: 51–53

Overall J, Gorham D 1962 The Brief Psychiatric Rating Scale. Psychological Reports 10: 799–812

Ritchie J, Dick D, Lingham R 1994 The report of the inquiry into the care and treatment of Christopher Clunis. HMSO, London

Inter-agency working in the UK

Peter Van Der Gucht

CASE STUDY: KEVIN

Introduction

Kevin was born in a rural area, the middle of three children. He describes an insecure childhood. His mother, the youngest of a large family, was orphaned at an early age and brought up in children's homes. They have a close but ambivalent relationship, primarily damaged by her misuse of alcohol, which can see her change from caring mother to vitriolic critic in a matter of hours. He considers his father to have been a rather remote, strict disciplinarian, who was rarely at home and had extramarital affairs which undermined his mother's confidence, contributing to her heavy drinking. At school, Kevin was a bright pupil, but constantly underachieved, and was often in trouble for breaking what he considered to be petty rules. At the age of 15, he was expelled from school for headbutting the deputy head master. As a result of this assault, he was sent for 21 days to a youth detention centre.

Kevin briefly attended technical college but did not gain any qualifications. He has often flirted with the idea of returning to college, but has never followed this through. From the age of 14, Kevin freely admits to misusing a wide range of illicit substances, commencing with glue sniffing. He has also smoked cannabis, taken magic mushrooms, LSD, ecstasy and amphetamines; he has occasionally tried cocaine and, more regularly, heroin. Although the evidence suggests the contrary, he insists he is in control of his drug use.

In 1989, Kevin, his mother and younger brother moved into adjacent caravans on a remote site with sparse provisions. Shortly afterwards, he was arrested for assaulting his mother. When he subsequently appeared at court, the probation officer, who had known him since his first offence, was concerned by his strange presentation, which he believed to be caused by drug misuse. He was therefore referred to the care of the local drug and alcohol team. The consultant for this team referred him on to the consultant psychiatrist for a more complete assessment of his mental state. Because he kept absconding, he was detained under section 35 of the Mental Health Act 1983 to ensure that the assessment could be completed.

The psychiatrist concluded Kevin was suffering from a schizophreno-form psychosis, possibly triggered by drug use, with several first-rank symptoms of schizophrenia, including thought disorder, paranoid delusions, as well as lack of motivation. He also considered there was evidence of an underlying personality disorder. Despite his lack of co-operation and persistent absconding, Kevin did agree to have a depot injection prior to discharge. I believe this reflected the intensity of his distress as he has always had strong reservations about medication and the involvement of the psychiatric services, which he perceives to be over-controlling.

In hospital, he had expressed delusional ideas which were influenced by his own pseudo-religious/spiritual ideas. He believes that at the age of 5 he met a man who recognised him as 'homo-cosmo', the next evolutionary stage of man. This man had stolen his 'inner eye, atom or spiritual essence' leaving chaos, emptiness and muddled thoughts. He talked of other out of body experiences and how three people were controlling his thoughts. These ideas largely receded with treatment, although he retained his alternative philosophical perspectives. This included an interest in Zen-Buddhism and black magic. He later related these delusional beliefs back to a childhood experience when he remembered being sexually abused by an older man.

His life remained chaotic and, on my recommendation, probation services arranged an interview at a Richmond Fellowship Home. Unfortunately, it became clear he was unwell and the placement was not pursued. Within days, his behaviour had become increasingly bizarre, threatening and self-neglectful. He had run up a local hill, naked for the last part, in freezing cold conditions. After being assessed at the probation office, he was detained under section 3 of the Mental Health Act. Kevin frequently returns to this episode. 'I had been about to answer a question the doctor asked me; I knew exactly what he meant and what I should say, when the probation officer dropped his pen and broke my concentration, that's why I answered incorrectly and ended up in hospital.' He has never fully accepted the grounds for his admission to hospital.

Later in the admission he was seen by a forensic consultant psychiatrist, who diagnosed Kevin as suffering from schizophrenia, complicated by drug abuse, and that he had a schizophrenic defect state, leading potentially to the disintegration of his personality. After several months, Kevin was transferred to the local rehabilitation unit. Although he was compulsorily detained, and his appeals to the managers and mental health review tribunal were turned down, he was rapidly discharged following frequent absconding and for head-butting a staff nurse. This was without prior planning, to his mother's caravan. Because of the highly emotionally charged atmosphere, I persuaded the local government housing department to place him in the homeless unit. This placement quickly broke down as a result of him misusing drugs, neglecting himself and placing others at risk. In addition, his manner appeared aggressive and threatening. He was re-admitted to hospital as an informal patient.

There have been further admissions, many brief, in reaction to crises in his life, others for a longer, planned duration. These have been affected by outside factors, in particular accommodation. The housing department, after the earlier problems, questioned his ability to manage independently. They initially offered him short-term, sub-standard lets, which Kevin saw as a form of discrimination. The low standard of this accommodation left him demoralised as he struggled to make it homely. This resulted in frequent returns to his mother's new housing association property. Matters were not helped by the fact that he allowed local drug users to use his flat. This, in turn, increased his own levels of drug use, leading to damage to the property, including an unidentified person setting fire to his first flat. This reinforced doubts in the neighbourhood that he could manage on his own.

In 1996 his increased drug use, combined with a deterioration in his mental state, resulted in Kevin committing a number of offences, including driving whilst disqualified and theft of £300 from a family friend. He was referred to the regional forensic consultant psychiatrist who confirmed the previous diagnosis and recommended a placement in a specialist cognitive therapy unit. There were no vacancies available and he was sentenced to 10 months in prison. On discharge, he returned to live with his mother and re-encountered all the familiar pressures. He quickly re-commenced drug-taking, and, although he committed no other offences, his antisocial behaviour caused persistent complaints and he was re-admitted to hospital. After several months, and lengthy negotiations, he was offered a new tenancy by the council to be managed by a housing association which works closely with the probation department. He was placed on the Supervision Register, but the decision was taken not to place him on section 25 of the Mental Health Act. He has coped in this flat for the past 7 months with a range of inter-agency support. Though he has continued to take heroin and has had some confrontations with neighbours because of his demanding behaviour, excepting a recent charge of driving a friend's car whilst disqualified, he has avoided committing further offences. This may reflect the fact he is maturing, is less stressed living on his own and his mental health symptoms are reduced with treatment. It also shows our intervention has been moderately successful in reducing the risks Kevin presents to himself and the local community.

Identified problems/needs

Kevin has multiple problems, which one could argue were caused largely by the failure to meet his needs in childhood. On the one hand, he was offered care and love; on the other, he was rejected and criticised by his mother or disciplined by his father. This inconsistency influenced his disruptive and chaotic behaviour. The school failed to cope with his increasingly antisocial behaviour, resulting in him underachieving and leaving without any formal qualifications. As with many youths in this situation, he drifted into misusing drugs. However, his excessive experimentation may well have been influential in triggering his psychosis, or at least in exacerbating an underlying disorder, contributing to his disinhibited, demanding and aggressive behaviour.

He has experienced a variety of symptoms of schizophrenia, such as episodes of thought disorder and delusional ideas of a pseudo-religious and grandiose nature, for example, the belief he has cosmic spiritual powers and an IQ of 800. He experiences paranoid ideas that his mind is being controlled by others and thoughts inserted. There is also evidence of disintegration of personality and a lack of motivation or ability to organise his life. This in turn appears to have exacerbated the deeply engrained personality traits he had demonstrated since adolescence. The features of this include his impulsivity, refusal to accept responsibility for his actions, failure to learn from his mistakes and inability to maintain a consistent course of action.

He has formed relationships with girlfriends, but these have proved short-lived. Despite his somewhat irresponsible and demanding behaviour, Kevin has a pleasant, caring side which means he is liked by many people, who, in turn, try to protect him. Sadly, their loyalty is repeatedly tested to the limit as he fails to meet his promises. His impulsivity means he spends any money he has as soon as he receives it. Many of his offences have been related to this fact and, when combined with his low tolerance and frustration level, have led to confrontations with family, friends and neighbours. In particular, this directly contributed to the assaults on his mother, beginning as arguments, fuelled by his drug use and her alcohol consumption, leading on to loss of temper and control. Such behaviour has alienated many people in his local community, which has caused problems in finding suitable accommodation, especially in a small market town.

Interventions

The interventions employed have involved facilitating close inter-agency collaboration between probation, social services, the health authority, housing, police, courts and, as necessary, the regional forensic psychiatric unit. There have been various strands to this co-operation, which has crystallised around the section 117 planning in the context of the Care Programme Approach (CPA) being instrumental in regularly bringing together representatives of the different agencies involved. The local mentally disordered offenders group, which has representatives from health, local authority, probation, courts and the police, has engendered better links and liaison between these potentially disparate agencies and professional disciplines.

The development of a housing referral panel for people with mental health problems provided a forum to put forward Kevin's needs, which were in danger of being lost against a backcloth of fears in the local community. Despite limited housing stock and doubts about Kevin's ability to manage, accommodation was found (albeit in an area with other people stigmatised as having mental health or other problems). The tenancy is managed by a specialist housing group with links to probation and there is a clear understanding that the other agencies regularly monitor the situation. Arguably this is 'building bridges' (Department of Health 1995) in action.

There has been a commitment to offer advice and support to maintain Kevin's independence in the community, diverting him from custody and avoiding unnecessary hospitalisation. However, he has still had numerous admissions to the local psychiatric unit. Framing this

positively, these have enabled Kevin's medication to be adjusted and stabilised, Kevin has been offered an opportunity to be largely free of illicit drugs and provided with a structured environment, where his demanding behaviour has been constructively challenged by staff and fellow patients alike.

In the community, his key-worker, the community psychiatric nurse (CPN), co-ordinates the care plan, within the rubric of the CPA, which is reviewed every 3 months. The needs identified are:

1. To work towards Kevin stopping taking heroin and getting out of a drug-related routine
2. To review medication
3. To continue to help manage his finances
4. To encourage him to become involved in other activities through the involvement of paid volunteers or friends
5. To oversee and support him in his accommodation
6. To monitor any indicators of relapse, such as increased drug-taking, or emerging paranoid ideas, which might in turn raise concerns about his behaviour, requiring urgent intervention, for example, re-admission to hospital.

Kevin has been on the Supervision Register for 3 years because he is identified as a significant risk to himself and others because of the severity of his mental health problems, exacerbated by his drug misuse and previous episodes of violence, particularly towards his mother.

His CPN gives Kevin his weekly depot injection, which often requires skilful negotiation because of his ambivalent feelings about medication. His probation officer has seen Kevin on a flexible basis, in a voluntary and statutory capacity, providing regular supervision sessions, looking to provide opportunities for involvement in various activities, such as motorbike scrambling, or motor mechanics, as well as providing a concerned, listening ear. Kevin has recently been placed on probation again, following another driving offence. He is getting to know a new officer after seeing the same worker for 16 years.

They are both having to work hard to establish their relationship.

As his social worker, I have called to see Kevin and his mother on at least a weekly basis. It was agreed with Kevin and my co-workers that I should act as appointee, to provide some structure and avoid him spending his benefit immediately. This has given him back some control and ensured his ability to regularly pay off bills and other debts and ensure his mother has money for fuel tokens and food. It reflects the strength of our relationship that this arrangement has continued, despite his reservations about being controlled.

I also provide regular support for his mother, who is vulnerable and isolated, backing her up when she is under pressure, but also challenging her when she drinks too heavily and becomes abusive. In the course of regular meetings she is able to explain her concerns and worries. I also attempt to ensure Kevin pays her for meals and other assistance she provides. In many ways, Kevin's mother remains his primary carer, providing help at all times of the day and night. She has, over recent years, despite occasional binges, decreased her drinking significantly, and this has greatly reduced the volatility in their relationship.

Despite a tense relationship with the housing department, close inter-departmental working has previously secured him two short-term tenancies. Most recently, the council has allowed a specialist housing association to manage one of their properties and sub-let it to Kevin. For the first time, he feels he has been given reasonable accommodation. He welcomes the support of the housing worker. Although there have been complaints from neighbours because of his demanding behaviour, the police have responded positively by doing a joint visit with me to reinforce the seriousness of these concerns.

A member of the rehabilitation team calls regularly but has been unable to interest him in anything other than occasional trips out. He is banned from the local drop-in facility and refuses to attend the day centre. I am trying to arrange for an experienced volunteer, paid from the Independent Living Fund, to offer him valued time, appropriate to his own wants.

The voluntary and statutory drug teams have been involved intermittently. His consultant introduced a methadone programme to try to wean him off heroin. It is too early to know how successful this will be.

We have been able to call on the expertise of the regional forensic psychiatrists, who have offered advice on diagnosis, dangerousness and vulnerability and contributed helpfully to treatment plans both for his mental health and his offending behaviour. In the past, Kevin has been too readily dismissed as someone with a personality disorder, a habitual offender and drug user who was not deserving of psychiatric services. Clarification of the diagnosis has helped various stakeholders understand that Kevin does indeed suffer from schizophrenia, which needs to be treated and addressed to avoid a total disintegration of his personality. Furthermore, it is realised that his tendency to impulsivity and disinhibition had been increased by his illness, and he needed a lot of support, care and protection to cope with these pressures. This has helped avoid his behaviour spiralling out of control into a state of anomie.

Outcomes

The key aim of our joint intervention has been to prevent escalation in Kevin's offending behaviour. There was a real danger that he would face periods of incarceration in prison or the regional secure unit because of his antisocial behaviour. Our approach has failed to prevent him from misusing drugs, in particular heroin. However, it may be unrealistic to expect him to totally abstain, as there are so many pressures for him to continue. He has a lack of satisfaction in his life that heroin briefly provides. His mother misuses alcohol and his brother, sister and brother-in-law are all heroin users. Other drug users tend to be the people that most accept him.

Depot medication has been partly successful in treating his thought disorder, agitation and distress, though it has also caused severe side effects. He stands and walks in an odd, rigid manner, which leads to further stigmatisation, as he looks different. Attempts to prevent side effects by reducing or changing his medication have not been entirely successful. His suspicions and agitation have increased as the medication has been reduced.

Social, emotional and practical support has proved important in reducing a further disintegration of his personality. He expresses intermittent anger that his life is being over-controlled by people in authority, yet he continues to accept his depot injection as well as myself as appointee. He resents this interference on one level, but on another recognises that it provides him with the control and structure he is unable to provide for himself at this time. The involvement of a range of workers has provided him and his mother with positive, but not uncritical, assistance. He largely experiences the world as a hostile, friendless place and our support has given him reassurance that, even though we may condemn some of his actions, he remains valued and respected as an individual. This, in turn, has had a beneficial effect for his mother, helping to limit her drinking and the volatility of their relationship.

Reflection on practice

This case study has described inter-agency working over a number of years. At times, there have been tensions between the different services involved. For example, Kevin has been discharged suddenly, without clear planning, on two occasions because of his disruptive behaviour. This reflected divisions of opinion between staff who, variously, see him on stages of a continuum between personality-disordered drug user through to an individual with multiple problems, including schizophrenia. The community team has strongly challenged this precipitative action and have insisted that no discharge should take place without paying attention to proper process, including convening a 117 meeting, with all the relevant personnel informed.

In reality, Kevin has a combination of all these characteristics. He has been damaged by a troubled childhood, which has been the root cause of his impulsive, demanding, drug-using behaviour, and, possibly, contributed to the development of schizophrenia. We have adopted a pragmatic approach, attempting to flexibly adjust and react to his situation, virtually on a daily basis. This has reduced and contained the excesses of his behaviour, by bringing some order to his life. Confronting Kevin about aspects of his behaviour, and encouraging reflection on how this undermines his relationships with others, has been linked to acknowledging how it is unacceptable to assault his mother however much feels provoked. Progress has been made in helping Kevin to manage his finances, rather than waste his money indiscriminately, which ironically gives him back some control.

A psychosocial intervention, combined with the treatment of his symptoms of schizophrenia, has helped him to mature, and to realise an independence he has wanted, but struggled to achieve. He remains dissatisfied with much of his life, using heroin as a simple route to gratification. Though he has committed further offences, like driving whilst disqualified, these have been less frequent or serious than in the past.

He has, in the main, been diverted from custody through the close collaboration between probation, social services, health authority, his solicitor and the courts who have worked to try to deal with his offending behaviour in the community rather than in prison. Even his one prison sentence did not prove as destructive as had been feared. He received a custodial sentence only because we were unable to find a vacancy in a specialist hospital unit, given the reluctance of the local psychiatric unit to admit him at this time. However, he has since been successfully re-admitted to this unit, with this facility now forming an important part of his overall package of care, if the need arises.

There have been critics of our approach who have argued that Kevin should have taken more responsibility for his actions, but I believe his treatment has more effectively helped him to face up to his responsibilities and the consequences of his actions. In some ways, prison provided him with an institutional setting where decisions were taken for him; in the community, he is being encouraged to think before he acts and to move towards increased independence. My view is that intervention has tried to meet the complexity of his individual needs. The prison system, at the present time, is designed as a punishment not as a treatment. After a prison sentence, he would return, as he did, having experienced containment, but not rehabilitation.

Conclusion

Inter-agency collaboration has succeeded, to some degree, in reducing incidents of Kevin's antisocial behaviour. He continues to be a troubled young man, who misuses drugs and whose behaviour can be both demanding and threatening. However, he has been living independently in pleasant accommodation for over 6 months, with relatively few complaints, although tensions undoubtedly exist. There is still a danger this could break down, leading to a further deterioration in his offending or aggressive behaviour. However, the close collaboration of individuals from the different agencies involved has provided a network for regular formal liaison, underpinned by section 117 after-care meetings. These should identify early warning signs and enable us to proactively manage any relapse or deterioration.

REFERENCE

Department of Health 1995 Building bridges: a guide to arrangements for inter-agency working for the care and protection of severely mentally ill people. HMSO, London

CONTENTS

Inter-agency working in the USA

Ute Goldkuhle

Introduction

I have been a criminal all my life, or most of my life, done drugs, drank, stole cars, broke into houses, beat up people, and a lot more. Started when I was about 10. I spent most of my teenage time in the locker, and twice in prison since then. Don't want to go back anymore; it's over for me. I have four kids; I want to be a better father to them. My dad beat me unconscious; he used a belt; my mom did drugs and the streets, then I helped her. My dad was always drunk and beat us kids, but I got it most. I don't know why. I started beating my kids, I don't know why. I beat my girlfriend and she beat me. But one thing, I never used a belt or cords, only hand and fist. I don't want that life anymore but I get such a rage sometimes, I don't know…

Sam was on parole and residing in an assisted-living programme. He and his family came to my attention as a result of teaching and clinical practice in community health nursing. Sam, his partner Judy, and their four children represent the profile of a high-risk population in communities throughout the USA. Such risk is a challenge to the delivery of effective health management in close co-ordination with correctional health, community health and supportive services.

Criminal activity takes place within an inter-related mesh of social factors that 'play significant causal, effectual, or augmenting roles with regard to the state of health or illness of the group or society' (Hanlon & Pickett 1979: 120). In this sense crime is violence against the community and a decade ago was identified by the Surgeon General as a major public health

317

Box 11.1 Examples of community-based initiatives since 1990

OFFICE OF JUSTICE PROGRAMS
Source. Robinson 1996a
Weed and Seed Programs
A neighbourhood-based, multi-agency approach to law enforcement and community revitalisation in high crime areas. Programme strategy integrates Federal, State and local law enforcement and criminal justice resources with corresponding human services to weed out crime and prevent it from re-occurring. By 1996, more than 76 communities across the country were implementing Weed and Seed.
Project PACT (Pulling America's Communities Together)
PACT builds on Weed and Seed strategy. Its goal is to empower local communities to address youth violence by developing broad-based, co-ordinated, anti-violence strategies that incorporate the resources of Federal, State and local government agencies, law enforcement, schools, businesses and community organisations. Programmes include a broad range of components, such as after-school, mentoring and family strengthening programmes; mental health services; gang prevention, intervention and suppression for schools; and initiatives for serious, violent and chronic offenders.
Safe-Futures Program (Office of Juvenile Justice and Delinquency Prevention)
The programme's specific focus is on youth violence. Efforts are community-based, multi-disciplinary to provide a continuum of broad range services, including after-school, mentoring and family-strengthening programmes; mental health services, gang prevention, intervention and suppression; and initiatives for serious, violent and chronic offenders.

PUBLIC HEALTH /CORRECTIONS COLLABORATIONS
Source. Hammett 1998
Rhode Island AIDS Services After Prison (ASAP)
Collaborations of the State Department of Health, the State Department of Corrections, academic medical center (Miriam Hospital, affiliated with Brown University) and approximately 40 community-based organisations. Agencies of AIDS service providers, case management (mental health, hospice), medical services, housing services, drug treatment programmes and State/Federal Agencies formed a structured partnership programme to case manage populations who are at high risk for HIV/AIDS, STDs and TB on a long-term basis in treatment, follow-up and prevention methods. Collaborations involve regular meetings, disease surveillance, policies, legislative proposals and union issues in the correctional facilities and after release in the community.
New York State's Model of Collaboration
Collaborations between the New York State Department of Health and the Department of Correctional Services on HIV/AIDS and TB involve almost constant interaction between the two agencies at both central office and facility levels. Collaborative services focus more on correctional facilities to provide disease surveillance, staff training, inmate education, clinical protocol development, testing, screening and follow-up of treatment when released to the community.

---

problem of epidemic proportions (Robinson 1996). The consequences of crime can rob the community of its vitality and deplete it of its healthful existence, with far-reaching consequences for the entire public. It signals illness in the community.

Over 10 years ago, the Attorney General's office recognised that the criminal justice system would fail to reduce crime without comprehensive, collaborative, community efforts. This stimulated many pioneering initiatives seeking broad-based, co-ordinated, anti-violence strategies at national, State and local levels. Communities responded by bringing together government officials, service providers, business people and residents themselves to attack crime, identifying crime-related problems and mobilising a broad spectrum of resources (Robinson 1996). Since that time, many more programmes have evolved, targeting drug treatment, mental health and young people, complementing community policing (see Box 11.1).

The medical community, particularly in the private sector, has largely remained distant from mental health, social services and other community efforts. Part of this reluctance may stem from a limited understanding of health-related issues surrounding crime, including the health risks and needs of the offenders, victims and their families. From the medical perspective, there is sparse discussion in the health science literature relating crime and violence in terms of a biopsychosocial profile. Only recently have some select health care providers and public health agencies recognised the importance of health interventions within judicial settings, or potential benefits of their services to the health of the larger community (Conklin et al 1998, Goldkuhle 1995, Hammett 1998).

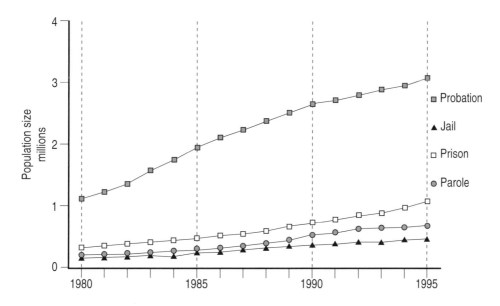

Fig. 11.1   Correctional populations in the USA 1980 to 1995.

Impact of the 'crime epidemic'

The USA is plagued by crime in nearly epidemic proportions. Sam is one of more than 5 million people who, in 1995, were under some form of correctional supervision. Over the past 30 years, the increase of the correctional population maintained an upward trend in all categories: incarceration, parole and probation (Fig. 11.1). The inmate population has doubled within a decade at an average yearly increase of nearly 8%, from 600 000 in 1988 to more than 1.7 million prisoners in 1998, which is close to 1% of the national population. Drug-use violations or related crimes and violent offences account for most of the convictions (Hammett 1998, US Department of Justice 1998).

The crime data beg some questions about whether correctional programmes are effective or whether incarceration is a sufficient deterrent to criminal activities. Reportedly, almost two-thirds of defendants charged with a felony in the 75 most populated counties, and released in May 1992, have since been re-arrested, either for a new offence or the violation of conditions regarding their pre-trial release (US Department of Justice 1998). Sam is representative of these statistics. Nearly all inmates return to the community. Without adequate and appropriate follow-up services, some will, most likely, place themselves or others in danger. When released from incarceration, they often return to harmful and unhealthy lifestyles or face rejection from family and friends. Infectious diseases among incarcerated populations are far more prevalent than in the general population, notably sexually transmitted diseases (STDs), HIV and tuberculosis (TB) (Hammett 1998). In the context of returning to community life, this is one more dimension to the cost of high-risk behaviours.

Health profile of the offender population

Sam's background typifies the profile of the majority of the offender population, being proportionally more likely to possess minority status, limited educational achievements, low income and impoverished circumstances, unemployment and homelessness. Disturbed family relationships, including experience of abuse and neglect, are common. Crime and misuse of alcohol, drugs and other substances are part of the life history of approximately 85% of the inmate population (ACA 1990, US Department of Justice 1996). The majority come from families of whom at least one member has a criminal record, or is incarcerated, and in most cases prisoners are associated with others involved in crime-related activities (US Department of Justice 1997).

With such complex social backgrounds, the overall health of the offender population is compromised, often severely. High rates of psychiatric disorder and psychological distress associated with exposure to traumatic events are common among the prison population (Jordan et al 1996, Levy 1997). Chronic medical problems such as diabetes, heart disease, musculoskeletal complaints, infectious diseases and multi-system involvements are again reported to be higher than the general population (Carp & Schade 1992, Peternelj-Taylor 1998, Weisfuse et al 1991).

Health impact of crime and violence on family members

Of great concern are the families and those closely linked with the offender population. They are a 'hidden' group in the community, not directly accounted for, and hardly discussed in the health science literature. Since nearly 94% of the offender population are male (US Department of Justice 1996) most of the offenders' affiliates are women and children. In 1994, women were about two-thirds as likely as men to be victims of violence compared to 20 years ago (US Department of Justice 1996).

It is no longer a surprise to the medical community that abused and battered women use increased medical resources. Victims of domestic violence, compared to a control population, scored consistently higher in the uptake of services: general, behavioural and psychiatric presentations (12% vs 3%); family/marital/sexual problems, anxiety and depression (19% vs 8%); and, of women using a psychiatric emergency service, 25% had a history of domestic violence (Stark & Flitcraft 1988). Between 10 and 32%

of obstetric patients have a history of abuse (Campbell et al 1992). Among the estimated 1.4 million hospital emergency department patients treated in 1994 for non-fatal injuries, 94% were injured during an assault, including rape and sexual attacks. Some 77% knew the perpetrator, either as a relative, friend or acquaintance (US Department of Justice 1997). Battering represents the single most common source of serious injury to women, accounting for more injury than automobile accidents, mugging and rape combined (Stark & Flitcraft 1988), and the frequency of abuse is a strong predictor of the number, and severity, of reported symptoms (Follingstad et al 1991, Salber & Taliaferro 1995).

Many children of the offending adult population are vulnerable and at risk of failure to thrive, permanent health and developmental damage and continuing the crime cycle. Emotional and cognitive problems, related to family deprivation, hinder healthy psychological, social, intellectual adjustment. Delinquent youths usually have a long record of criminal misconduct (Altschuler & Armstrong 1996). Offenders or their affiliates may not be in a position to evaluate, or clearly articulate, their health care needs, nor may they understand their condition. Problems often reflect examples of ignorance, neglect, self-harming behaviour (including substance use problems), poor nutrition and health habits, or indifference (Ross & Fabiano 1986).

Several information gaps seem to be the strongest barriers to developing effective community-based, inter-agency collaborations. For instance, health care providers may not understand the scope of inter-related factors to do nwith violence and health. Equally, a marginalised population are unlikely to see their risk behaviours and health neglects in a wider context. Thus, the crime-affiliated population is disconnected from the protective shield of the community that maintains the health and vitality of its members.

Community defined

Community can be described from a variety of perspectives, not necessarily geographical.

Political boundaries, for example, demarcate a district, city, county or neighbourhood. Phenomenological boundaries, on the other hand, are made up of special populations who have a sense of belonging (Green & Kreuter 1991, Smith & Maurer 1995), with a complex, inter-related structure of interaction patterns on the basis of which certain relevant functions are performed (Trotter et al 1995: 300). These shared values, norms, communication and helping patterns (Green & Kreuter 1991) are significant factors to be considered in community resource management and service interventions.

Community through the eyes of a community health practitioner

From the perspective of a community health practitioner, a community refers to people living in the context of their environment as they continuously interact with each other and the environment (Kleinberg et al 1998). Here, community captures all aspects of living and social institutions within which people interact: home, school, hospital, prison, church and government. The interaction is dynamic and maintaining community health should be a seamless process from a total living perspective. The strength and functionality of linkages between people and resources, the unique patterns of environmental living, and how people utilise the community resources, all reflect a collective sense of belonging. That identity is the 'pulse' of the community in its vitality and health. Conversely, a community in distress brings about struggles in dealing effectively with the social ills. When protective mechanisms of resource linkages weaken, or break down, groups of people become isolated and disconnected from their own community. That is when a community no longer enjoys its full health. No single or quick fix method will suffice to control the complex health issues surrounding crime.

Ex-offenders and their families exemplify a disconnected group within the community. Most have limited, fragmented or no access to appropriate follow-up. Many cannot pay for any care needed. If care is offered, it is usually short term and focused on individuals, their crime and

addiction problems, but not on the family. There are, however, indications of change. Some public health service agencies are moving towards comprehensive collaborative care with social services and criminal justice programmes, forging inter-agency alliances in an effort to strengthen, protect, or reclaim the health of communities (see Box 11.1).

Inter-agency collaboration

Inter-agency collaboration is a relatively new direction within the American health care system as part of a managed care delivery concept, yet models of case management have been proposed since the turn of the century. To better understand the barriers in building viable inter-agency collaborations, the current era of overall changes in the American health care system needs to be realised. The system is known to be, organisationally, a loose structure in a competitive social environment (Lasker 1997). For decades, it has excelled in acute care interventions, specialisation and the development of high technology diagnostic and treatment modalities. However, American society can no longer afford spiralling health costs. Pressure for change has filtered down to every level of health care delivery. Managed care delivery methods as a system of cost containment evolved, shifting the emphasis from illness and acute care specialisation to health and wellness promotion, though many emerging health service programmes are driven more by competition than collaboration, with increasing fragmentation of services (Lasker 1997).

This is not surprising. Competitive programmes enforce independent functioning, for profit or prize, while collaborative services depend on interdependent joint efforts to survive. Thus, strong barriers of resistance, or hesitance, exist among agencies and providers towards the development of a more comprehensive unified care system, especially in community settings. This is even more pronounced in the application of health promotion for under-served and vulnerable populations who, typically, are unable to pay. Barriers of access, data gathering and information exchange, finance and structural/

organisational provisions are but a few common considerations in anticipation of successful collaborations (Hammett 1998).

Emerging collaborations and model development

Bringing together the perspectives, resources and skills of diverse health professionals and organisations in a competitive social environment is a difficult undertaking, which explains the slow development to date. Unrelenting forces of declining government funding for health care over the past decade, and mounting community pressures to regain some measure of health, have brought about new incentives in multi-disciplinary partnership building (see Box 11.1). In the absence of a guiding framework to bring together criminal justice, social and health services to collaborate effectively with community efforts (Green & Kreuter 1991, Hammett 1998), much can be learned from these efforts of the past decade.

In Box 11.1, two different approaches of community-based initiatives are presented. One, a Federal initiative, was developed by the Office of Justice Programs (OJP), with financial and technical assistance in programme development. The other initiative evolved from within State or community jurisdictions, in most cases from the Departments of Health (DOH) and Departments of Correction (DOC) with resource sharing of funding, staffing and expertise. Though diverse, both initiatives and their respective programmes share the same vision, to restore and protect the health of communities and direct their attention toward the offending population or those at risk. Most of their collaborations involve intensive psychosocial, mental health and criminal justice efforts.

While the OJP approaches focus on issues of crime and violence control, that is, public health safety issues, the DOH/DOC concentrate on infection control (HIV/AIDS, STDs, TB), while Hampton County Correctional Center (HCCC) stands out in their approach to include problems related to chronic illness or biopathology. Conklin et al (1998) indicated that the 152 known

HIV-seropositive patients at HCCC had a recidivism rate of 46% versus 72% among the general offender population. They stated that 'offenders who are involved with their health care may view themselves more positively and be less inclined to engage in criminal or unhealthy behaviors when they return to the community'. Though empirical evidence needs to show that health care involvement may contribute to a decline in recidivism, the fact that health care providers have begun to link health behaviour with criminal behaviour is promising.

The benefits of these partnerships to the health of the larger community are already evident. Specifically, a 1997 National Institution of Justice (NIJ)/Center for Disease Control (CDC) national survey examined the extent and nature of public health/correction collaborations in the prevention and treatment of HIV/AIDS, STDs and TB. Responses were received from 50 State Departments of Correction, 41 of the largest city/county jail systems, and the Federal Bureau of Prisons. In addition, 11 site visits were conducted to six States and five city-county-level jurisdictions. In the final evaluation report, Rhode Island and New York State were considered 'model' examples, having the most comprehensive and structurally organised collaborations (Hammett 1998).

From a public health perspective, this survey is significant because: it includes health care for the offender population; it is the most up-to-date and comprehensive survey on the subject; and it is the only national evaluation report on diverse interagency collaboration developments to look at administration and infrastructure, policy development and service delivery. The study also revealed that virtually all correctional systems examined had at least some collaborative ventures with public health agencies related to disease surveillance, staff training, legislation and policy development, education/prevention programmes, testing/screening and follow-up and treatment services. Effects were seen in decreased morbidity in STDs, improved case finding and registry for follow-up and continuity of treatment interventions and social support when inmates returned to the community. Most importantly, the correctional facilities became permeable to the community in service interventions and resource sharing, which made the transitions for the inmates back to the community easier.

Aside from the model programmes and the HCCC, discharge planning and continuity of medical services from correctional facilities to the community were mostly inadequate across services. Although public health and correctional agencies have complementary missions in the health and safety of the larger community (Hammett 1998), the difficulty in overcoming

respective differences in perspectives, philosophies and priorities remains a strong barrier to collaboration.

Common facilitative and limiting factors

What facilitated the aforementioned successful collaborations? Hammett (1998) identified three key elements: strong commitment, willingness to open facilities to outside agencies and sensitivity to the concerns of both corrections and public health. Negative personal attitudes to crime or institutionalised positions can impede deeper levels of analysis. This author was once told by a community health nurse supervisor that her agency was not prepared to offer services to men on parole because 'the safety of the nurses comes first'. Similarly, the director of a leading hospital stated that nurses should not be concerned about this population, 'after all, they are criminals and have harmed others'. Yet, the majority of the population with a criminal history and their affiliates belong to high-risk and vulnerable groups in communities, with a complex set of psychosocial and physical needs, as indicated in Box 11.2.

Box 11.2   Population at risk

Offenders/ex-offenders
Addicted
Impoverished
Disabled, brain-injured
Families (violent, abusive)
Homeless
Immigrants/refugees
Teen mothers/parents
Children
Ethnic minorities
Unemployed
Women
School dropout
Suicidal
Mentally ill/disturbed

Box 11.3   Facilitative and hindering factors in inter-agency collaborations

FACILITATIVE FACTORS
Human
- Attitudes, perceptions and philosophies
- Clear vision of potential benefits of collaborative interventions to the larger community
- Acceptance of strength, limitations, capacities of various resources

Structural
- Time allocation to planning, co-ordination
- System for: assessment, data collection, tracking, evaluation, information exchange, oversight
- Funding mechanism for resource exchange, e.g. staff, liaison, expertise
- Formalised collaborative agreement
- Inter-agency relationship

Procedural
- Demonstrating a need for collaboration
- Use of adequate information technology
- Common-ground intervention approach
- Regular meetings

HINDERING FACTORS
Human
- Attitudes, perceptions, philosophies
- Level of knowledge, understanding of causal factors or problems
- Resistance to change, innovations
- Level of community acceptance or resistance

Structural
- Different organisational structures
- Insufficient, inappropriate or inequitable funding, staff, expertise, or support systems, time allocation
- Inadequate information technology/exchange
- Level of efficiency and effectiveness
- Programme comprehensiveness and efficiency

Procedural
- Inadequate planning, evaluation
- Limited to no follow-up
- Lack of supervision of special projects
- Level of comprehensive programme strategies

In planning or developing inter-agency collaborative strategies for health interventions, positive and negative factors need to be considered. Box 11.3 presents an organised summary of facilitative and hindering factors as to whether an intervention plan fits with the structural system of other possibly participating agencies, and whether a plan is compatible with procedural systems, human commitment and attitudes. Another critical factor to be highlighted is 'time', which 'is inflexible in its supply and affects the availability and cost of all other resources' (Green & Kreuter 1991: 190).

An intervention plan or collaboration strategy must either adapt to the existing policy of the organisation or be changed. If neither is workable, another agency must be considered for partnership. This is critical when community health service agencies plan to link with judicial services. Often, strict safety rules, restrictions and structured living arrangements have to be followed in correctional facilities, or parole agreements in the community. These security issues can become difficult barriers to overcome for community health care providers, given the potential effect upon therapeutic relationships, privacy or confidentiality, and individual's freedom of movement.

Practitioners of medicine and community health, generally, are not educated in areas of criminal justice, criminality, violence and victimisation. Nor do most officers within judicial systems adequately understand the therapeutic relationship between the client and practitioner. As such, many have to rely on personal perceptions which, to some extent, typify the barriers that are most difficult to overcome. The following description of an attempt by a community health nurse to case manage Sam provides some practical insight of the challenges involved.

CASE STUDY: SAM

Sam is a 28-year-old young man, healthy looking, slender and well groomed. He was released from prison on parole. As part of a parole agreement, he has to undergo an intensive drug rehabilitation programme in a structured, assisted-living transition home for 6 months. He suffers from severe post-traumatic stress disorder and requires drug treatment and intensive therapy. The assisted-living programme is designed for mentally or emotionally disturbed ex-offenders on parole who have a history of severe chemical dependency. The overall programme involves intensive rehabilitation services in mental health, substance abuse and vocational rehabilitation to prepare for a more healthful, self-sufficient re-integration into community life.

Sam has a crime history of repeated theft, burglary and assault to support his drug dependency of over 15 years and a record of domestic violence. Throughout his life, he has spent time in various correctional facilities: youth facility, jail and twice in prison. He is unemployed and is struggling to find a job to provide for his family. Though he earned his graduate-equivalent degree during his last imprisonment, he has not developed any marketable skills. In the past, he has had various short-lasting jobs as a labourer between incarcerations but was unable to develop any special skill. He comes from a family background of crime, substance misuse, battering and neglect. Father and mother were drug users; father has a criminal record of multiple incarcerations for assault and attempted murder; mother was a prostitute.

Sam is married and has four children, ages 9 and 8 years, and 20 and 11 months. His wife, Judy, unemployed, resides in a state-supplemented housing project and receives public assistance to care for the children. Judy did not complete high school. She has a history of alcohol misuse but no background of illicit drugs or crime involvement. Both Sam and Judy grew up in homes where violence and substance use were witnessed and experienced.

Case management: Sam and his family

While residing in a transition home, after release from a correctional facility, Sam had his first contact with a community health nurse (CHN).

The transition home provides a structured, supportive living skills programme for ex-offenders on parole who are recovering from substance addictions. Though mental health services are provided, other health care services like community health or public health nursing have not been involved.

The role of the CHN, in relation to a high-risk population, is to explore case management strategies (see Box 11.4). Crime and judicial involvement, however, brings a very different perspective to Sam's case and his place in the community. Special knowledge and skills in clinical forensic practice would be required to accurately identify the family's needs and supportive resources within the considerations of the justice system's responsibilities. A clinical forensic nurse, a rapidly evolving practice role, specialises in high-risk populations who have been afflicted with some type of violence as victim or perpetrator. There is a focus on victims of physiological and psychological trauma, criminal and interpersonal violence, evaluation and treatment of perpetrators and the families of both (Lynch 1993). Currently, only a few CHNs are prepared for clinical forensic work.

Assessment at the transition home

Though the CHN in Sam's case was not a clinical forensic nurse specialist, she approached Sam with a knowledge base of multi-disciplinary case management principles that apply to especially complex cases. One of the principles is that neither an overwhelming plan for the client nor overlooked needs will bring about hoped-for outcome results (Smith & Maurer 1995). Sam must be able to tell his story freely, if possible, to bring out in his own words a health profile and his understanding of life and living.

I have two brothers in prison; one did worse than me, he shot somebody. My dad is dead, was shot; I don't know, maybe drugs. My mom, I don't know, lost track; she always did the streets. I have a sister, she is nice but haven't seen her for a long time. I guess she got tired of me. You are all people who get education. My dad or mom beat me if I did not hustle some money or food. I am a criminal, why would you want to mess with me? People will not want to get me a job, I have to figure this out. Do you know what it means? If I do drugs, I can get $1000 bugs easy. Who would pay me $1000 bugs a night for work? You don't understand this. I get drug rehab., but this is a thing they don't understand and can't help. I only know people who do drugs. The only one I know who does no drugs is my wife. But she drinks every few days or once a week. I don't want her to drink, it's not good for the kids; we fight when she drinks. Me, at least I don't do drugs when my kids are around. She doesn't know what it is to be in the slammer, but she always sticks by me, I have to say that, and she is good with the kids. You look like me, right? But when you know I was in prison, most don't want to talk to me. I feel shame because I don't know how to talk to you. The other day we came to a dental clinic. I was all wet from sweat and nervous. I have never been there. But all were so nice, I couldn't believe it. I get all shook up over it. I couldn't say nothing. But, you see what I mean, when I talk to my guys, no sweat.

Box 11.4 Community health nursing: role and scope of practice

Definition
Community health nursing (CHN) is an umbrella term for all nurses who work in the community, including public health nursing. CHN is a synthesis of nursing and public health practice, applied to promoting and preserving the health of the community and populations. The practice is general, continuous and comprehensive with a dominant responsibility to the population as a whole, while interventions may be directed to individuals, families or groups at risk. The heart is primary prevention of illness and promotion and protection of health.
Scope of practice
The community health nurse:

- identifies sub-groups which are at high risk of illness, disability or premature death
- represents and negotiates exchanges between community and multi-disciplinary team members to effect a health care plan
- co-ordinates the assessment, planning, implementation and evaluation processes and creates alliances for the improved health of the community
- serves as communication link
- facilitates transitions between systems of care.
Sources. American Nurses Association 1980, American Public Health Association, 1980.

It is important in complex community health situations to immediately organise all information that is received from a free-flow, open-ended, dialogue. Many organising frameworks, or assessment tools, have been developed but experienced CHN practitioners eventually adopt their own organising method. Regardless of practitioner style, assessment of health, behavioural and risk factors need to consider all biopsychosocial aspects. These concepts are defined in Engel's (1977) 'health behaviour model', a structuring of interacting factors between the biological state (health status and risks), psychological processes (interpersonal relations) and social functioning (socio-demographics such as age, sex, marital status, employment). 'In this [biopsychosocial] model the biological, psychological and social context are considered as equally important dimensions, with none having a priori superiority and understanding of the nature of human behaviour in health and disease' (McHugh & Vallis 1986: 1). This model has been found to be particularly suited to an exploration of health needs and stress factors in women offenders (Goldkuhle 1995).

The rich profile provided by Sam offers insights into his perceptions of himself and his family. To demonstrate an initial organising assessment process, and the unfolding of health and support needs, specific factors can be highlighted:

Biological dimensions. Sam appears to be in good physical health. However, his health risks are numerous, related to a long-standing history of substance use: street drugs, alcohol and smoking. There is a history of physical and emotional childhood abuse. His father beat him unconscious with a belt. Both his parents had a history of drug and alcohol abuse. It is alleged that Sam's wife also misuses alcohol and that she has attacked him. His children are at high risk of physical abuse and neglect.

Psychological dimensions. Sam has difficulty with interpersonal relationships. He has physically abused his wife, children and other people and is disconnected from his mother, sister and two brothers. He feels 'shame' and has very low self-esteem. Sam perceives physical abuse as using an object, say a belt or cord. Though he wants to be a better father, ideas of responsible parenting are limited to not 'doing drugs in front of my kids'.

Socio-demographic dimensions. Sam is married and has four children. His mother's and sister's whereabouts are unknown. His father was shot dead and his two brothers are in prison. He has had minimal education and was forced to 'hustle' for money or food as a child. His income has largely been through 'stealing and dealing'.

Family interview and assessment

The next step in the assessment process involved a home visit to assess the health state of the family, specifically their strength and capacity for healthy behaviour and lifestyle changes. In most cases, problems in families can seem more obvious to the CHN than the family's actual and potential strengths, which might empower them to cope (Kleinberg et al 1998). To ensure assessment in all areas of functional patterns, family dynamics and patterns of daily living, the use of a detailed family health assessment guide is suggested as a helpful tool. Box 11.5 represents an example of such an assessment tool, adopted from the Family Wellness Assessment Guide (Kleinberg et al 1998).

The first difficulty arose in trying to contact Sam's wife, Judy, to arrange a meeting. She did not have a telephone and lived approximately 6 miles away from the transition home. Sam depended on someone else to drive him home to participate in a family assessment, aimed at developing a case management health plan. There was no friend, or family member, that Sam wanted to ask for transport because, 'all are on drugs and I don't want them around anymore.'

The family home is situated in a remote rural area, where Judy and their four children lead a socially isolated and economically disadvantaged existence. They are far from the bus station and rely upon friends or neighbours for contact with food stores, health clinics and general services. Though other family members or

---

Box 11.5   Family health assessment guide

I. Family unit
A. Family members living in household – identifiers (name, age or date of birth, sex, occupation or school)
B. Other members, significant others or friends living in household – identifiers
C. Family members not living in household – identifiers
D. Other individuals or families closely connected with the family

II. Patterns of daily living
A. Nutrition – status of members, meal preparation, financial considerations
B. Sleep/wake/rest – patterns, adequacy of sleeping arrangements, safety
C. Work/leisure – balance work with recreation, adequacy and sources of financial support
D. Physical activity and fitness – patterns, types, motivation
E. Sexuality – satisfaction, expression, safety
D. Education – status, goals and values of members

III. Intra-family dynamics
A. Patterns of communication
   1. Relationships between each dyad and of family as a unit
   2. Extra-familial – friends, neighbours, organisations, social activities
B. Role functions
   1. Roles assumed by each member
   2. Nature of role functions: flexible, complementary, reciprocal

   3. Identified unmet role functions
C. Patterns of decision-making – consensus, accommodation, de facto, unilateral, indecision
D. Norms and values – culture, religion, spirituality, priority placed on health
E. Distribution of power among members – personal and shared power
F. Patterns of conflict management – issues of importance and sources of stress, resolution
G. Energy to accomplish tasks and goals – patterns of flow, blockages, endurance, weaknesses
H. Capacity of family to change and grow over time – identification of goals and resources

IV. Environment
A. Housing – type, condition, context in community
B. Resources available – bathroom, kitchen, refrigeration, water supply, heat
C. Safety – hazards
D. Use of community resources

V. Impact of illness on family – what happens when illness strikes, when chronic or terminal

VI. Analysis of family function
A. Family health risks
B. Family health problems
C. Family health strengths

VII. Family self-assessment – capacities for self-care

Source. Kleinberg et al 1998

---

friends come and go, their activities and whereabouts are unclear; none are employed and Judy hesitantly alluded to possible drug involvement. Her two daughters, aged 9 and 8 years, were in school, a 20-month-old daughter was asleep, and her son, a healthy-looking, 11-month-old infant, was asleep in her arms. The children are reportedly in good health, doing well in school, but the two young ones are significantly behind in their immunisation schedule. Their first child was born when Judy was 16. Thereafter, each child was conceived between Sam's incarcerations, but born while he was in prison. Judy tearfully said; 'I can't do this no more,' but revealed that she is not on any precautionary birth control measures.

Pills make me sick; it's hard to go to the clinic with the kids, it's so far; the bus takes too long, the babies are too active and heavy, then I have to wait at the clinic, then I am too late to pick up the others from school.

Judy is amiable, but cautious, articulate and attentive to her children. She is overweight and feels dizzy much of the time. Every Friday night, she 'binge drinks' with girl friends after the children are asleep, consuming 15 to 20 cans of beer. She is unemployed but expressed a desire to go back to school and become a pre-school teacher.

But Sam wants to go to school, the state will pay for him, so I can't go; but I don't know how we feed the kids; food stamps are not enough; we don't want any more drugs in the house or make money on it. I love Sam. He is so good with the kids; we love our kids and want them to go to school; sometimes I talk to the teacher and school counsellor, but every day the teacher sends notes home with the kids; they are nice but they don't know about Sam; the kids cannot play until they done their homework.

There is no immediate support network. Judy's father is not in the locality and her mother is an alcoholic. When he is around, Judy's brother drives her into town to collect groceries, but he is a heavy drug user. A church is close by but Judy expressed shame to attend. She has not seen a social worker for several months and she does not know the name of the social worker responsible for her supplement services.

There is always someone else coming, when someone comes; I think I am late with my papers; I get so tired; I am happy and afraid when Sam comes home; he is good, but when he has that temper, boy … Each time he promises to do good, but then he is in prison again. I can't do it any more, I am stuck with the kids. Don't get me wrong, I love my kids.

Judy has never been offered a 'family re-adjustment programme' or some support system from either the judicial or public health nursing or social service sectors.

When asked the question: 'What do you think you can do to strengthen your family situation and what do you think would be most support-ive to you to achieve your goal?' Judy said that she wants the children go through school and be healthy:

If someone who is safe, not on drugs, and I can trust, will watch the little ones, I want to get more involved with the school; or, if someone is home when they come from school, then I don't mind taking the bus to the doctor.

Sam said that for now, he would take any job as long as he can feed the family, but '*I need to get to the job.*'

Sam and his family's strengths and capacities, their health risks and needs, when summarised from a biopsychosocial perspective, show the need for inter-agency collaboration of various service systems: health, social and judicial.

Biological dimensions

Strengths. Family members have no known illness; responsive to health guidance, open to behaviour change.

Capacities. Both parents are physically able to work, learn a new skill, or continue education if opportunities are available.

Health risks. Another unintended pregnancy; younger children not fully immunised. Sam's relapse to drug misuse. Health effects of long-standing drug use for Sam, alcohol misuse for Judy and childhood abuse for both. The children are at risk of abuse and neglect. Judy's unknown cause of dizziness and general health

problems around nutrition and body weight; insufficient money for quality diet.

Health needs. Medical health attention, immuni-sation update, family planning, drug and alcohol treatment programme; evaluation of food supply.

Psychosocial dimensions

Strengths. Willingness to make behaviour changes. Both parents openly share their family history and concerns. Expressed love for their family and desire to raise their children better than their own childhood experience. Good con-nections with school counsellor and teacher. Sam's intent to no longer connect with his friends on drugs.

Capacities. Able to communicate with mem-bers of community agencies. Willing to improve interpersonal relationship, stopping the physical abuse.

Health risks. Sam's rage. Judy's fear of Sam's relapse. Both are shy and have a feeling of shame; isolation from extended family. Potential isolation from supportive services once Sam comes home (the mental health social worker was connected with the transition home and arranging anger management and drug treat-ment programmes for Sam, but without a family focus). Risk of children's neglect.

Health needs. Family support group, involv-ing help with parenting, communication and socialisation.

Socio-demographic dimensions

Strengths. Both parents have strong desire and intent to work and support the family by legal means and desire to go to school; bus trans-portation available. School and church close by. Older children doing well in school. Judy wants to connect with a church in the neighbourhood.

Capacities. Sam and Judy are able to drive a car if available.

Health risks. Limited transportation, no car and Sam has temporarily lost his driver's licence. No telephone and limited access to community resources, shops, health clinics and social services because of distance and restricted bus schedule; all of which jeopardises service utilisation. Limited financial support (public assistance) and no savings. No vocational skills.

Health needs. Social service assessment of financial status and supportive interventions. Vocational training and job placement. A means of transportation for necessities and a system of communication.

Without doubt, the whole family has become victim to Sam's incarceration. They present a high risk of failing to achieve a healthier life. Sam's perception of responsibilities is marred by a lifelong dysfunctional existence. Risks of continuing the abuse cycle, getting involved again with illegal activities and neglect of his children are apt to totally overwhelm him once he leaves the protective environment of the transition home. Judy is in need of special support. Her alcohol problems are of great concern, but she may not be able to deal with this until some basic needs are met. These might include family planning, medical care and child immunisations, stable income from paid employment and means of transportation and communication.

Community resources and health services

The final stage of the assessment process was an exploration of the health, social and judicial service systems that were needed. Self-care initiatives have become a social institution variously expressed as self-help, self-sufficiency or improvement to encourage and empower people to take charge of their own health and become partners in their health management (Green & Kreuter 1991). Yet Sam and his family may not be in a position to conceptualise, or even understand, the self-care concept in promoting health and its long-range benefits. The family will need extensive attention and a resource network of multi-disciplinary interventions and support services. If the barriers, however, that were encountered are not overcome, the family will have minimal chance of strengthening to a level of self-sufficiency.

Prior to Sam's leaving prison, there had been no discharge planning or any connection with his family, nor was there any referral made to health or social services to assist in the transition to re-unite with the family. The parole officer was keen to collaborate with the CHN, but this was compromised by case-load responsibilities and limited resources. Owing to difficulty contacting the family, and their failure to keep home visit appointments, the case had been accorded a 'low priority' status with social services. There was no family physician; the family clinic and public health services were unaware of the domestic situation. The family's interest in the nearby church was explored for possible beginnings of resocialisation into the local community and to possibly help overcome the expressed sense of shame. The church offered some volunteer transportation, but expressed some concern regarding drug trafficking in the neighbourhood.

Conclusion

It was a challenge to test the role of a CHN by becoming the 'self-proclaimed' case manager for Sam and his family. It was an even greater challenge to test the community's readiness for collaborative efforts to provision of 'seamless' community-based health interventions; from prison, to transition home, to family and community. Ex-offenders typically experience multiple chronic conditions, severe chemical dependency, abuse, violence and neglect. Many suffer from disability, mental disorder and long-standing unhealthy lifestyles, coupled with rejection from family and community. On release, most inmates have limited, fragmented or inadequate access to appropriate follow-up because of failed service co-ordination, inefficiencies in delivery and inadequate financing.

Protecting the community and its members from the complex health effects of crime requires a comprehensive public health service commitment that includes medical health interventions and collaborations with psychosocial and judicial services. From a public health perspective, the status of this special group reflects the state of health or illness of the community of which the group is a part. Correctional facilities and community health resources rarely collaborate with services in preparation for inmate release to assure co-ordinated service

continuity or effectiveness. Efforts to enhance the health of this population can also contribute to crime prevention, by dealing with adverse social pressures, addiction, violence and risk behaviours.

REFERENCES

Altschuler D, Armstrong T 1996 Intensive aftercare for high-risk juveniles: a community care model. US Department of Justice. Office of Juvenile Justice and Delinquency Prevention, Washington DC

American Correctional Association (ACA) 1990 The female offender: what does the future hold? ACA, Laurel, Maryland

American Nurses Association (ANA) 1980 A conceptual model of community health nursing. ANA, Washington DC

American Public Health Association (APHA) Public Health Nursing Section 1980 The definition and role of public health nursing in the delivery of health care. APHA, Washington DC

Campbell J, Poland M, Waller J, Ager J 1992 Correlates of battering during pregnancy. Research in Nursing and Health 15: 219–226

Carp S, Schade L 1992 Tailoring facility programming to suit female offenders' needs. Corrections Today: 152–159

Conklin T, Lincoln T, Flanigan T 1998 A public health model to connect correctional health care with communities. American Journal of Public Health 88: 1249–1250

Engel G 1977 The need for a new medical model: a challenge for biomedicine. Science 196: 129–136

Follingstad D, Brennan A, Hause E, Polek D 1991 Factors moderating physical and psychological symptoms of battered women. Journal of Family Violence 6: 81–95

Goldkuhle U 1995 Stress factors and response effects on health services utilization among women in prison. UMI Dissertation Services, Ann Arbor, Michigan

Green L, Kreuter M 1991 Health promotion planning: an educational and environmental approach. Mayfield Publishing, Monlo Park, California

Hammett T M 1998 Research in brief: public health/corrections collaborations: prevention and treatment of HIV/AIDS, STDs, and TB. National Institute of Justice, Centers for Disease Control and Prevention, Washington DC and US Department of Justice, Office of Justice Programs, NIJ, NCJ 169590.

Hanlon J, Pickett G 1979 Social pathology and public health. Public health administration and practice. Mosby, St Louis, p 111–129

Jordan K, Schlenger W, Fairbank J, Caddell J 1996 Prevalence of psychiatric disorders among incarcerated women. Archives of General Psychiatry 53: 513–519

Kleinberg M, Holzemer S, Leonard M, Arnold J 1998 Community health nursing: an alliance for health. McGraw-Hill, New York

Lasker R 1997 The Committee on Medicine and Public Health 1997 Medicine and public health: the power of collaboration. The New York Academy of Medicine, New York

Levy M 1997 Prison health services. British Medical Journal 315: 1420–1424

Lynch V 1993 Forensic aspects of health care: new roles, new responsibilities. Journal of Psychosocial Nursing 31(11): 5–6

McHugh S, Vallis T 1986 Illness behaviour: operationalization of the biopsychosocial model. In: McHugh S, Vallis T (eds) Illness behaviour: a multidisciplinary model. Plenum Press, New York

Peternelj-Taylor C 1998 Care of individuals in correctional facilities. In: Glod C (ed) Psychiatric-mental health nursing: a psychobiological approach. F A Davis, Philadelphia

Robinson L 1996a Communities: Mobilizing against crime, making partnerships work. National Institute of Justice Journal, Washington DC, US Department of Justice, Office of Justice Programs, National Institute of Justice, August 1996, NIJ 231

Robinson L 1996b Linking community-based initiative and community justice: the Office of Justice Programs. National Institute of Justice Journal, Washington DC: US Department of Justice, Office of Justice Programs 231: 4–7

Ross R, Fabiano E 1986 Female offenders: correctional afterthoughts. McFarland Jefferson, North Carolina

Salber P, Taliaferro E 1995 A physicians' guide to domestic violence. Volcano Press, Volcano, California

Smith C, Maurer F 1995 Community health nursing: theory and practice. W B Saunders, Philadelphia

Stark E, Flitcraft A 1988 Violence among intimates: an epidemiological review. In: Van Hasselt V, Morrison L, Bellack A, Hersen M (eds) Handbook of family violence. Plenum Press, New York, p 293–318

Trotter J, Smith C, Maurer F 1995 Community assessment. In: Smith C, Maurer F (eds) Community health nursing: theory and practice. W B Saunders, Philadelphia, p 299–339

US Department of Justice 1996 Female victims of violent crime. Bureau of Justice Statistics, Selected Findings, Washington DC

US Department of Justice 1997 Violence-related injuries treated in hospital emergency departments. Bureau of Justice Statistics, Special Report, Washington DC

US Department of Justice 1998 Correctional trends. Bureau of Justice Statistics, Washington DC. Available World Wide Web: http://www.ojp.usdoj.gov/bjs/glance/htm#Crime

Weisfuse I, Greenberg B, Back S et al 1991 HIV-1 infection among New York City inmates. AIDS 5: 1133–1138

Key issues in forensic care

Social assessment of risk: the Behavioural Status Index

Phil Woods

Introduction

This case study describes a behaviourally based assessment instrument that has been developed to be part of a battery of tools to assist in the evaluation of social risk. The instrument is described before offering an example of its use in the assessment and planning of intervention strategies within a high-secure psychiatric setting.

It is without doubt that the fundamental principle underpinning care in forensic psychiatry is the assessment and management of risk. In essence, the process is concerned with three inter-related parts. First, an assessment of the risk that was posed in the past. Second, the risk posed now. Third, some indication of probable risk posed in the future. Generally speaking, mental health professionals are expected to be able to adequately assess the risk that their patients pose to both themselves and others and while this task previously lay solely on the shoulders of the forensic psychiatrist, this is certainly not the case today (Duggan 1997). It has been suggested that risk assessment is a key skill of many mental health professionals (Bingley 1995) and this relies heavily on clinical judgement from a multi-disciplinary perspective, as no single measurement device is currently available (Chiswick 1995).

Conceptual arguments exist between the differing camps of practitioners in the risk assessment field, particularly between researchers and theoreticians. Whilst one camp promotes the use of an actuarial or statistical approach to the assessment process, the other prefers a clinical emphasis. In general terms, the former has been found to be the more reliable. However, these assessments are based on static or historical variables, grounded on the assumption that an individual, coming from a population within which a certain type of behaviour is common, is more likely to display this form of behaviour (Pollock & Webster 1990). Therefore, if an actuarial approach alone is used, this can have few, if any, implications for treatment planning with mentally disordered offenders, since such approaches are essentially not about individuals, but about populations (Vinestock 1996).

Consequently, we run the risk of the 'risky individual' becoming a 'non-person' in therapeutic terms and his or her perceived risk becoming based solely on previous recorded violent incidents. Such an individual may well become static on the continuum of 'risky/non-risky' or 'non-person/person' (Hepworth 1982). Indeed, the clinician at the front line of forensic care is likely to see little importance in distant historical variables, for example, the age at which the first violent offence occurred, as having any bearing on the patient's daily treatment planning. Webster et al (1994) inform us that clinical judgment can be improved through utilising an actuarial estimate of risk as an anchor but clearly see the relevance of involving both approaches.

Following this brief look at research and theoretical difficulties, we are left with the thorny question of how to prepare mental health clinicians for this onerous task? To hinder us further, little effort has been made, to date, to develop research frameworks which can be applied alongside clinical practice (Borum 1996).

Pollock & Webster (1990) and Monahan & Steadman (1994) assist us in this enterprise by highlighting the need for assessments to be systematic and based on the population directly undergoing the assessment. Identified risk factors are required to be broken down into more manageable components, further recorded through effective treatment planning and outcomes evaluated through recovery status. In essence, we want to 'achieve the best possible grasp of the likely behaviour of an individual and to elicit detail sufficient for risk factors to be minimised and appropriately managed' (Vinestock 1996). Once we have completed our risk assessment, a risk management plan is then implemented which focuses on the likelihood of the outcome actually occurring. Vinestock (1996) describes this as a method of balancing probable consequences of decisions which formalises the decision-making process in relation to the risk of harm to self or others.

A description will now be given of a behaviourally based assessment instrument which is intended to assist in daily risk-assessment planning. This instrument represents a move towards meeting the needs of professionals seeking an appropriately operationalised version of constructs commonly relied on in multi-disciplinary planning of individualised treatment within forensic care (Robinson et al 1996).

The Behavioural Status Index

The Behavioural Status Index (BSI) is a behaviourally based assessment instrument which views risk assessment from a therapeutic standpoint (Woods & Reed 1998). This comprises key areas of cognitive–affective adjustment and skill performance and includes:

a. behaviours normally associated with 'risk' in a forensic context
b. the degree of insight into causality and current status shown by the patient
c. assessment of the patient's current communication and 'social' skills.

Through the model which the BSI proposes, these then become the three main focal areas for treatment planning in forensic mental health care. The theoretical propositions underpinning this combination are that such variables are essentially inter-related and that they are in some sense predictive of one another.

The risk sub-scale of the BSI (see Box 12.1) measures such constructs as supportive family links, elements of violence to others and self, and verbally directed aggression.

The insight sub-scale (see Box 12.2) examines an individual's cognitive constructs of reality and the communication and social skills sub-scale (see Box 12.3) principally examines social skills or adaptive social behaviour.

Identification of problems and needs using the BSI

All 70 scalar items within the BSI are scored from 1 (worst case) through to 5 (best case). Of interest

---

Box 12.1   Risk sub-scale

No.	Item.	No.	Item.
1	Family support	10	Attacks on objects without apparent trigger event
2	Serious violence to others without apparent trigger event	11	Attacks on objects following trigger event
		12	Breaches of security
3	Serious violence to others following trigger event	13	Disruptive episodes
4	Minor violence to others without apparent trigger event	14	Imitative disruption
		15	Inappropriate sexual behaviours
5	Minor violence to others following trigger event	16	Sado-masochistic behaviours
6	Serious self-harm	17	Macho gear and adornment
7	Superficial self-harm	18	Obsessive–compulsive behaviours
8	Verbal aggression without apparent trigger event	19	Substance abuse
9	Verbal aggression following trigger event	20	Psychiatric disturbance

---

Box 12.2   Insight sub-scale

No.	Item	No.	Item
1	Awareness of tension	11	Attributes liked in others
2	Description of tension	12	Events producing insecurity
3	Tension-reducing strategies	13	Events producing security
4	Recognition of negative or angry feelings	14	Antecedent events leading to treatment
5	Tension-producing thoughts	15	Ascription of responsibility
6	Tension-producing events	16	Self-appraisal
7	Personal strategy for reducing tension	17	Prioritisation of problems
8	Identifying relaxing thoughts	18	Goal-planning
9	Identifying relaxing activities	19	Compliance with therapy
10	Attributes disliked in others	20	Expectations

Box 12.3   Communication and social skills sub-scale

No.	Item.	No.	Item.
1	Facial expression	16	Conversational topics
2	Eye contact	17	Egocentric conversation
3	Orientation to others	18	Frankness
4	Body posture	19	Expressing opinions
5	Expressive gestures	20	Disagreement
6	Social distance	21	Arguments
7	Tone of voice	22	Making requests
8	Voice modulation	23	Assertiveness
9	Verbal delivery	24	Self-presentation
10	Conversational initiative	25	Social activities
11	Amount of speech	26	Emotional control
12	Fluency	27	Relationship with others
13	Turn-taking	28	Ease of communication
14	Listening skills	29	Sociability and support
15	Response to questions	30	Deferring to others

> **Box 12.4 Example of BSI item-rating scale**
>
> **3** Tension-reducing strategies
> **3.1** Has no constructive personal strategy for relieving tension and anxiety
> **3.2** Aware of problem and seeks advice or *attempts* to develop such a strategy
> **3.3** Co-operates with therapist to develop such a strategy
> **3.4** Follows the developed strategy *with encouragement and support*
> **3.5** *Spontaneously* follows an insightful and constructive personal strategy

here is that this is opposite to the scoring of existing risk scales which tend to rise as 'risk' worsens. The BSI examines behavioural performances viewed within a *normative*, rather than a *sociopathic*, frame of reference. Consequently, a higher score indicates the achievement of a more socially adaptive or 'acceptable' behavioural performance.

Assessment using the BSI is undertaken through behavioural observation and from everyday social as well as therapeutic contact with the individual. Scores are entered on a single sheet for each of the three sub-scales, allowing for visual comparison of the rating from 1 through to 5 given for the items, both within the scales and also between scales. Extensive manual and fully descriptive rating scales are used for scoring. An example of one of the item-rating scales is provided in Box 12.4. There is also a glossary of commonly used terms such as frequently and occasionally, so that raters can be more specific in their measurement. The manual has been prepared so raters have all information at hand that relates to the item which is being rated. The completion of the BSI takes anything up to 45 minutes. However, it is not necessary to complete a rating all at once.

As lower scores are indicative of poor functioning or problematic areas, these should be the main focus of concern. This is probably best explained through an example assessment that was undertaken in high-secure forensic care.

CASE STUDY: FRED

Fred is a man in his late 40s with a mental illness and a mild cognitive impairment. His illness is long standing, with the first signs having appeared in his late teens. Since the onset of his illness, Fred has been institutionalised in some way or another. Currently, he is detained in high-secure psychiatric care, where he has been for some 20 years. He has been described as a 'schizophrenic of the paranoid and violent type'.

Generally over the years, his clinical presentation has not altered significantly. He has a fixed and rigid personality, complex delusional system, lack of coping skills, refuses to accept ownership for his own actions, lacks insight and generally is not accepted as a member of any ward community. He has a long history of violent and impulsive behaviour which eventually resulted in the death of another person. It was at this point that he came into contact with the high-secure psychiatric services via the courts. He was admitted under section 37 of the Mental Health Act 1983 with section 41 restrictions for discharge. Over his stay in the services he has been troublesome and disruptive, and has had one failed attempt at rehabilitation through medium-secure services.

The above history paints a bleak picture. However, this is a not untypical presentation of a problematic individual in high-secure care; someone with complex needs, an element of treatment resistance and difficult to rehabilitate to areas of lesser security.

Although there are many items rated as less than optimal functioning (i.e. scored less than 5), to aid clarity, and as these could be seen as the most urgent areas for intervention, only the items receiving the minimum scores are reported. From the base-line assessment, we note that five items that form the BSI risk sub-scale indicate poor functioning. We find that there is frequent occurrence (regularly and predictably at intervals of less than 1 month) of minor violence to others, verbal aggression and attacks on objects, all following trigger events. There is frequent evidence of disruptive episodes and the issuing of threats to others. Although this gives us a clear picture of a man who is considered 'risky', further examination of related items which form the other two sub-scales highlights possible areas for the focus of intervention.

Tension items on the insight sub-scale indicate possible intervention areas. Fred is unable at any time to express awareness of increased tension (insight item 1), has no constructive personal strategy for relieving tension or anxiety (item 3) and is unable to articulate a strategy for preventing or reducing feelings of irritation or anger (item 7). Furthermore, he cannot identify any thoughts which are personally relaxing and pleasurable (item 8) and cannot identify any relaxing activity (item 9). He is completely unable to make a realistic appraisal of current behavioural or emotional problems (item 16), cannot decide on relative priority or urgency of problems (item 17) and finally cannot decide on a realistic goal-planning action (item 18).

From the communication and social skills sub-scale, we note a number of items that are pertinent to our above observations. Fred is very tense and cannot sit still for long (item 4), never appears to listen to others (item 14), usually argues in an aggressive but never physically violent manner but (item 21), unable to stay on good terms with others (item 27), never gives in gracefully and manifests anger and violence (item 30).

Interventions

Of course, once we have carried out our baseline BSI assessment, one can ask what exactly does this tell us, and how can our interventions focus around this? We can see from the above items that have been highlighted as problem areas that what we have is a volatile man, who at present is displaying risky behaviours. However, through focusing our thoughts around other areas of individual functioning, such as insight and communication and social skills, we have opened up the possibility of therapeutically working with Fred to reduce his risky behaviours. This is the thrust behind the BSI which logically links items that are specific to the individual to form meaningful and measurable intervention strategies.

In formulating a plan of intervention to focus on Fred's risky behaviours, we firstly focused around some of the items on the insight sub-scale. One-to-one sessions between Fred and his primary nurse were the vehicle for the interventions. Sessions lasted for approximately 1 hour and would take place once a week. If an incident occurred between sessions, the next pre-planned session was brought forward to the next available opportunity.

The focus of the sessions was to examine in detail aggressive incidents that had taken place recently as well as in the past. Specific coping strategies that Fred had employed were examined and discussion was moved towards what would have been more appropriate responses. Examination was also undertaken into what needs Fred thought had been met by his course of action, and how a different coping strategy for frustration and anger may more satisfactorily meet these needs. Furthermore, identifiably unacceptable coping strategies were examined in relation to Fred's original offending behaviour, resulting in his admission to high-secure care and how his coping strategies and behaviours at that time were not too dissimilar to the ones portrayed now.

Outcomes

Outcome measures that relate to the BSI assessment are built within the item scales themselves. Therefore, this allows us to develop our interventions and outcome measures alongside any systematic evaluation of progress or otherwise.

In practice, this can be illustrated by taking, for example, item 3 from the insight sub-scale (tension-reducing strategies) where Fred was rated as functioning poorly. Within the scale, there are five possible scores:

- Score 1 (where Fred was rated) – has no constructive personal strategy for relieving tension and anxiety
- Score 2 – aware of problem and seeks advice or attempts to develop such a strategy
- Score 3 – co-operates with therapist to develop such a strategy
- Score 4 – follows the developed strategy with encouragement and support
- Score 5 (the optimal behaviour) – spontaneously follows an insightful and constructive personal strategy.

Ideally, of course, we would want Fred to function at the score 5 behaviour, but more realistically he may never achieve this. Fred was rated at the least score possible (score of 1), therefore, we may firstly focus interventions based on score 2, but always working towards higher scores. It is possible, given the global assessment of Fred's behaviour, that a score of 4 is the optimal behaviour that we can expect him to function at, at least for the foreseeable future. The above example, albeit simplified, shows how the BSI can be used as an outcome measure to focus our interventions. Thus, the scales assist us in relating outcomes through reassessment of behaviours, which logically links up to the baseline measure which initially identified areas of poor functioning.

Initially, outcomes resulting from the above interventions were negative and there was a drastic increase in observed incidents. However, after 1 month his behaviour became more settled. He appeared to benefit from the one-to-one sessions and following an incident would actively seek out his primary nurse to discuss his coping strategies. Eventually, over a period of a number of months, critical items showing deficit on the BSI risk sub-scale were showing improvement at re-assessment.

More specifically, for the insight items that the intervention strategy was addressing, improvement was also noted. For item 1 (awareness of tension), Fred actually had moved two points on the rating scale between assessments. Initially, he was rated as unable at any time to express awareness of increased tension, whereas now he was occasionally spontaneously identifying feelings of increased tension. For item 2 (description of tension), Fred had been originally rated as 'unable to describe feelings of tension', however, again he had jumped two points on this scale and was now 'occasionally spontaneously describing such feeling reasonably clearly'. Item 7 (personal strategy for reducing tension) was originally rated as 'unable to articulate a strategy for preventing/reducing feeling of irritation or anger' but now could be rated as one point higher towards more adaptive behaviour, such as 'appears able to work out such a strategy given appropriate support'. Finally, for item 16 (self-appraisal), originally rated as 'completely unable to make a realistic appraisal of current behavioural and/or emotional problems', he also showed improvement and can now be rated as, 'with help identifies at least one initial problem to be tackled early in therapy'.

Discussion

What we have seen is how the BSI can be used to focus assessment and interventions for a man who is currently displaying risky behaviours. In our case example improvement was noted over the few months that are described. Moreover, this behaviour has been maintained and although incidents do occur, they are rare and their ferocity has greatly diminished. However, only time will tell if Fred can maintain more acceptable coping responses in times of stress and frustration. Regular assessment using the BSI will help to monitor this.

It appears quite clear, to those working with the BSI, as to why it should be included in the risk-assessment process, and indeed as a measure of managing risk through its therapeutic properties. It is the individual's behaviour which initially got him or her into trouble; and it will undoubtedly be his or her subsequent behaviour that will limit or extend that trouble (Woods & Reed 1998). Expressed otherwise, an individual is required to alter or modify behaviours in order to effectively function within, or be accepted by, society.

Monitoring within the closed hospital environment should provide useful data for assessment of future risk. Clark et al (1993) endorse its value, provided that (1) there is a selection of appropriate variables to monitor; (2) there is actual sound and objective monitoring of these; and (3) that monitoring is tailored to the therapeutic needs of the individual patient. Clinically, the logic underpinning the BSI is that there may exist certain patterns or behavioural 'diatheses' which predispose to (i.e. increase the risk of) occurrence of offending behaviour. Such a 'diathesis' may consist of behavioural elements or skill repertoire, allowing for assessment of base-lines, appropriate interventions which are designed to ameliorate specific deficits, or promote insightful adjustment and social

learning, and, importantly, the evaluation and re-measurement of data (Woods et al 1999).

REFERENCES

Bingley W 1995 Assessing dangerousness: protecting the interests of patients. British Journal of Psychiatry (Suppl) 170(32): 28–29

Borum R 1996 Improving the clinical practice of violence risk assessment. American Psychologist 51(9): 945–956

Chiswick D 1995 Dangerousness. In: Chiswick D, Cope R (eds) Seminars in practical forensic psychiatry. Gaskell, London

Clark D A, Fisher M J, McDougall C 1993 A new methodology for assessing the level of risk in incarcerated offenders. British Journal of Criminology 33: 436–448

Duggan C 1997 Assessing risk in the mentally disordered (Introduction). British Journal of Psychiatry (Suppl) 170(32): 1–3

Hepworth D 1982 Influence of the concept of 'danger' on assessment of danger to self and others. Medicine Science and Law 22(4): 245–254

Monahan J, Steadman H J (eds) 1994 Violence and mental disorder: developments in risk assessment. University of Chicago Press, Chicago

Pollock N, Webster C 1990 The clinical assessment of dangerousness. In: Bluglass R, Bowden P (eds) Principles and practice of forensic psychiatry. Churchill Livingstone, Edinburgh

Robinson D, Reed V, Lange A 1996 Developing risk assessment scales in psychiatric care. Psychiatric Care 3: 146–152

Vinestock M 1996 Risk assessment: 'A word to the wise'? Advances in Psychiatric Treatment 2: 3–10

Webster C D, Harris G T, Rice M E, Cormier C, Quinsey V L 1994 The violence prediction scheme: assessing dangerousness in high risk men. University of Toronto, Toronto

Woods P, Reed V 1998 Measuring risk and related behaviours with the Behavioural Status Index (BSI): some preliminary psychometric studies. International Journal of Psychiatric Nursing Research 4(1): 396–409

Woods P, Reed V, Robinson D 1998 The Behavioural Status Index: therapeutic assessment of risk, insight, communication and social skills. Journal of Psychiatric and Mental Health Nursing 6(2): 79–90

CONTENTS

Clinical supervision for nurses in a learning disability forensic service

Christopher Minto and Maureen Morrow

Introduction

The purpose of this case study is to examine a range of issues related to clinical supervision and its relevance to nurses working in a forensic learning disability service. A review of the current literature has identified a multitude of aims relating to how clinical supervision is utilised in practice situations. Our objective was to explore practitioners' previous experiences of clinical supervision, at both professional and personal levels. Issues identified as important by staff were explored in depth, in the course of interviews and subsequent reflections. The implications that this might have in relation to the implementation of a clinical supervision framework are discussed.

Arguably, clinical supervision can be explored from both macro (organisational and professional) and micro (personal and practitioner) levels. Although our work was inevitably more concerned with micro perspectives, it cannot be ignored that wider structural issues are influential and important.

Background

In the widest sense, the current interest in clinical supervision can clearly be regarded as professionally driven. The central aim of clinical supervision should be to support the delivery of optimum care by safeguarding standards and also by developing professional expertise in practice. Developing and sustaining practice should be a high priority for the whole profession, as the role of the skilled nurse evolves to adapt to the changing socio-political priorities which face the National Health Service.

The nursing profession has been relatively slow to accept that nurses at all levels, from students to senior clinicians, need a relationship which focuses on the process and experience of nursing. This view is not, in any way, intended to undervalue the contribution of unqualified staff. Faugier (1992) argues that nursing is nothing if it is not practice and yet nurses have been quite prepared to practise without being properly clinically supervised. Regrettably, there has been a tendency to rely upon 'hands on' experience.

The importance of implementing formalised systems of clinical supervision has been stressed by both the Department of Health and nursing's professional regulators (NHS Executive 1995, UKCC 1995a). Significant drivers have included the UKCC Code of Conduct (1992b) and the Scope for Professional Practice (1992a). A recognition of the importance and value of clinical supervision for the development of nursing resulted in extensive consultation and culminated in the UKCC's (1995b) Position Statement. Clinical supervision, however, is not only about professionalism. It is also about what we do for patients, what the outcomes are, what the clinical effectiveness of nursing practice is and the issue of linking ourselves constantly with the group of people that we care for. Effective supervision of practice is a process that must be based on clinically focused professional relationships between the practitioner and the clinical supervisor.

Given our concern with examining the process of developing and introducing a clinical supervision framework within a forensic learning disability service, it is worth spending some time to briefly describe this practice context. Successive reports addressing security in the NHS (DHSS 1974) and mentally disordered offenders (DoH 1975) were instrumental in providing a blueprint for the future development of forensic services. This was consolidated by the more recent Reed (1992) report. It has been estimated that there has been an eight-fold increase in practitioners working in forensic settings within the Northern and Yorkshire Regional Health Authority (Minto &

Graham 1998). This marked increase begs some important questions. First, where have all the experienced 'forensic staff' come from? Second, how have they been prepared in terms of academic and practice background? Finally, how will future developments be dealt with? The answers to these questions have strong implications for clinical supervision in terms of who conducts the supervision, and how.

The hospital in this study provides a wide range of services for learning disability clients and has recently developed specialist services for a forensic learning disability population. This unit is a purpose-built, medium-secure facility situated within the Northern and Yorkshire Regional Health Authority. It provides a service for patients with a learning disability who are detained under the Mental Health Act 1983 and who have also been convicted of a range of offences. Those admitted to the medium-secure unit (MSU) are mainly diagnosed as having 'borderline learning disability'. The index offences of the population can be broadly categorised into three main divisions:

1. Sex offences
2. Firesetting/arson
3. Violent offences.

It appears obvious that the difficult and sensitive nature of the work requires a formalised system of clinical supervision (Pritchard 1995). Practitioners who provide a multi-disciplinary service within the unit include nurses, psychiatrists, psychologists, social workers, occupational therapists, specialist educationalists and a range of support staff. The issues facing practitioners in a learning disability forensic setting are many, varied and complex. Clearly, clinical supervision should be high on the agenda in providing efficient, effective and clinically credible services to patients and their families.

Clinical supervision

The literature examines a range of issues relating to the introduction of formalised clinical supervision systems. Examples include the development of models and frameworks for clinical supervision, the nature of clinical supervision, local service needs and practitioner requirements. However, Severinson (1995) argues that there are, in fact, few studies which focus on clinical supervision from a nursing research perspective, citing Paunonen (1991), Hallberg & Norberg (1993) and Hallberg (1994).

It has also been claimed that clinical supervision is often viewed as a negative experience. Power (1994) argues that such experiences for practitioners conjure up memories of threatening and unsupportive seniors standing over them, 'ever watchful, ever critical'. It is hardly surprising that those who have been subject to this sort of negative encounter would wish to avoid it. We need, therefore, to be able to clearly demonstrate the purpose and potential benefits of clinical supervision for patients and practitioners.

Exploring nurses' views of clinical supervision

Amongst our group of nurses we wanted to explore their perceptions of both the need for, and the nature of, clinical supervision. Given that a clinical supervision framework was being explored for the unit anyway, we sought to find out individual viewpoints of the nurses relating to their previous exposure to clinical supervision and to identify their current perceptions and expectations for the implementation of a formalised clinical supervision framework. This was achieved using a phenomenological view of nursing research, suggesting an approach, rather than a strict method. The enquiry was shaped by our specific interest in engaging with personal perspectives on clinical supervision from the standpoints of potential supervisees and supervisors within a newly established forensic setting. In the course of interviews, three broad exploratory questions, and the relationships between them, provided a focus:

- Can you tell me about your previous experience of clinical supervision, both formal and informal?
- What issues do you think you might bring to clinical supervision at both a practice and personal level?

- What do you think your expectations of clinical supervision are?

A qualitative framework was utilised for analysis of the responses. Taylor (1994) proposes that phenomenology is suitable for researching nursing questions about nursing phenomena. She believes a positive feature of this approach 'is the ability to focus on the experiences of nurses and clients existing in a health care attainment/maintenance environment, seeking to understand practical concerns.' Munhall (1994) further suggests that care planning requires an understanding of the various lived experiences which arise from persons telling their descriptions of live events. Thus, it is hard to imagine that the role of nursing in the care planning process within a forensic learning disability setting can be undertaken effectively without some involvement of clinical supervision.

A purposive sampling framework is seen to be valid in this type of research. Our small study included clinical practitioners who would eventually have both a supervisory and supervisee role in any proposed clinical supervision framework and who also had a range of clinical experiences. The nurses who volunteered to take part were reassured about confidentiality and anonymity. These nurses were also aware that a framework for clinical supervision was being discussed by managers, both on the unit and more widely within the hospital. Each participant was a first-level registered nurse, working within a forensic learning disability service. Three men and one woman agreed to be involved. The breadth of professional experience since qualifying was 2 to 15 years.

The nurses' perceptions and experiences were explored during thematic, open-ended, semi-structured interviews, using the questions referred to earlier to guide and direct discussion. The interviews lasted approximately 30 to 50 minutes and were audio-taped. The interviews took place on the unit and in work time and were transcribed verbatim.

Clarkson & Aviram (1995), using a content analysis, identified six facets which they believe capture the experience of clinical supervision.

These are 'structuring', 'teaching', 'nurturing', 'supervisor as person', 'supervisor as colleague' and 'the triangle' (client, practitioner and supervisor). We were interested to see whether the content of our interviews with staff could be located within the same six facets.

CASE STUDY: THE NURSES' ACCOUNTS

Although the practitioners interviewed had experienced a range of differing organisational structures and practice models, common themes did emerge.

Can you tell me about your previous experience of clinical supervision?

From this question relating to *formal* experience of clinical supervision, several organisational issues and constraints were highlighted:

...the experience of clinical supervision, what I interpret clinical supervision to be is your PDP, your personal development plan, appraisal... (1)

...not really, when I first qualified we had a period straight after coming out of nurse training school called staff nurse development... (2)

...it was formal, it was there, it was not compulsory but you went. You didn't actually change your times and it was actually evaluated as part of the course at the end. (3)

I think the experience that comes to mind is possibly when I was a student, you know, when you have different placements. It could be the deputy charge nurse, they would take and involve you in whatever was going on. (4)

It appears from these responses that the previous formal experiences of practitioners had been varied and, arguably, influential in framing their individual perceptions of clinical supervision. However, this is not to say that some practitioners cannot still have a positive perception of clinical supervision, even though they had had a negative experience from an organisational point of view.

A second element of our question related to *informal* experiences of clinical supervision. It could be suggested that nursing has always operated informal support strategies and many nurses do not see the need to formalise these arrangements. The information collected appears to demonstrate both the 'teaching' and 'nurturing' roles within the experience of supervision:

...good role models who involved you, encouraged you, maybe took time out to explain why something happened, why they were going to do a particular thing. It could be anything from why a patient behaves in a particular way, why they managed them in a particular way ... you knew you were being bestowed this tablet of stone which you were not entitled to. (4)

...since then it has been more informal with the other four managers, when we are on together we get together, sound things out, chat things through. (2)

The informal experiences of previous clinical supervision indicated that the sharing of experiences, and positive support offered, were identified as being important.

What issues do you think you might bring to clinical supervision at both a practice and personal level?

Question 2 asked the practitioners to indicate what issues they felt that they would take to formalised clinical supervision sessions. The responses appeared to support facets of 'supervisor as person' and 'supervisor as colleague':

...what I would bring with me is my personal development portfolio file, courses, and things like that. I'd have a plan of what I would like to achieve and improve ... my knowledge base, courses and things that are available to me in-house and out-house, health and safety, environmental issues, staffing levels, shift hours, any concerns about patients. (1)

...I think I'm quite experienced now as a nurse. I've worked in different areas within the psychiatric side, and I've learned on each. I've hopefully learned new skills in each area where I've worked. Coming up here and working on this Unit, the fact is that I've had to develop that knowledge and learn new skills. I'm working with a different group of people in a strange environment where I would say everybody has been in the same boat, there's none of us come from a secure hospital background. We've had to develop most of our practices and procedures ourselves, and, thankfully we've got most things right. But we've also got things wrong and I think there are still areas where we possibly struggle, which is probably what you're getting at. I feel personally I haven't, or I'm not, developed as a nurse to the extent that I could be because I don't feel I have as much knowledge. I've got all the patient management skills that I need, and the skills that involve organising staff and the day-to-day business of the ward. (4)

...I suppose I would like being a manager. I would assess, I don't know if assess is the right word, but certainly think back over time since the last session of supervision and try and decide what had gone well, what things had gone badly during my working time. To try and relate those to how I was feeling and just come to my supervisor with the idea that we could talk them through, identify good areas and learning experiences from them. I suppose I would look for reassurance and support, maybe wanting to know that you had done the right thing. Wanting to know if there are alternatives... (3)

...I would possibly take things to supervision that had been raised from my team during their supervised sessions with me, if it wasn't deemed confidential or personal to them. Any areas of concern, or areas that might need action, that I didn't have the autonomy to action. Ideas, suggestions, or just concerns. (2)

An attempt was made to differentiate between clinical practice concerns and personal difficulties in relation to caring for patients with complex and difficult problems. The nature of forensic practice is, undoubtedly, a domain where especially complex and sensitive issues need to be dealt with every day. It is unreasonable to assume that practitioners will not be affected by the nature of this work, particularly in terms of the very serious offences that many patients will have committed or the extremely difficult behaviours that often present. In implementing a clinical supervision framework it would appear imperative to acknowledge these personal issues:

...if there is something, a personal problem, I would feel very comfortable discussing it with my manager. But, having said that, it would have to be a great problem to the extent that it was affecting my ability to carry out my duty... (1)

I think it would be very difficult to talk to somebody who I didn't trust, or who I didn't know. I think it is a bit ludicrous to ask anybody to do that... (4)

I think it would depend on personalities, and how formal it is. If you are feeling particularly stale in your work area you might be able to discuss secondments and your career. That's not patient related, but it is personal to you and where you are heading. (2)

It is interesting to note that none of the nurses verbalised the difficult nature of their clinical practice, but it is not difficult to conjecture why this might be. First, clinical supervision in learning disability nursing remains a relatively novel concept. Second, the specific service location in question is a very new one with practitioners brought together from other areas of the organisation. Finally, it should not be assumed that it is easy for practitioners to readily immerse themselves into the prospective clinical supervision roles.

What do you think your expectations of clinical supervision are?

Regarding practitioner expectations of clinical supervision, Clarkson & Aviram (1995) argue that it is 'perceived through the prism of one's own theoretical framework, beliefs and attitudes'. Thus, the expectations of clinical supervision for individual practitioners will be influenced by factors such as grade, experience and the nature of the work:

...I would like to be told with no strings attached, but obviously you are dealing professional to professional, so there is professional courtesy. If I was not fulfilling my role correctly and those areas were highlighted, brought to my attention, which I am sure they would be, and how I could improve on those areas... (1)

...initially I would be a bit concerned because I don't know if I've got the skills. To begin with, I don't know enough about clinical supervision, so I don't know if I would be capable of that role or function. (4)

I probably have more expectations downwards of the effect it will have as opposed to affecting me upwards, if that makes sense. What I mean is that if it's done right and carefully, then the idea of support, help, guidance, some new learning, some rationalisation, some change of practice should filter through at all levels. I suppose stress is the buzz word and I think within an environment such as this, a locked environment, you're physically enclosed, you're in close proximity for long hours with patients who can be very, very difficult. The stress levels are immediately raised, no matter what level of stress an individual can tolerate. Then, even if you can dissipate some stress within the environment, and whether it's the idea of getting away for an hour if that helps, then it has a role. (3)

...the time, the recognition, that it is a valuable service for people. Training and insight for supervisors so that they are doing it properly, and making sure that it is not being abused. Done properly to avoid people feeling under pressure or people being under misconceptions of what it is all about. I think the whole thing needs to have its profile raised before we move forward with it. (2)

Discussion

The practitioners in this case study had previously experienced, within different organisational structures, a range of supervision arrangements. Each of the nurses appeared to view the formal experience of clinical supervision as a managerial responsibility. However, the UKCC suggests that the function of clinical supervision should not be the exercise of managerial responsibility; neither should it be seen as a system of formal individual performance review, nor should it necessarily be hierarchical in nature (Farrington 1998).

Practitioners had experienced a range of very positive informal experiences of clinical supervision, including:

- The sharing of skills
- Identification with good role models and positive attitudes
- The opportunity to integrate theory with practice
- Being able to share and discuss individual strengths and weaknesses.

These areas could all be used as goals for supervision, allowing the opportunity to facilitate reflective practice and drive the notion of patient-centred quality care. The nurses described a range of issues which they felt that they would be able to bring to clinical supervision. In the absence of a formalised system, it has to be asked whether these are being adequately addressed.

With regard to professional issues, previous experience and knowledge of clinical supervision inevitably influenced how the practitioners responded. Farrington (1998) suggests that there are clear levels through which a supervisee progresses. The first stage is often characterised by supervisee dependence on the supervisor. For example, in this study, one nurse (a junior staff nurse) responded predominantly in terms of broad organisational issues. More senior members of staff were eager to concentrate on the development of micro skills relating to practice. This again is supported in the literature, identifying a need to confront personal and professional problems. Often supervisees become supervisors themselves, yet the process of transition from one role to another is rarely articulated.

In terms of working with clients who present with particularly complex and difficult problems, this could have the potential to cause both distress and stress for practitioners. It is particularly problematic to separate professional and personal issues within the parameters of clinical supervision. All of the nurses seemed to indicate that bringing personal issues to clinical supervision would depend on the relationship between supervisor and supervisee. Key characteristics of a therapeutic alliance such as openness, trust and thoughtfulness could be identified as positive elements of a good supervisory style. What cannot be established are the complexities involved in moving between the roles of supervisor and supervisee. The need to constantly improve and re-define professional skills and to consider new professional challenges indicates a commitment to lifelong learning.

The expectations of practitioners may be very different in relation to clinical supervision and it is important that these matters are considered by supervisors involved in setting up a clinical supervision contract. Issues of boundaries, rights and responsibilities, confidentiality, setting, time, professionalism and ethical dilemmas are deserving of attention. Dimond (1998) notes that, even though the professional elements of clinical supervision are important, there is also a legal dimension.

Scrutiny of the nurses' accounts offered in this case study provides supportive material to argue for the general recognition of clinical supervision as a valid construct. However, the lived experience of a small number of practitioners, within a very specific service, also indicates that the process involved in establishing a clinical supervision framework may not be so straight-forward. Practitioners' previous experience, knowledge and expectations need to be acknowledged and validated before the process can be implemented effectively. Aside from individual experience, UK health care provision is increasingly embroiled within the predominant culture of market forces. Here, managerial imperatives may impede, or even contradict, certain philosophies of care delivery.

There are obvious limitations to this exploratory and descriptive case study, which restrict any unreasonable generalisations. We felt that a crucial prerequisite to the implementation of a clinical supervision framework was that the views and experiences of some nurses in this setting were accessed. The sample was very small and comments are only valid in terms of the lived experience of the participants. The context of the caring environment also has to be recognised as exerting a major influence. It does reveal, though, a range of issues that vary from practitioner to practitioner. These include differing prior experiences of organisational structures, positive and negative experiences of clinical supervision, varying personal and professional expectations and, finally, the complex and problematic nature of clinical concerns which practitioners indicate they would bring to clinical supervision sessions.

An important implication of listening to the nurses themselves addresses the issue of whether formal structures of clinical supervision should be developed at the level of the practitioner, the organisation or both. Whichever approach is adopted, the articulation and validation of the practitioners' previous experiences and perceptions are recommended prior to the implementation of any selected model of clinical supervision.

REFERENCES

Clarkson P, Aviram O 1995 Phenomenological research on supervision: supervisors reflect on 'being a supervisor'. Counselling Psychology Quarterly 8(1): 63–80

Department of Health 1975 Report of the Committee on Mentally Disordered Offenders (Butler Report) Cmnd 6244. HMSO, London

Department of Health and Social Security 1974 Report of the Department of Health and Social Security Working Party on Security in NHS Psychiatric Hospitals (Glancy Report). HMSO, London

Dimond B 1998 Legal aspects of clinical supervision 1: employer vs employee. British Journal of Nursing 7(7): 393–395

Farrington A 1998 Clinical supervision: issues for mental health nursing. Mental Health Nursing 18(1): 19–21

Faugier J 1992 The supervisory relationship. In: Butterworth C, Faugier J (eds) Clinical supervision and mentorship in nursing. Chapman and Hall, London

Hallberg I 1994 Systematic clinical supervision in a child psychiatric ward: satisfaction with care, tedium, burnout, and the nurses' own report on the effects of it. Archives of Psychiatric Nursing 1: 44–52

Hallberg I, Norberg A 1993 Strain among nurses and the emotional reactions during one year of systematic supervision combined with implementation of individualized care in dementia nursing. Journal of Advanced Nursing 18: 1860–1875

Minto C, Graham F 1998 The development of forensic services in the former Northern Regional Health Authority. Forensic Practice Research Unit, UNN, Newcastle

Munhall P 1994 Revisioning phenomenology. Nursing and Health Science Research, National League for Nursing Press

NHS Executive 1995 Clinical supervision: a resource pack. Department of Health, London

Paunonen M 1991 Promoting nursing quality through supervision. Journal of Nursing Staff Development Sept/Oct: 229–233

Pritchard J 1995 (ed) Good practice in supervision: statutory and voluntary organisations. Jessica Kingsley, London

Power S 1994 A unique source of support and advice: the benefits of supervision in clinical practice. Psychiatric Care 1(3): 105–108

Reed J 1992 Review of health and social services for mentally disordered offenders and others requiring similar services: Final summary report. HMSO, London

Severinsson E 1995 The phenomenon of clinical supervision in psychiatric health care. Journal of Psychiatric and Mental Health Nursing 2: 301–309

Taylor B 1994 Being human: ordinariness in nursing. Churchill Livingstone, Melbourne

United Kingdom Central Council for Nursing, Midwifery and Health Visiting 1992a The scope of professional practice. UKCC, London

United Kingdom Central Council for Nursing, Midwifery and Health Visiting 1992b Code of conduct for the nurse, midwife and health visitor. UKCC, London

United Kingdom Central Council for Nursing, Midwifery and Health Visiting 1995a Clinical supervision for nursing and health visiting. Registrar's letter: 4/95. UKCC, London

United Kingdom Central Council for Nursing, Midwifery and Health Visiting 1995b Position statement on clinical supervision for nursing and health visiting. Annexe to Registrar's letter: 4/95. UKCC, London

CONTENTS

Practitioner training, future directions and challenges for practice

Arlene Kent-Wilkinson, Mick McKeown, Dave Mercer, Ged McCann and Tom Mason

Introduction

In this final section, we offer four brief cases of different education initiatives which exemplify various aspects of meeting forensic training needs. The courses we comment on do not constitute a comprehensive account of the availability of forensic practice training. Though the number of institutions offering such training is limited, there are many examples of excellence in the field, and the volume of such training is likely to expand as practitioner groups mature and develop their knowledge and practice base. Rather, the selected examples are included to allow us to address some key issues in education and training and, ultimately, service development. From Canada, there is a distance-learning package, available internationally over the Internet, which facilitates student's critical engagement with 'on-line' case examples and scenarios. Then there is the post-graduate diploma, leading to a Masters degree, in forensic behavioural science, a traditional academic course taught at the University of Liverpool. From the University of York is a course in psychosocial interventions for severe and enduring mental health problems, which brings together forensic and mainstream mental health practitioners and embraces experiential approaches to skills acquisition and ongoing supervision of clinical practice. Finally, we comment on a small-scale training and development programme working with a team of staff in the context of their actual workplace, where the emphasis is on the interaction between trainers and practitioners, aimed at producing lasting changes in real-life practice. We conclude with some reflections on possible future directions and challenges for forensic care.

National contexts

Given the fact that our examples are drawn from the UK and North America, it may be helpful to briefly outline the development of forensic practice education from the different sides of the Atlantic. In the USA, the establishment of forensic practice disciplines has been closely linked to the correctional (prisons) system. Issues in education can be exemplified with recourse to the development of forensic psychiatric nursing, having its origins in the US Federal corrections system in the early 1930s (Furman 1973, Hufft & Fawkes 1994). In 1946, the first detailed policies governing nursing activities in Federal prisons was initiated by the US Prison Health Services (Hufft & Fawkes 1994).

It can be argued that, historically, US schools of nursing were less than responsive to the health needs of inmate populations in their education of nurses. Then, the Civil Rights Movement of the 1960s and 1970s created an awareness of prisoners' rights as members of an identified minority (Felton et al 1987). The subsequent jailing of civil rights activists helped to usher in legislative changes which resulted in the recognition of a right to treatment and a focus of attention on health care delivery within correctional facilities (Bernier 1986). Nursing's professional interest in prison settings began to emerge concurrently with increasing societal concerns (Dubler 1979). Progressive changes in correctional health care, beginning in the late 1970s, supported a role change for nurses to become the major provider of primary health care in correctional facilities (AMA 1978, Droes 1994).

In the early 1980s, the literature began to cite the use of correctional institutions for clinical learning experience by students in community mental health nursing (Bridges 1981). Of note, the Catholic University of America School of Nursing was awarded a grant in 1986 from the National Institute of Mental Health to prepare forensic psychiatric nurses as clinical nurse specialists at graduate level to function in all areas of the correctional system (Bernier 1986). In 1984, correctional nursing was recognised as a specialty by the American Nurses Association (ANA) and the Scope and Standards of Nursing Practice in Correctional Facilities was passed (ANA 1984, Hufft & Fawkes 1994).

In 1990, a survey of forensic psychiatric nurses supported the acknowledgement of forensic nursing as a distinct clinical sub-specialty and sought special credentialing for practice. Recent research in the USA indicated that there were at least 2000 registered nurses working in psychiatric forensic facilities (Scales et al 1993). Forensic nursing was formally recognised as a distinct discipline during the 1991 Annual Meeting of the American Academy of Forensic Sciences in Anaheim, California (Lynch 1995); then, in 1995, forensic nursing was recognised as a specialty by the ANA and standards of nursing practice were approved (ANA 1995). There are now numerous elective courses in the forensic psychiatric correctional area, dispersed throughout the USA. Specific forensic correctional nursing programmes of study are being developed, or are now offered, at Vanderbilt University School of Nursing in Nashville, at the University of Maryland in Baltimore and at Rudgers University in New Jersey.

In Canada, forensic psychiatric services have been provided federally by Correctional Service Canada since 1973 (Conacher 1993) with guidelines for professional conduct of health professionals established in 1977 (Lehmann 1983). Commencing in 1980, there has been the opportunity for students to gain practical, clinically based work experience in the correctional setting and in the forensic psychiatric unit in Calgary, Alberta. Phillips' (1983) survey indicated an identified need to educate the public regarding the mentally ill offender and to convince government to allocate more funds for the provision of forensic psychiatric services. In 1988, Correctional Service Canada developed Standards of Health Care (CSC 1988). Presently there are over 400 correctional forensic psychiatric nurses in Correctional Service Canada (CSC 1997), with approximately identical numbers in provincial forensic psychiatric services.

Canada's geography, with forensic practitioners scattered throughout the country across provincial and Federal forensic and correctional services, has led to feelings of isolation for clinicians. These circumstances provided the inspiration for harnessing the technology of the Internet to education and aimed at bringing some presence of connectedness to forensic practice as a whole. Distinct forensic educational courses are becoming popular for students wanting to work in the field and are also of interest to those already established in practice. The value of accessing and utilising forensic people and resources internationally on the World Wide Web is just beginning to be realised for future collaborations, with a greater degree of international links promised.

In contrast with the North American experiences, the British forensic domain, until recently, has been largely dominated by the historical tradition of the Special Hospital. The first of these, Broadmoor, was established in the mid 19th century. Since that time, three other maximum secure psychiatric institutions have opened in England, with a comparable State Hospital in Scotland. Until recently, these institutions were centrally managed by the government, in parallel with the prison system, despite their manifest function of care and treatment for mentally disordered offenders. More recently, their management has been incorporated into the National Health Service, and a range of lesser secure units and community initiatives has emerged.

Given the lengthy history of forensic provision, formal initiatives to develop specialist practice training have arrived only relatively lately on the scene. Large practitioner groupings such as nurses have been subject to the professionalisation agenda which spread through the general asylums, but little in the way of focused training was available to forensic nurses. As such, preregistration training for mental health nurses need not pay any attention to the needs of forensic service users. Ironically, even though the Special Hospitals operated their own schools of nursing, they were bound to use the nationally validated curriculum. Arguably, they were training nurses to work in a specialised environment without offering them an appropriate knowledge and skills base. Conversely, perhaps because of forensic services' isolation from the mainstream, resident practitioners could find themselves insulated against progressive developments in practice and training available elsewhere in the health service. In more recent times, a number of interesting multi-disciplinary education developments have been designed to better meet the contemporary needs of specialist forensic practitioners.

CASE STUDIES

1. Mount Royal College

The need to develop forensic health studies courses was identified in 1996. Stimulated by advances in the field of practice and an escalating incidence of violence and trauma, Mount Royal College began an exciting journey to develop a unique series of courses for professionals seeking preparation in the forensic health and justice fields. The courses were developed for distance study using digital technology to provide maximum access to learners across Canada and around the world.

Examples of course content are illustrated in Box 12.5.

The authors of the material and clinical experts are highlighted by hyper-linking reference to their photographs. Images of flags denote the countries internationally represented by the research, case studies and articles. The historical firsts, facts, laws and acts presented in each unit of study are time-lined for each country. Interview clips are added on-line using steaming audio in a macro-media director programme. Animation is used to give a three-dimensional effect to frameworks for conceptual models of practice and courtroom depictions. Unit interactivities are facilitated by a discussion board on-line, where forensic issues and clinical practice are described and debated.

The use of computer technology in health care education has proliferated. Not only is it now a

---

Box 12.5   Distance study course examples

Mount Royal College – Internet: Forensic Health Studies

Introduction to theories, concepts and issues in forensic populations
- This multi-disciplinary theory course focuses on prevailing social and ethical forensic issues where health care overlaps with the law. Roles of the forensic sub-specialties are outlined, together with the target forensic populations they serve. Historical roots, principles and professional practices of emerging specialties are examined, while current and future career opportunities are presented. A larger systems overview of criminal justice and health care shows the societal influence and legal dimensions of forensic practice. This course also explores victims of physical and/or psychological trauma, abuse, or neglect, the assessment and treatment of perpetrators, and the families and communities of both.

Health care in forensic psychiatric and correctional populations
- This multi-disciplinary course addresses the roles and career opportunities for health care professionals in correctional and forensic psychiatric areas. Assessment, intervention and prevention are explored for various forensic 'at risk' populations. Relevant ethical and legal practice issues in the correctional and forensic psychiatric setting are debated with the opportunity to access international forensic resources on the World Wide Web.

---

part of patient care in many settings, its use continues to grow in undergraduate programmes, continuing education and post-entry level nursing education (Hawley & Desborough 1998). There are many advantages to integrating computer-assisted learning into the curriculum. Since such learning does not depend on teacher availability, learning can occur at times that are convenient for the student (Hawley & Desborough 1998). A possible disadvantage with the use of on-line case material would be threats to confidentiality for subjects. Hence, vigilance about maintaining client anonymity is required (Lewis & Kaas 1998).

Since 1994, the World Wide Web and related Internet resources (e.g. e-mail, chat and news groups) have become an increasing viable component in higher education pedagogy. This has led to significant interest in the implementation of Internet-based virtual teaching (Schutte 1998). In the past, distance education was considered a pre-packaged text or audiovisual course, with little or no interaction between the student and the instructor. Today, the evolving interactive communication technology allows learning experiences to occur at any time between instructor and student, student and student, and student and expert.

Incorporating computer technologies into a forensic behavioural science curriculum may at first seem problematic, given that the practice core of the specialty has traditionally been the face-to-face development of therapeutic relationships. However, this can be addressed through the interaction of various different methods: tutorial, drill and practice, simulation, problem-solving, games and testing. Case studies, for example, often use simulations in presenting situations that the student might encounter in practice and the student makes decisions about what action to take (Joos et al 1992).

2. Diploma and Masters in Forensic Behavioural Science

The Diploma and Master of Science Degree Course in Forensic Behavioural Science was set up in 1991 by the University of Liverpool, and the Special Hospital Service Authority, under the stewardship of a steering group comprising many eminent practitioners and researchers in the forensic field. More recently, the establishment at the university of a research grouping in investigative psychology, led by Professor David Canter, an internationally recognised forensic specialist, has supported the further development of this course. The course arose out of a concern that the complexities of forensic services and systems are such that they often fail to deliver services that achieve their own stated goals. In 1990, a multi-disciplinary group was formed to consider how a course could be developed which would meet the needs of the main professionals in the relevant agencies. Agreement was reached by the group that such a course should gather students from a variety of professional backgrounds and provide them with teaching from all of the disciplines that are involved in the criminal justice, mental health and social services systems. Since its inception, participating students have been drawn from a wide range of professional backgrounds, representing a range of forensic and related services. The course continues to attract a large number of applicants and has developed an excellent reputation at a national level.

The aims of the course include:

1. To equip practitioners at the meeting point of the legal, clinical and social services professions with the specialised knowledge and skills they need to become more effective in their work
2. To improve their understanding of the different perspectives of the professional groups in terms of the concepts they use, the approaches they adopt, the assumptions they make and the perceptions they have of each other
3. To facilitate a better understanding of the links between theory, research and practice and, in the light of this, to enable practitioners to critically examine their own work practices.

Students can choose to accept the award of Diploma in Forensic Behavioural Science after 1 year. Alternatively, if they perform adequately in this first year, they may elect to proceed to a second year MSc, which is a research degree by thesis. The Diploma is divided into seven modules which represent distinct but overlapping areas of knowledge including:

- The legal framework
- Criminology, offenders and offending
- Approaches to mental disorder
- Self-harm and harm to others
- Behavioural concepts in law
- Systems of services
- Skills for forensic behavioural work.

Teaching on the diploma course takes the form of lectures, seminars and workshops with considerable emphasis placed on active participation by students. The MSc provides training and experience in basic research methods via formal teaching input, including 1-week residential study block, and from the students' allocated academic supervisors.

3. Postgraduate Diploma/Masters Degree in Psychosocial Interventions

This course, taught at the University of York, UK, involves a 2-year, part-time, multi-disciplinary training programme which aims to equip professionals to work more effectively with the severely mentally ill, either within community settings, in-patient environments or forensic settings. The curriculum is based upon programmes established in the UK by the THORN initiative, which was a developmental and research project concerned with clinical effectiveness in the care of the severely mentally ill (Gamble 1995). The learning content is focused upon the practical delivery of care, accurate assessment of need, the involvement of families and the psychological management of specific symptoms.

The forensic dimensions of the course draw heavily on research and practice developments in implementing psychosocial approaches to the forensic arena, previously undertaken by the course director and colleagues in the UK (McCann 1993, McCann & McKeown 1995a 1995b, McCann & Clancy 1996, McCann et al 1996, McKeown & McCann 1995). The course planning, direction and teaching are shared between personnel from the university and Stockton Hall, a local, independent, medium-secure unit. A novel feature of the course is that it brings together forensic and mainstream practitioners, helping to challenge some of the past isolation of forensic practice insulated from external developments.

The programme is open to nurses, occupational therapists, social workers, psychologists and medical staff, or any mental health professional wishing to focus more specifically on the needs of the severely mentally ill. Students complete four modules in the first year for the postgraduate diploma (PGDip) and a further period of study and a dissertation in the second year for the Masters Degree (MSc). Students studying for the MSc will be able to opt for either a community- or forensic-focused period of study. Clinical work with six clients is assessed at key stages during the course by reviewing audiotaped recordings of clinical sessions. In addition, students attend weekly clinical supervision sessions integral to the course programme. The course is accredited by the THORN Steering Group based at the University of Manchester and the Institute of Psychiatry, London.

4. Training for whole teams in the workplace

This case discussion draws on developmental work undertaken with multi-disciplinary staff at Rathbone High Dependency Unit (HDU) on Merseyside, and referred to in Finlayson and Forster's case study in Chapter 11. The training dimension of this project presents the opportunity for some interesting reflections, allowing us to make a case for innovative models of training geared towards effecting service level change across whole teams. We have rehearsed arguments elsewhere for such a shift, taking learning from the classroom directly into the workplace (McKeown et al 1998). The philosophical underpinnings of this approach are akin to Corrigan & McCracken's (1995) polemic in favour of an interactive dimension to practitioner training. This strategy attempts to focus not just on the content of training, though this is important, but also on the process. As such, lessons are learnt from the field of organisational psychology which suggest that enduring positive changes to working practices will only occur if the training is conducted with whole teams together, in the context of where the translation of new knowledge into practice must take place. That is, training at the 'line-level', in the everyday clinical setting. Crucially, the training has to acknowledge both the special expertise of the facilitators and the special knowledge of the participants, as experts in their own working environment. Hence, changes to working practices are negotiated in the workplace in

ways which are more likely to actually work in practice.

A small-scale version of such an approach has been undertaken at Rathbone HDU, resulting in many positive changes. The content of the training was broadly concerned with the implementation of psychosocial approaches to the management of psychosis. This allowed the adaptation of techniques of family therapy, largely developed for community settings, for use by the staff in their routine interactions with people at ward level. In the course of the project, it became clear that it was not only staff–patient communication and problem-solving which could be addressed from a psychosocial perspective, and the attention of the team members became focused on their own professional communications. This led to new systems of working, resulting in multi-disciplinary care planning meetings and the introduction of unitary case notes for the use of all disciplines. An evaluation of the training demonstrated a significant impact upon practitioner knowledge about schizophrenia, reported levels of stress amongst the nursing staff and the overall quality of the care planning documentation (McKeown et al 1997, Savage & McKeown 1997).

The Rathbone project has demonstrated positive outcomes despite the relatively low levels of trainer input of around 4 hours per week. We would envisage a more substantial impact if a model of training could be established whereby the trainers became integral to the team for appreciably longer periods of time. This would enable greater attention to be given to ongoing clinical supervision and the delivery of problem-based learning sessions.

Problem-based learning can be used as a basis for imparting clinical skills as well as basic knowledge. For example, a scenario may be presented concerning distressed relatives. This would lead to discussion around the concept of 'expressed emotion' and reading materials concerning particular family intervention techniques. A small group presentation may describe a case study of family intervention in detail. However, in the case of clinical skills, problem-based learning elements will be followed by a structured programme of clinical experience and supervision tailored to the needs of the trainee. For example, trainees may be asked to act as a co-therapist in a family intervention carried out by one of the facilitators. This may lead to the trainee taking the lead role in a therapeutic intervention with another family.

CHALLENGES IN TRAINING

Training is important in improving not just the knowledge and skills base of practitioners, but ultimately in enhancing the quality of services to benefit the recipients of forensic care and interventions. We are interested in both the content and the process of training as crucial features in the effectiveness of what is delivered. The need to ground educational curricula and learning objectives in interventions known to be clinically effective is taken as axiomatic, yet forensic practitioners face a relatively thin evidence base, with much systematic research, especially into outcomes, needing to be undertaken. The dilemma of what is known to work in practice is thus a perennial problem in forensic care. Notwithstanding these difficulties, there remains a problem in applying systematically and comprehensively those interventions or approaches which are known to be effective. Some of the possible reasons for this may lie in the quality of training and continuing education opportunities available to practitioners and organisations.

The context and style of any learning experience will be influential in terms of the impact of training upon individuals and the extent to which this extends into real-life practice. A general obstacle to any training initiative, whatever the learning content, is the limited extent to which an impact at the level of individual knowledge or skills translates into enduring changes in practice. Similarly, most training usually commences with an appraisal of what the participants already know, before attempting to extend this in the chosen direction. Often in forensic care, these issues may not be particularly clear. Practitioners may have accumulated a wealth of grounded, practical awareness and skills, useful in negotiating their daily

interactions in the field. However, they may find it more difficult to explain what it is they do, let alone rationalise why certain approaches seem to be effective.

This 'latent' knowledge base of what works at grass roots levels also needs to be the subject of more systematic inquiry. Interestingly, such contingencies are supportive of the desire for practitioners to develop a reflective approach to their own activities and experiences, in an attempt to delineate more sophisticated understandings of the processes of therapeutic engagement and intervention in forensic settings. This ought to enable individuals and groups of staff to explore what factors are influential on outcome, how positives can be emphasised, reflect on their use of self and enhance consistency in approaches within teams. Such reflections are at the core of the case material presented in this volume, which it is hoped will connect with the tangible concerns of 'line-level' practitioners. Such a systematic approach ought to be realisable in the context of clinical supervision or peer support groups. This raises an important issue in forensic care: the need to work through the personal impact for practitioners working with highly emotive patient behaviours or offending histories.

CHALLENGES FOR THE FUTURE

Several of the contributing case studies in the book have raised the issues of whole systems in impacting upon client outcomes. Hence, the potential for training to address systems and not just individuals is again highlighted. One approach to achieving systemic change and efficiencies in care delivery involves making improvements to case management. This involves systems of multi-disciplinary care, planning, implementation and evaluation and, crucially, co-ordination of multi-agency inputs. Typically, forensic case management takes place in a context of risk and concerns for public safety. Commentators such as Rose (1998) have suggested that the entirety of mental health care is now dominated by an obsession with risk, which may be detrimental in the long term, especially for the overwhelming majority of mainstream service users who do not pose severe levels of risk. Hence, there is a need for forensic practitioners to focus on the minority of dangerous and vulnerable individuals and attempt to resist any trends for the forensic domain to be forever extended, increasingly colonising hitherto untouched territory within mainstream psychiatry or criminology. This is not to say that certain specialised knowledges and skills cannot be employed or adapted to more generic settings, or challenging behaviours, to overall benefit. The management of violence, or the possibilitity of opening up more effective means of managing the care of persons with concurrent substance use problems, would be just two examples. Similarly, it is possible that better informed practice in mainstream services could actually prevent the cross-over into forensic patient careers for many individuals.

The role of training in taking forward a progressive agenda of practice development needs to be cognisant of a number of perennial challenges in forensic care. These include the extent to which custodial care implicitly compromises the effectiveness of interventions. It is also imperative for educationalists and practitioners to respond constructively to the consistent findings and recommendations of various critical reviews of services and inquiries into service failings. Not least of these is the need to develop effective systems of co-ordinated and systematic case management, involving diverse agencies and practitioner disciplines. Finally, the rights of individuals not to be abused, neglected or discriminated against within forensic services needs to be a fundamental concern. It is likely that where the extreme failures to achieve this have occurred, training on its own, however sophisticated, will not succeed in the absence of other material and political change.

REFERENCES

American Medical Association 1978 AMA Pilot project to improve medical care and health services in correctional institutions. AMA, Chicago, p 2–8

American Nurses Association 1984, 1995 Scope and standards of nursing practice in correctional facilities (Publication # NP–104)

Bernier S 1986 Corrections and mental health. Journal of Psychosocial Nursing and Mental Health Services 24(6): 20–25

Bridges M 1981 Prison: a learning experience. American Journal of Nursing 81: 744–745

Conacher G 1993 Issues in psychiatric care within a prison service. Canada's Mental Health 3: 11–14

Correctional Service Canada 1988 Standards of health care. CSC, Ottawa

Correctional Service Canada 1997 Basic facts about corrections in Canada. CSC, Ottawa

Corrigan P, McCracken S 1995 Psychiatric rehabilitation and staff development: educational and organisational models. Clinical Psychological Review 15(8): 699–719

Droes N 1994 Correctional nursing practice. Journal of Community Health Nursing 11: 201–210

Dubler N 1979 Depriving prisoners of medical care: a cruel and unusual punishment. Hastings Centre Report 9(10): 7–10

Felton G, Parsons M, Satterfield P 1987 Correctional facilities: a viable community health practice site for students. Journal of Community Health Nursing 4: 111–115

Furman B 1973 A profile of US public health service 1798–1948. DHEW, Washington DC

Gamble C 1995 The Thorn nurse training initiative. Nursing Standard 9(15): 31–34

Hawley P, Desborough K 1998 The computer as tutor. The Canadian Nurse 94(4): 31–35

Hufft A, Fawkes L 1994 Federal inmates – a unique psychiatric nursing challenge. Nursing Clinics of North America 29(1): 35–42

Joos I, Whitman N, Smith M, Nelson R 1992 Computers in small bytes: the computer workbook. National League for Nursing Press, New York

Lehmann A 1983 Nursing's last frontier: our Canadian prisons. The Canadian Nurse 79(7): 37–39

Lewis M, Kaas M 1998 Challenges of teaching graduate psychiatric-mental health nursing with distance education technologies. Archives of Psychiatric Nursing 12: 227–233

Lynch V 1995 Forensic nursing: what's new? (Guest Editorial) Journal of Psychosocial Nursing 33(9): 6–8

McCann G 1993 Relatives' support groups in a special hospital: an evaluation study. Journal of Advanced Nursing 18: 1883–1888

McCann G, Clancy B 1996 Family matters. Nursing Times 92(7): 46–48.

McCann G, McKeown M 1995a Clinical management: a special case. Journal of Nursing Management 3: 115–120

McCann G, McKeown M 1995b Applying psychosocial interventions within a forensic environment. Psychiatric Care 2: 133–136

McCann G, McKeown M, Porter I 1996 Understanding the needs of relatives of patients within a special hospital for mentally disordered offenders: a basis for improved services. Journal of Advanced Nursing 23: 346–352

McKeown M, McCann G 1995 A schedule for assessing relatives: the Relative Assessment Interview for Schizophrenia in a Secure Environment. Psychiatric Care 2: 84–88

McKeown M, Finlayson S, Roberts K 1997 Implementing a psychosocial model of practice within a ward environment. Paper presented to the second international conference on psychological treatments for schizophrenia, Oxford, October 2–3

McKeown M, McCann G, Bentall R 1998 Time for action: a new system of training mental health practitioners. Mental Health Care 1(5): 158

Phillips M 1983 Forensic psychiatry: nurses' attitudes revealed. Dimensions in Health Service 60(9): 41–43

Rose N 1998 Living dangerously: risk thinking and risk management in mental health care. Mental Health Care 1(8): 263–266

Savage L, McKeown M 1997 Towards a new model of practice for a high dependency unit. Psychiatric Care 4: 182–186

Scales C, Mitchell J, Smith R 1993 Survey report on forensic nursing. Journal of Psychosocial Nursing 31(11): 39–44

Schutte J 1998 Virtual teaching in higher education: the new intellectual superhighway or just another traffic jam? Available: http://www.csun.edu/sociology/virexp.htm

Index

Index